CONTENTS

CONTRIBUTORS

James C. Agre, MD, PhD
Ministry Medical Group, Eagle River, Wisconsin

Dorothy D. Aiello, PT, MS
Senior Physical Therapist, Spaulding Rehabilitation Hospital, Framingham, Massachusetts

John R. Bach, MD
Professor and Vice Chairman, Department of Physical Medicine and Rehabilitation; Professor of Neurosciences, University of Medicine and Dentistry of New Jersey–New Jersey Medical School; University Hospital, Newark, New Jersey

Brent Bernstein, DPM
Department of Podiatry, Staten Island University Hospital, Staten Island, New York

Kristian Borg, MD, PhD
Associate Professor and Head, Department of Rehabilitation Medicine, Karolinska Institute; Huddinge University Hospital, Stockholm, Sweden

Neil R. Cashman, MD
Professor, Department of Medicine, University of Toronto Faculty of Medicine; Director, Neuromuscular Clinic, Sunnybrook and Women's Health Sciences Center, Toronto, Ontario, Canada

Maria H. Cole, OTR
Senior Occupational Therapist, Spaulding Rehabilitation Hospital, Framingham, Massachusetts

Deborah Da Costa, PhD
Assistant Professor, Department of Medicine, McGill University; Medical Scientist, McGill University Health Center, Montreal, Quebec, Canada

Marijke Dallimore, PT
Clinical Associate, Post Polio Clinic, University of British Columbia, Vancouver, British Columbia, Canada

Elizabeth Dean, PT, PhD
Professor, School of Rehabilitation Sciences, and Coordinator, Post Polio Clinic, University of British Columbia, Vancouver, British Columbia, Canada

Lois Finch, MSc
School of Physical and Occupational Therapy, McGill University, Montreal, Quebec, Canada

Anne C. Gawne, MD (deceased)
Director, Post-Polio Clinic, Roosevelt Warm Springs Institute for Rehabilitation, Warm Springs, Georgia

Lauro S. Halstead, MD, MPH
Clinical Professor, Department of Medicine, Georgetown University School of Medicine; Director, Post-Polio Clinic, National Rehabilitation Hospital, Washington, District of Columbia

Claire Z. Kalpakjian, PhD
Research Fellow, Department of Physical Medicine and Rehabilitation, University of Michigan Health System, Ann Arbor, Michigan

Beth Kowall, MS, OTR
Post-Polio Resource Group of Southeastern Wisconsin, Milwaukee, Wisconsin

Frederick M. Maynard, MD
Department of Physical Medicine and Rehabilitation, Marquette General Hospital, Marquette, Michigan

Pima S. McConnell, PT, ATP
Director, Seating and Wheeled Mobility Clinic, Roosevelt Warm Springs Institute for Rehabilitation, Warm Springs, Georgia

Sunny Roller, MA
Program Manager and Research Associate, Department of Physical Medicine and Rehabilitation, University of Michigan Health System, Ann Arbor, Michigan

Laura A. Ryan, OTR
Occupational Therapist, Spaulding Rehabilitation Hospital, Framingham, Massachusetts

Julie K. Silver, MD
Assistant Professor, Department of Physical Medicine and Rehabilitation, Harvard Medical School, Boston, Massachusetts; Medical Director, Spaulding Framingham Outpatient Center; Director, International Rehabilitation Center for Polio, Framingham, Massachusetts; Associate in Physiatry, Massachusetts General Hospital; Associate in Physiatry, Brigham and Women's Hospital, Boston, Massachusetts

Kathryn A. Smith, BS, MPT
Aquatic Program Director, Roosevelt Warm Springs Institute for Rehabilitation, Warm Springs, Georgia

Barbara C. Sonies, PhD
Chief, Oral Motor Function Section, Department of Rehabilitation Medicine Clinical Center, National Institutes of Health, Bethesda, Maryland; Adjunct Professor, Speech and Hearing Department, George Washington University, Washington, District of Columbia; Adjunct Professor, Hearing and Speech Science Department, University of Maryland, Baltimore, Maryland

Denise G. Tate, PhD
Professor, Department of Physical Medicine and Rehabilitation, University of
Michigan Health System, Ann Arbor, Michigan

Daria A. Trojan, MD, MSc
Assistant Professor, Department of Neurology, Montreal Neurological Institute,
McGill University Faculty of Medicine; Physiatrist and Director, Post-Polio Clinic,
Montreal Neurological Hospital, McGill University Health Center, Montreal, Que-
bec, Canada

Jose Vega, MD, PhD
Department of Physical Medicine and Rehabilitation, University of Medicine and
Dentistry of New Jersey–New Jersey Medical School; University Hospital, Newark,
New Jersey

PREFACE

During the course of working on this book, my co-editor, Dr. Anne Gawne told me that she would like to write the preface. She said, "There are some things I want to say." I readily agreed, knowing that whatever she wrote would be thoughtful and insightful. Unfortunately, Anne died suddenly in the middle of publishing this book, and none of us will ever know what exactly she had in mind.

I have found it a difficult process to sit down and write something meaningful in her place. I know for a fact, however, that one of the things that Anne would want me to say is a heartfelt thank-you to the people who contributed to this volume. The polio health care community is a small one. Most of us know each other, and we work together, collaborating and sharing ideas. So, thank you to all of the authors who wrote chapters for this book. Thank you for your willingness to devote your time and energy yet again to helping polio survivors.

Anne and I published this book with a focus on evidence-based medicine. The authors who contributed to this text are all extremely knowledgeable and have based their recommendations on what the current polio research reveals. Whenever I write or edit a book, I always ask myself two questions: (1) Will this book help people? and (2) Will I learn something from working on this project? With respect to this book, the answer to both questions is a resounding yes. I am confident that this text will help health care providers sharpen their skills in order to provide state-of-the-art medical treatment for polio survivors. Polio survivors, too, can benefit from reading this book—even if some of the writing is rather technical. Moreover, I have learned a great deal from my colleagues who collaborated with me on this project.

I sincerely wish that Anne was here to write this preface. She did, however, write several chapters in this book. I encourage you to read her work and to consider the wonderful contribution she made to helping polio survivors throughout the world.

For those of us who continue our work with polio survivors, we will remain steadfast in our goal to improve their health and quality of life through excellence in medical care and thoughtful research that is evidence based.

Julie K. Silver, MD

DEDICATION

To Dr. Anne Gawne, who cared deeply about the health and
well-being of polio survivors.

—JKS

ACKNOWLEDGMENTS

As with any authoritative work, there are many people who are responsible for the final text and who are deserving of recognition. In this case, I first want to recognize those individuals who have designed and conducted the research studies that are the basis for this publication. It is true that we need more research on polio-related issues, but there are many clinicians and scientists who are adding to our current knowledge about the late effects of polio and postpolio syndrome. For those of us who treat polio survivors, we are grateful for the diligent efforts of these investigators.

The authors who wrote chapters for this book have provided not only an insightful review of the scientific literature, but also their own clinical and research experiences that make the chapters vibrant and relevant. These contributors are heroes to many polio survivors—and for good reason. They are compassionate, intelligent, and extremely knowledgeable. They understand the research and know how to translate it into a clinical approach that makes sense. I am deeply grateful to all of them.

Lauro Halstead has long been a teacher, mentor, and friend to me. His expertise on polio-related issues is unsurpassed. Daria Trojan and her colleagues, Lois Finch and Deborah Da Costa, have made wonderful contributions to this text and to the polio literature in general. Daria did a lot of pinch hitting for me in getting this book together, and she is someone that many of us in the polio health care community know we can count on. Neil Cashman worked with Daria, and having collaborated extensively in the past, they continue to make a fine team. Fred Maynard is highly respected by all of us. His contribution to this book is extremely valuable. Kristian Borg is an amazingly intelligent and gracious man. It was a pleasure to work with him. John Bach is always the doctor I go to with my most complicated polio pulmonary issues. John is the foremost authority on respiratory complications in neuromuscular diseases, and his chapter on postpolio pulmonary dysfunction, with colleague Jose Vega, is an important section in this book. I am grateful to Barbara Sonies who took time out of her busy schedule at the National Institutes of Health to write a terrific chapter on speech and swallowing issues in polio survivors. Jim Agre is currently pursuing a number of other interests but still took time out to write a chapter on exercise. This is a complicated topic in the polio literature, and Jim wrote a thoughtful and insightful analysis for this text. Elizabeth Dean and Marijke Dallimore are experts on physical therapy and exercise in polio survivors, and their chapter is outstanding. Kathy Smith contributed an excellent chapter on aquatic therapy that I found truly enlightening. Brent Bernstein worked closely with Anne Gawne and provided a very informative chapter on polio foot and ankle problems. Dorothy Aiello is one of the physical therapists at my center, and she is incredibly knowledgeable. Her writing reflects a deep understanding of polio-related issues from both a research and clinical perspective. Pima McConnell was extremely kind to write a chapter quickly as my deadline loomed. She did a great job, and I am very thankful for her hard and fast work. Beth Kowall is an occupational therapist whose work many of us refer to on a regular basis. Her chapter is an important part of this volume. Maria Cole and Laura Ryan are both occupational therapists at my center. I am regularly impressed by their skill and empathy. Claire Kalpakjian, Sunny Roller, and Denise Tate wrote an insightful chapter on the psychological well-being of polio survivors—an often overlooked subject. To all of you who contributed: thank-you!

I am also grateful to the many polio survivors who have supported my work at the International Rehabilitation Center for Polio at Spaulding Rehabilitation Hospital. In particular, I am thankful for the wonderful support of David Rubin and his wife, Arlene. David Rubin is a successful businessman who contracted polio at 9 years of age. Although he is still very active, he is suffering from postpolio syndrome. David is determined to help not only himself, but other polio survivors who are similarly struggling with the late effects of this disease. The Rubin Family Fund for Polio Research helped to make this book possible.

A number of people at Spaulding have been extraordinarily helpful as well. Anna Rubin is the polio outreach and education coordinator at my center and is an amazing person to work with. Lori McCrohon is the clinical coordinator and is a gentle, compassionate, and capable woman. Lynn Forde expertly manages my center and has helped raise the level of skill of all of the clinicians on my team, including those who contributed to this book. Terry Cucuzza and Terry O'Brien are research librarians at Spaulding who help me on a daily basis with finding the important information that I need. I often wonder if they know how many lives their hard work touches. Walter Frontera is the Chairman of my department (Physical Medicine and Rehabilitation) at Harvard and has been my biggest supporter and finest mentor throughout my academic career. He is highly respected for his intelligence and thoughtful analysis of clinical, administrative, and research issues. Diana Barrett is the Chair of Spaulding's board, and her energy and enthusiasm are infectious. It is an honor and a pleasure to watch Diana in action. David Storto has been a wonderful leader and visionary for Spaulding. I appreciate his insight and support.

This book was published at a time when Elsevier acquired Hanley & Belfus, Inc. Therefore, I have several editors to thank for their hard work on this volume. I have worked with Bill Lamsback on several books, and I always appreciate his perceptive opinions. Tom Stringer and Cecelia Bayruns helped me start and finish this book, respectively. Linda Belfus was a big support behind the scenes.

And finally, I am grateful to my colleague, Anne Gawne, without whom this book would not exist. Thank you and may God bless you.

                                                                    Julie K. Silver, MD

Diagnosing Postpolio Syndrome: Inclusion and Exclusion Criteria

Lauro S. Halstead, MD, MPH

tarting around 1970, reports began to appear in the medical literature that persons who had paralytic poliomyelitis many years earlier were experiencing new health problems related to their prior illness.[4,11,35,37,42] Initially, one of the most common terms to describe these problems was *the late effects of polio*.[15,34] This term refers to all of the musculoskeletal and neuromuscular complaints that affect these individuals, many of which are no different from the symptoms experienced by anyone who has lived with a chronic neuromuscular condition for many decades. However, within this broad category of symptoms, it soon became clear that there was a smaller group of symptoms that was more specific and discrete.[3,22,31] Although no diagnostic test exists for these symptoms, most experts agree that they share a common pathophysiology primarily involving a dysfunction of polio-affected motor units.[49] These symptoms are now widely known as *postpolio syndrome* (PPS). This chapter describes the natural history of polio, the historical background of PPS, and how PPS is currently diagnosed using both inclusion and exclusion criteria.

THE NATURAL HISTORY OF POLIO

Historically, polio has been divided into three fairly distinct stages: acute illness, period of recovery, and stable disability. By the mid-1980s, however, clinicians and researchers began to realize there was a distinct fourth stage characterized by the onset of new symptoms related to the original polio attack.[13,23,30] This stage has been described by various terms, including *the late effects of polio, postpolio sequelae, postpolio progressive muscular atrophy, postpolio muscle dysfunction,* and *postpolio syndrome*.[18,21,50,56] The names *postpolio muscle dysfunction* and *postpolio progressive muscular atrophy* emphasize abnormal muscle function. This narrow focus makes these terms more appropriate for research. By contrast, PPS is broadly defined, making it more practical for clinical purposes. In addition, PPS has been widely used in the medical and lay literature for many years. For these reasons, PPS is used in this book.

Figure 1 shows the typical course for the three traditional stages of paralytic polio as well as the beginning of stage IV. The data for these health and functional changes are based on the acute and chronic polio experience of a group of persons evaluated at The Institute for Rehabilitation and Research Post-Polio Clinic in Houston, Texas.[31]

STAGE I: ACUTE ILLNESS

The symptoms at the onset of polio are similar to many other viral illnesses: they include mild fever, headache, sore throat, diarrhea or vomiting, and malaise. In the great majority of individuals, these symptoms are gone within 2 or 3 days. For fewer than 5% of the people who contract polio, however, the symptoms are more severe, reflecting a viral invasion of the central nervous system (CNS).[46] Infection of the CNS results in a sharp escalation of symptoms with high fever, stiff neck, severe headache, and muscle pains. In some individuals, the disease stops there and no weakness or paralysis ever occurs. In others (approximately 1–2% of those affected), the infection continues to spread, producing variable amounts of muscle paralysis or weakness in the limbs, trunk, and even the face and neck. During the large epidemics of the 1940s and 1950s, roughly 12% of those who developed acute paralytic poliomyelitis died from breathing or swallowing complications.[24,43,65,66]

STAGE II: PERIOD OF RECOVERY

Recovery begins as soon as an individual's temperature returns to normal and the other symptoms subside. This stage can last from weeks to years, depending on the severity of involvement and age at onset. Persons who contract polio as children or infants and have extensive paralysis take the longest time to recover. During this period, individuals usually begin an intensive program of rehabilitation in the hospital or home with the goal of strengthening and retraining weakened muscles and learning

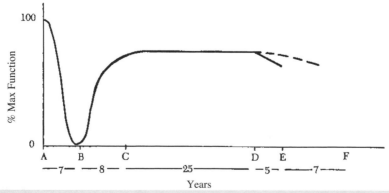

Figure 1. Natural history of polio. Health and functional changes showing the four stages of polio for 132 individuals with PPS at the Post-Polio Clinic in Houston, Texas. A = birth; B = onset of acute polio (average age of 7 years); B to C = period of recovery (an average of 8 years); C to D = maximum recovery and period of neurologic and functional stability (an average of 25 years); D = onset of PPS (B to D an average of 33 years); E = time of clinic evaluation (D to E, an average of 5 years); F = death (E to F, unknown). Dashed line = projected course without PPS.

to regain lost function. For the group of persons shown in Figure 1, the average length of stage II was 8 years.

STAGE III: STABLE DISABILITY

Stage III begins when a person reaches a plateau of maximum recovery of strength and stamina. The precise time when this stage starts may be hard to determine, especially if the individual is still growing and changing developmentally or is undergoing reconstructive surgery to enhance strength and function. Despite these difficulties, most people have a general idea about when their recovery was complete.

STAGE IV: POSTPOLIO SYNDROME

The third stage of polio lasts indefinitely for many individuals, perhaps for the majority who had paralytic polio. For as many as 50% of individuals, the stage of stable disability ends and stage IV or PPS begins with the onset of new weakness, which is often accompanied by other symptoms, such as fatigue, pain in the muscles or joints, and decreased function.[2,10,49,68] For the individuals shown in Figure 1, stage III lasted an average of 25 years. Stage IV began, on average, 33 years after the acute onset of polio. A similar interval is found in other studies, but the range has been reported to extend from 2 to 8 decades.[1,27,30]

THE HISTORY OF POSTPOLIO SYNDROME

The late effects of polio have been recognized for more than a century with the first descriptions appearing in the French medical literature in 1875.[12,17,51] These cases involved three young men who had paralytic polio in infancy and developed significant new weakness and atrophy as young adults. These new problems occurred in muscles previously affected by polio and in muscles thought to be spared. All of the subjects had physically demanding jobs that required strength and repetitive activities. In a commentary on one of the cases, the great 19th century French neuropathologist Jean Martin Charcot suggested several hypotheses for these changes.[51] He believed an initial disease of the spinal cord (e.g., polio) might leave some individuals more susceptible to a subsequent spinal disorder. He also hypothesized that the new weakness was caused by overuse of the involved muscles. His observations are surprisingly relevant to our current understanding of PPS.

After those initial reports, there was only sporadic interest in the late effects of polio for many decades. In the century after Charcot's observations, fewer than 35 published reports appeared, describing fewer than 250 cases.[67] As with the first subjects, these reports described new problems that included weakness, atrophy, and fasciculations, occurring up to 71 years after an attack of paralytic polio.

It is unclear why these aftereffects of polio remained an obscure and largely unexplored area of medicine until recently. Few diseases are as widely prevalent in the world or have been as intensively investigated as polio. Because of the rapid and dramatic onset of symptoms, polio was viewed as a classic example of an acute viral infectious disease. As a result, most of the scientific energy and resources were directed at early management and prevention with virtually no research into long-term seque-lae.[43] Until recently, medical textbooks classified paralytic polio as a *static* or stable neurologic disease.[36]

With widespread use of the vaccines, polio quickly became a medical oddity in the industrialized world; interest and funding in polio-related problems waned. However, polio and its complications only *appeared* to have been defeated. Because the major epidemics occurred in the 1940s and 1950s and new neurologic changes appeared 30–40 years later, many thousands of polio survivors in this country did not begin to experience new problems related to their polio until the late 1970s and early 1980s.

By sheer weight of numbers, persons experiencing PPS finally started attracting widespread attention in the early 1980s. The term *postpolio syndrome* was coined at about the time of the first International Post-Polio Conference at Warm Springs, Georgia, in May 1984.[13,33] In the intervening years, there has been a marked increase in the attention focused on PPS by researchers and clinicians, leading to a more pre-cise definition, a better understanding of possible causes, and development of more effective management.[20,60]

EPIDEMIOLOGY AND RISK FACTORS FOR POSTPOLIO SYNDROME

Accurate numbers of Americans who had paralytic poliomyelitis are not available and probably never will be. There is no national registry of persons who had polio. Also, there is no way, after all these years, to compile accurate figures from state and local health departments. The best estimate is based on data from the government's National Center for Health Statistics, which conducts a National Health Interview Survey each year. This survey collects data from a random sample of the U.S. popu-lation regarding various health and disability issues. In 1987, surveyors specifically asked questions about the number of persons who were given a diagnosis of po-liomyelitis with or without paralysis. Based on the results of this survey, the Center calculated slightly more than 1.63 million polio survivors. Of these, 641,000 (39.2%) persons had paralytic polio; 833,000 (51%) had nonparalytic polio; and 160,000 (9.8%) did not know which they had.[45] Unfortunately, some of these data have been miscopied or misrepresented and then erroneously published in the medical literature as fact. The most common error is the statement citing 1.63 million persons with par-alytic polio when the correct estimate is really 641,000 as cited above.

The latter figure, however, is based on a survey conducted more than 15 years ago. Since then, it has been estimated that 5–10% of the polio population has died. This attrition has been offset in part, at least, by the recent recognition that a number of persons who had nonparalytic polio (or no history of polio at all) had sufficient inva-sion of the CNS early in life by the poliovirus to cause PPS many years later.[32] As a result, both the numbers of individuals with PPS and those at risk for developing it are unknown. Based on a review of the literature, a consensus statement by the Post-Polio Task Force noted, "On the basis of symptoms (from questionnaire and clinic studies), PPS will develop in about 50% of survivors of acute paralytic polio (APP). Retrospective studies using objective criteria have estimated that PPS will develop in

20% to 40% of APP survivors."[49] Using these figures, the number of persons currently experiencing PPS is probably in the range of 200,000–400,000 individuals. However, it is important to note that the majority of polio survivors who have residual paralysis will need medical treatment as they age regardless of whether or not they have PPS.

A number of studies have found that the persons most at risk or most likely to develop PPS were those who experienced severe polio initially and, more particularly, those whose original losses were largely regained during the period of recovery.[31] *It is not unusual, however, to see individuals with typical postpolio symptoms who had seemingly very mild acute polio followed by an excellent recovery.*[32,52] Besides severity at onset, other risk factors identified in research studies include a greater length of time since the onset of polio, the presence of permanent impairment after recovery, a recent increase of weight or physical activity, and being older at the time of diagnosis.[2,38,39,58,62,68] Several studies also found that women are more likely to develop PPS than men.[50,63] Most commonly, the onset of new problems is gradual, but in many persons, the outset may be triggered by specific events, such as a minor accident, a fall, a period of bed rest, or surgery. Typically, individuals report that a similar event experienced several years earlier would not have caused the same decline in health and function.[30]

MAKING A DIAGNOSIS OF POSTPOLIO SYNDROME

PPS is a *neurologic* disorder that produces a cluster of symptoms in individuals who had poliomyelitis many years earlier. Typically, these problems occur after a period of functional and neurologic stability of *at least 15 years* after the initial episode of polio and include new weakness, fatigue, decreased endurance, and loss of function.[1,2,10,18,25,56] Some researchers also add pain as part of the syndrome, especially in muscles and joints.[39,54] Less commonly, the symptoms include muscle atrophy, breathing and swallowing difficulties, and cold intolerance.[6,21,34,55] Some of the symptoms (e.g., weakness, fatigue, and atrophy) appear to be caused by a progressive degeneration or impairment of motor units. Other symptoms (e.g., muscle and joint pain) are more likely the result of excessive wear and tear on different parts of the musculoskeletal system, although this wear and tear can be brought on or made worse when muscles become weaker.

The percentage of new health and functional problems reported by persons evaluated in several studies is listed in Table 1.[1,14,15,31,50] The most common problems are fatigue, weakness, and pain in the muscles and joints. The new weakness is located in muscles previously affected by polio as well as in muscles believed to be *unaffected* by the original illness. At first glance, the phenomenon of "unaffected" muscles becoming weak seems contradictory but, in fact, is well known. Usually, it means that the polio was so mild in those muscles at the time of the original illness that the individual, as well as health care professionals, was unaware of any polio involvement in those particular limbs. However, there was enough loss of motor neurons that after many years of overuse, new weakness developed. The most common new functional

Table 1. NEW HEALTH AND FUNCTIONAL PROBLEMS IN PATIENTS WITH PPS	
SYMPTOM	**PATIENTS, %**
Health Problems	
Fatigue	86–87
Muscle pain	71–86
Joint pain	71–79
Weakness	
• Previously affected muscles	69–87
• Previously unaffected muscles	50–77
Cold intolerance	29–56
Atrophy	28–39
ADL Problems	
Walking	64–85
Stair climbing	61–83
Dressing	16–62

problems include increased difficulty in walking, climbing stairs, and dressing—activities that require repetitive muscular contractions.[2,14,16,31]

In the absence of a pathognomonic test, the diagnosis of PPS has traditionally been based on inclusion criteria that are essentially subjective in nature. This subjective information is often supplemented with objective clinical and electrodiagnostic data that are helpful but nondiagnostic. Because no diagnostic test exists, the inclusion criteria require that other disorders with similar symptoms be *excluded* by history, physical examination, and appropriate laboratory testing. For this reason, PPS has often been called a diagnosis by exclusion even though specific exclusion criteria have never been defined.[30,49]

The current criteria for diagnosing PPS are listed in Table 2.[49] *New weakness is the cardinal symptom of PPS.* Without a clear history of new weakness, the diagnosis cannot be made. When diagnosing PPS, several other considerations need to be kept in mind. First, symptoms such as pain and fatigue are fairly common and nonspecific. Ruling out *all* possible causes, therefore, is not practical and can be prohibitively expensive. Second, coexisting medical, orthopedic, and neurologic conditions may be present and can produce very similar symptoms. Deciding which symptoms are caused by PPS and which symptoms are caused by another condition can be difficult for even the most experienced clinician. As shown in Figure 2, after a problem such as weakness or pain occurs—regardless of the underlying cause—it may initiate a chain reaction of other complications that makes the original problem difficult or even impossible to identify. A common example occurs when new weakness (see Fig. 2A) develops in the quadriceps. The loss in strength may decrease the stability of the joint, leading to knee pain (Fig. 2B). To minimize the pain, the individual then uses that leg less frequently (Fig. 2C), which, in turn, may lead to disuse weakness and increased pain. If the cycle continues, the original problem of new weakness is often ob-

Table 2. CRITERIA FOR DIAGNOSING POSTPOLIO SYNDROME		
ORIGINAL CRITERIA[42]	**CURRENT CRITERIA**[49]	**PROPOSED CRITERIA**
1. Credible history of prior poliomyelitis	1. Prior episode of paralytic polio with residual motor neuron loss (which can be confirmed through a typical patient history, a neurological exam, and, if needed, an EMG exam)	1. No change
2. Partial recovery of function	2. A period of neurologic recovery followed by an interval (usually > 15 years) of neurologic and functional stability	2. No change
3. Minimum of 10 years of stabilization	3. A gradual or abrupt onset of new weakness or abnormal muscle fatigability (decreased endurance), with or without generalized fatigue, muscle atrophy, or pain (period of stabilization changed to 15 years in #2 above)	3. A gradual or abrupt onset of *progressive* new weakness with a duration of *at least 12 months* (the rest unchanged)
4. Subsequent development of *progressive* muscle weakness	4. Exclusion of medical, orthopedic, or neurologic conditions that may be causing the symptoms mentioned in #3 above	4. No change
		5. Confirmation of the diagnosis by reevaluation of the patient and clinical course *at least 3 to 6 months* after the original diagnosis

scured by time and the presence of other symptoms. To clarify the initial symptom takes patience and persistence.

EVALUATION: GENERAL PRINCIPLES

The evaluation of postpolio individuals with new health problems presents a challenge because of the general nature of many of the symptoms and the absence of special diagnostic tests. This challenge is further complicated by the continuing uncertainty of the underlying cause and the lack of any medications or treatments that might result in a cure.[20] In light of these circumstances, it is important that even the most knowledge-

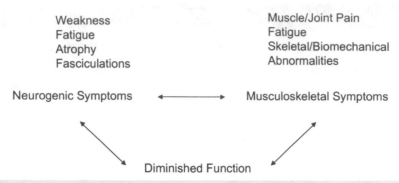

Figure 2. Perpetuating cycle of postpolio symptoms.

able health professional follow a systematic step-by-step approach to the evaluation of every individual who might have PPS. These steps are outlined in Table 3.[49]

Confirming the original diagnosis of paralytic polio has to be based on the medical history and physical examination. If these are inconclusive, a standard electromyogram (EMG) should be performed to look for the characteristic changes associated with a prior anterior horn cell disease (AHCD). These typically include giant motor units, an increase in polyphasic potentials, and decreased recruitment on voluntary muscle contractions.

To determine the extent and severity of current deficits, it is extremely helpful to obtain a *quantitative history* of a patient's function over a number of years. Because new weakness is manifested by decreased muscle endurance, this quantitative history should emphasize activities that require repetitive or sustained contractions such as walking, climbing stairs, or standing. A typical example is a 48-year-old man who was evaluated in the National Rehabilitation Hospital (NRH) Post-Polio Clinic with a

Table 3. STEP-BY-STEP APPROACH TO EVALUATING INDIVIDUALS WITH POSSIBLE POSTPOLIO SYNDROME*	
1. Confirm the original diagnosis of paralytic polio. 2. Determine the extent and severity of current deficits of strength, stamina, function, and so on. 3. Develop a list of reasonable alternative explanations for each symptom.	4. Perform diagnostic tests to exclude or confirm non-PPS causes for each symptom. 5. If other causes diagnosed, treat and then assess need for remaining rehabilitation or medical interventions. 6. If no additional causes diagnosed, establish an objective baseline of function and a plan for rehabilitation or medical interventions.

*Adapted from the Post-Polio Task Force Recommendations (unpublished).

6-year history of progressive new weakness in both legs. He had paralytic polio at age 16 months and eventually made a good recovery. As an adult, he walked with a limp but used no assistive devices. Ten years before his evaluation, he was able to walk approximately 2 miles and climb three flights of stairs without difficulty. Five years before his initial visit (and 1 year after the onset of his new weakness), his endurance dropped to approximately 1 mile of walking and 2 flights of stairs using a banister. At the time of his evaluation, his walking was limited to several blocks and climbing was limited to one flight of stairs, which he avoided whenever possible. In the absence of other illnesses that might explain his decline in function, this kind of historical information is almost diagnostic of PPS. Nonetheless, it is still critical to perform a thorough physical examination as part of the process of excluding other diagnostic possibilities.

This examination should emphasize a careful neurologic evaluation and attention to muscle and skeletal abnormalities such as scoliosis, a leg length discrepancy, a decrease in range of motion in major joints, and irregular patterns of walking. Deep tendon reflexes are generally diminished proportional to muscle strength; sensation should be normal. A limb that has been severely paralyzed may have *increased* sensitivity to light touch and pinprick; any *decrease* in sensation indicates some problem other than polio.

Because of the number, diversity, and complexity of the problems presented by many postpolio individuals, we have found it beneficial in the NRH Clinic to supplement, when appropriate, the standard medical history and physical examination performed by the physician with evaluations by other members of the rehabilitation team. Typically, this interdisciplinary team includes a nurse educator, physical and occupational therapists, and social worker or psychologist. Depending on the specific problems, an orthotist, respiratory therapist, dietitian, or vocational counselor may also be involved. Referrals to pulmonologists, orthopedists, neurologists, and other specialists are made as needed. Of prime importance is the fact that, for many individuals, the evaluation in an established postpolio clinic is the first assessment done by a group of specialists that is knowledgeable and comfortable with polio and the features of PPS.[29,53]

In addition to evaluations by members of the interdisciplinary team, an electrodiagnostic evaluation is helpful in evaluating limbs or muscles *thought* to be spared by the original infection but which, in fact, sustained subclinical polio. The information obtained by these studies can also be helpful in prescribing appropriate exercise programs. In addition, this examination can provide clues that assist in diagnosing or excluding a number of other neuromuscular disorders. A summary of abnormalities found on EMG and nerve conduction study (NCS) in 108 subjects evaluated at the NRH Post-Polio Clinic in Washington, D.C., is listed in Table 4.[28]

Based on the initial evaluation, a differential diagnosis is developed for each of the major symptoms of PPS. As a rule, we have not found it helpful to order a standard battery of screening tests for all individuals. Specific tests, such as complete blood count, hemoglobin A_{1c}, creatine kinase (CK), and thyroid function tests, are obtained when indicated by the medical history and physical examination. This applies to expensive imaging studies as well, such as a computed tomography scan or mag-

Table 4. ELECTRODIAGNOSTIC FINDINGS IN 108 POSTPOLIO INDIVIDUALS

FINDINGS	PATIENTS, %
Carpal tunnel syndrome (CTS)	32
Ulnar neuropathy at the wrist	2
CTS and ulnar neuropathy	3
Peripheral neuropathy	3
Brachial plexopathy	1
Tibial neuropathy	1
Radiculopathy	4
Subclinical polio	45

netic resonance imaging to evaluate for nerve root entrapment, spinal stenosis, or a spinal cord abnormality. Whether it is useful to monitor CK levels on a regular basis to assist in determining long-term prognosis or as an aid in clinical management is still not clear.[23,44,60,64]

Persons who initially had respiratory involvement and have a history of pulmonary disease, smoking, or scoliosis should have pulmonary function studies, including arterial blood gases. Individuals with significant spinal curvature should be evaluated with a weight-loaded scoliosis radiograph. If degenerative joint disease or other skeletal abnormality is suspected, plain films of the appropriate joints are ordered. A recent study by Trojan and colleagues using magnetic resonance spectroscopy demonstrated a significant decrease in N-acetylaspartate (NAA) and the NAA-to-creatine ratio in the reticular activating system of postpolio individuals with significant fatigue compared with normal subjects.[59] This finding is in an investigative stage, and it is unknown how it will eventually be applied in clinical settings. Another provocative finding was recently reported by Borg and associates.[7] They found that inflammatory cytokines were elevated in the spinal fluid and serum of individuals with PPS in the same range as persons with multiple sclerosis. The significance of this observation is still unclear but may imply that there is an inflammatory component associated with the pathogenesis of PPS.

To sum up, the assessments provided by special diagnostic testing are generally more fruitful in *excluding* certain conditions than assisting in the diagnosis or management of patients with PPS. Despite the growing body of evidence suggesting motor unit deterioration as the cause of new weakness, there is still no objective method to predict who might develop PPS in the future or to monitor the progression of the underlying cause in those who are already becoming weaker. Specifically, no radiograph, blood test, or muscle biopsy, singly or in combination, can diagnose PPS. Instead, a careful, detailed clinical history must be relied on to distinguish between individuals who have *no new weakness* (stable polio) and those who are experiencing *progressive new weakness* (unstable polio) after a period of stability of at least 15 years.

INCLUSION AND EXCLUSION CRITERIA

The original criteria for PPS were proposed by Mulder and colleagues in 1972 and are shown in Table 2.[42] Although they did not use the term *postpolio syndrome*, they described 34 individuals seen at the Mayo Clinic who had a history of paralytic polio followed many years later by new polio-related health problems. They labeled these problems a "late progression of poliomyelitis" and speculated that they might represent a variant or *forme fruste* of amyotrophic lateral sclerosis (ALS). Although they were not the first to propose a link between ALS and polio, it has since been shown in a number of studies that there is no relationship between ALS and a history of poliomyelitis.[9,48] However, the criteria Mulder and colleagues identified for the late progression of poliomyelitis or PPS are still relevant today and have been modified only slightly over the years.

In 1995, the Post-Polio Task Force proposed several changes to the earlier criteria (see Table 2).[49] Although not specifically called inclusion criteria, they have become the accepted standard by which PPS is currently diagnosed. Although these recommendations are still valid, further clinical experience suggests that the Task Force criteria need to be reconsidered and several modifications should be added (see Table 2).

The first change concerns the term *new weakness*. Although most practitioners may already assume *progressive* weakness is meant when discussing this symptom, there is merit in making the concept explicit and requiring there be a *progressive* component to the history of new weakness, as illustrated in the case history described earlier. As shown in Table 2, *progressive weakness* was part of the initial criteria; therefore, this recommendation can be simply seen as a return to the original proposal.

The second recommendation would require that the symptom of progressive new weakness be present for a minimum period of time, for example, at least 12 months. Although proposing the interval of 12 months is arbitrary, adding a dimension of time is very deliberate. Finally, the third proposed change also includes a dimension of time. In this case, the interval of time comes *after* the initial diagnosis. The specific proposal is that the diagnosis be confirmed by reassessing the patient and the clinical course at least 3–6 months *after* the original diagnosis. The rationale for this proposal is described in the next section under the discussion of the different subtypes of PPS.

In addition to the inclusion criteria discussed, it is useful to consider certain exclusion criteria to facilitate an accurate diagnosis of PPS. A preliminary list of exclusion criteria is outlined in Table 5. These criteria, although helpful, should be used with caution. They are not absolute except perhaps for number 3, the absence of findings on EMG consistent with prior anterior horn cell disease, and number 4, no history of new weakness. A number of individuals evaluated had a negative history of acute polio and yet, at some point early in their lives, were exposed to the poliovirus and had typical symptoms consistent with a diagnosis of PPS.[32] We have also seen persons who had no obvious polio stigmata on examination; however, in these cases, the history and electrodiagnostic findings confirmed the presence of prior polio and a diagnosis of PPS.

Finally, when the symptoms can be explained by another diagnosis, the differential reasoning may be very straightforward or quite subtle. Here are two examples. The first case is a 45-year-old man from Nigeria who had polio at age 10 years involving the right leg more than left. As an adult, he had no difficulty walking until 18 months before his NRH Clinic evaluation, when he sustained a compound fracture of his left leg in a motor vehicle accident. This injury required several operations and a prolonged period of bed rest and rehabilitation that lasted for nearly 6 months. When seen in the NRH Clinic, he gave a history of 14–16 months of new weakness in his injured leg. Was it PPS or disuse weakness? Fortunately, we were able to follow-up with him in the clinic for the next 6 months, during which time his strength gradually improved until he was back to his preinjury level of strength. Applying the inclusion criteria listed in Table 2 and the exclusion criteria listed in Table 5, it was clear he did *not* have a diagnosis of PPS. His 14–16-month history of new weakness was not progressive; follow-up evaluation at 6 months showed he had regained his baseline strength; and finally, there was a clear alternate explanation (disuse weakness) for his decreased strength that turned out to be temporary.

The second case is a 52-year-old woman evaluated in the NRH Clinic with a history of progressive diminished walking endurance over the preceding 8 years. She had a convincing history of paralytic polio at age 3 years with a good recovery that allowed her to walk with a right short leg brace. She also had a 40-pack-year history of smoking that resulted in a diagnosis of chronic obstructive pulmonary disease. Although she had stopped smoking a number of years before her visit to the clinic, her pulmonologist confirmed that her lung function was deteriorating and produced progressive shortness of breath on walking. Although the qualitative history of walking endurance reflected an obvious downward trend, it was difficult to determine with confidence how much, if any, of her progressive new weakness was polio related and how much of her decline in function was caused by her pulmonary disease. Using the inclusion and exclusion criteria, she met three of the five proposed inclusion criteria (see Table 2). However, we thought she also fulfilled the last exclusion criteria listed in Table 5 and that her decline in walking and apparent new weakness was not polio related but instead caused by her chronic lung disease. Was this the correct diagnosis? It is difficult to know for certain, and until there is a diagnostic test, we will have to rely in such cases—as is true in many other areas of medicine—on the experience and clinical judgment of the examining physician.

Table 5. EXCLUSION CRITERIA IN THE DIAGNOSIS OF PPS
1. No history of acute polio
2. Absence of stigmata on physical examination
3. No findings on EMG consistent with prior anterior horn cell disease (AHCD)
4. No history of progressive new weakness
5. Other diagnosis explains symptoms

MISDIAGNOSIS

A number of challenges confront even the most experienced clinician when making a diagnosis of PPS. One of these challenges is the tendency toward misdiagnosis (either under- or overdiagnosis). Despite the thoughtful and carefully crafted criteria proposed by the Post-Polio Task Force, many clinicians believe PPS is still misdiagnosed.[5] Some of the factors that contribute to this phenomenon are listed in Table 6. In addition, diagnostic uncertainty tends to be inherent in dealing with many syndromes generally, and PPS has unique circumstances, including the persistent demands of informed consumers who want an explanation for their multiple symptoms; the tendency of polio survivors to be well educated and skillful in obtaining information in this age of the Internet; and the fact that after years of disability, many may feel a certain sense of entitlement to a new diagnosis that explains their otherwise undiagnosed symptoms as they age.

But other possible explanations also exist as to why PPS is probably misdiagnosed. The first is based on biological reasoning, and the second on clinical observation. The biological reasoning is as follows: virtually every disease or disorder has a spectrum of biological or pathological severity—from extremely mild (in fact, so mild it is difficult to detect) to very severe.[26,41] Although we may all acknowledge this fact intuitively with regard to PPS, there is no proposed taxonomy that takes this into account. Patients either meet the criteria and have PPS or they do not. Even for disorders that do have specific diagnostic tests, there are still issues of *sensitivity* and *specificity* that invariably lead to false-positive and false-negative results.[26] The logical conclusion is that in a disorder such as PPS, in which there is no diagnostic test, we all must encounter occasional false-positive and false-negative results. By definition, these encounters must inevitably result in an unknown number of misdiagnoses and, at least, *raises the possibility* of over- or underdiagnosing.

The second reason PPS is probably misdiagnosed is based on the clinical observation that there appears to be a *differential progression* of symptoms in individuals given the diagnosis of PPS. Table 7 summarizes these informal observations and outlines four proposed subtypes of PPS based on their clinical courses.

Type I, or an "indeterminate" diagnosis, represents approximately 5–10% of individuals seen in the clinical setting. Generally, their involvement was not severe at onset and their symptoms are relatively mild. They may make a few modifications in

Table 6. FACTORS THAT INFLUENCE THE MISDIAGNOSIS OF PPS

1. Subjective diagnosis based on:
    • Patient report
    • Nonspecific symptoms
 2. Overlay of physical and psychological factors
 3. Highly dependent on experience or bias of examiner
 4. No diagnostic test
 5. No definitive cure or treatment
 6. Diagnosis by exclusion

their lifestyle and upgrade their bracing, start using a cane, or start an exercise program. These interventions are typically followed by the individuals' regaining their lost strength and then remaining stable. The vast majority of this group probably has disuse weakness or else a very mild form of PPS.

Type II is the largest group and represents approximately 50–60% of persons diagnosed with PPS. The clinical course of this group is best categorized by the term "stair step." After interventions, they may stabilize for a period of several months or even several years. This is followed by additional loss of strength and function that prompts the individual to make more interventions to accommodate to the new level of weakness. Over the years, this cycle is then repeated. It is likely that these people have true PPS, and their clinical course simply manifests on a macro level a reflection of the constant modeling, remodeling, and dropout of the motor units on a cellular level.[59]

Type III is the smallest group and represents somewhere between 3% and 5% of persons with a diagnosis of PPS. They usually had fairly severe polio at onset and then made a good neurologic recovery. They have often led very active lives. Despite conscientious efforts to implement interventions, they tend to pursue a mostly benign but relentless progressive downhill course. These individuals also have PPS and are probably similar to the group reported by Mulder and colleagues in 1972.[42] If there is an immunologic component to PPS, it would most likely be present in this group.

Finally, type IV, which affects approximately 25–35% of persons diagnosed with PPS, is a miscellaneous group that experiences some combination of the other three types. Perhaps one of the reasons that explains the presumed existence of these subtypes is the presence of fluctuating pathology of the giant motor units as proposed by Dalakas in analyzing the failure of drug trials.[19]

Figure 3 shows the clinical course for types I–III for four time periods. As suggested earlier, by adding a period of observation of at least 3–6 months *after* the diagnosis has been made, a number of persons with type I who are currently carrying a *false-positive* diagnosis would no longer be considered to have PPS. Although these three

Table 7. PROPOSED SUBTYPES OF PPS BASED ON CLINICAL COURSE	
SUBTYPES	**CLINICAL COURSE**
I	After interventions, they regain lost strength and remain stable; **most of these patients probably do not have PPS.**
II	After interventions, they have a stair-step course. They stabilize for several months or years and then lose more strength and function, only to restabilize again. **Most of these patients probably have PPS**.
III	Despite interventions, they have a benign but relentless and progressive downhill course; **all have PPS and are probably similar to the patients reported by Mulder** et al.[42]
IV	These patients experience some combination of the clinical courses described above.

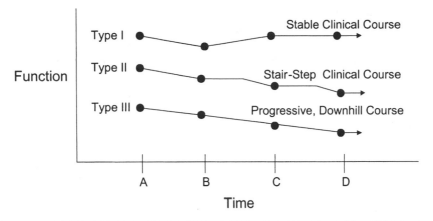

Figure 3. The clinical course for postpolio syndrome subtypes I, II, and III before and after diagnosis. A = 12 months prior to diagnosis; B = time of diagnosis; C = 3–6 months after diagnosis; D = future clinical course.

proposed subtypes of PPS are based on a description of their clinical course, any attempt to imply that there might be an etiologic basis as well is purely hypothetical. At this stage of our knowledge, a number of other descriptive labels might be equally apt. For example, one alternative nomenclature for these subtypes might be something as simple as "mild," "moderate," and "severe" forms of PPS, a taxonomy widely used to describe clinical variations among other disorders in medicine.

These suggestions are based on theoretical considerations and clinical experience. Their intent is to strengthen the current inclusion criteria with the goal of improving the accuracy and reliability of diagnosing PPS. The most important of these modifications concerns the dimension of time. Although this adds a level of complexity to making the diagnosis, there are numerous precedents for including the dimension of time in diagnosing other disorders. For example, each minor criteria of chronic fatigue syndrome (CFS) must be present for 6 or more months[47]; the Mayo Clinic's diagnostic criteria for tension myalgia requires that certain symptoms be present for more than 3 months[57]; and Jones and Hazleman's criteria for polymyalgia rheumatica requires that certain symptoms be present for two or more months.[8]

Another modification of the inclusion criteria involves obtaining follow-up information on the patient's clinical course. The proposed four subtypes shown in Table 7 illustrate a hypothetical scenario for three of these subtypes. It is entirely possible that there may be others as well or none at all. A third reason for misdiagnosing PPS is the absence of any studies that document the reliability of making the diagnosis. Clinicians and researchers have been debating the problems associated with diagnostic reliability for years about a wide variety of conditions; some of the more notable examples in recent years include polymyalgia rheumatica, attention deficit hyperactive disorder, CFS, and fibromyalgia (FM). In many of these conditions, the first step was for investigators to develop consensus criteria that then were refined over the years.[8,40,47] Sometimes these criteria became adopted by various professional organizations and then subjected to multicenter trials—not treatment trials but *diagnostic* trials with control groups and blinded examiners. At least two such studies have been reported that evaluated the criteria for FM.[69,70]

The field of PPS has begun to pursue a similar course. The work of the Post-Polio Task Force represented an important initial effort to develop consensus criteria.[49] Those criteria were then used as a basis for a multicenter trial of the medication pyridostigmine.[61] Unfortunately, because the results did not demonstrate significant benefits, the manufacturer of pyridostigmine withdrew its support for any further trials, either of the drug or of the criteria. However, in the absence of a diagnostic test, it is exactly this kind of investigation— a multicenter PPS inter-rater reliability study similar to those conducted for FM—that remains the next challenge in improving the clinical diagnosis of PPS.

CONCLUSION

Polio is on the brink of extinction and yet, ironically, both in the United States and around the world, it remains an illness that continues to be the source of widespread disability and suffering. It is now more than 40 years since the last dramatic epidemics occurred in the United States, but polio still remains the second leading cause of paralysis (approximately 600,000 individuals) after stroke. Many of these people—perhaps most—experience the aches and pains and loss of function common to other chronic musculoskeletal conditions.[16] These symptoms represent the late effects of polio. However, within this broad group of symptoms, a smaller cluster of disabling symptoms (affecting ≤ 50% of polio survivors) exists that have been accepted by the medical community as PPS. *The hallmark of this syndrome is progressive new weakness and is best diagnosed by a quantitative history of declining muscle endurance, a thorough physical examination, and a thoughtful exclusion of other diseases or disorders that might explain one or more of the PPS symptoms.* The inclusion and exclusion criteria discussed in this chapter are intended to facilitate the process of making what can often be a challenging diagnosis even for clinicians working in the field. It is important to remember, however, that these criteria are simply guidelines and were not developed as a surrogate for a diagnostic test; that will have to wait for additional research. As with many other syndromes in medicine that rely on subjective information for a diagnosis, there is, in the final analysis, no substitute for old-fashioned clinical experience.

ACKNOWLEDGMENT

I am grateful to Daria A. Trojan, M.D., for her helpful suggestions in reviewing the manuscript.

References

1. Agre JC, Rodriquez AA, Sperling KB: Symptoms and clinical impressions of patients seen in a post-polio clinic. Arch Phys Med Rehabil 70:367–370, 1989.

2. Agre JC, Rodriguez AA: Neuromuscular function: Comparison of symptomatic and asymptomatic polio subjects to control subjects. Arch Phys Med Rehabil 68:86–90, 1990.
3. Alter M, Kurland LT, Molgaard C: Late progressive muscular atrophy and antecedent poliomyelitis. In Rowland, LP (ed): Human Motor Neuron Diseases. New York, Raven Press, 1982.
4. Anderson A, Levine S, Gilbert H: Loss of ambulatory ability in patients with old anterior poliomyelitis. Lancet 2:1061–1063, 1972.
5. Aurlien D, Strandjord RE, Hegland O: The post-polio syndrome—a critical comment to the diagnosis. Acta Neurol Scand 100:76–80, 1999.
6. Bach JR, Alba AS: Pulmonary dysfunction and sleep-disordered breathing as post-polio sequelae: Evaluation and management. Ortho 14:1329–1337, 1991.
7. Borg K: Personal communication, 2002.
8. Brooks RC, McGee SR: Diagnostic dilemmas in polymyalgia rheumatica. Arch Intern Med 157:162–168, 1997.
9. Brown S, Patten BM: Post-polio syndrome and amyotrophic lateral sclerosis: A relationship more apparent than real. In Halstead LS, Wiechers DO (eds): Research and Clinical Aspects of the Late Effects of Poliomyelitis. White Plains, NY, March of Dimes Birth Defects Foundation, 1987, pp 83–98.
10. Bruno RL, Cohen JM, Galski T, Frick NM: The neuroanatomy of post-polio fatigue. Arch Phys Med Rehabil 75:498–504, 1994.
11. Campbell AMG, Williams ER, Pearce J: Late motorneuron degeneration following poliomyelitis. Neurology 19:1101–1106, 1969.
12. Carriere M: Des amytrophies spinales secondaire: Contribution a l'etude de la diffusion des lesions irritaves du systeme nerveu. These de Montpeleliere, France, 1875.
13. Cashman NR, Raymond CA: Decades after polio epidemics, survivors report new symptoms. JAMA 255:1397–1404, 1986.
14. Chetwynd J, Hogan D: Post-polio syndrome in New Zealand: A survey of 700 polio survivors. N Z Med J 106:406–408, 1993.
15. Codd M: Poliomyelitis in Rochester, Minnesota, 1935–1955. Epidemiology and long-term sequelae: A preliminary report. In Halstead LS, Wiechers DO (eds): Late Effects of Poliomyelitis. Miami, Symposia Foundation, 1985, pp 121–134.
16. Collet F: Perceived Health and Physical Performance in Postpoliomyelitis Syndrome. Amsterdam, PrintPartners Ipskamp BV, 2002.
17. Cornil V, Lepine R: Sur un cas de paralysie generale spinale anterieure subaigue, suivi d'autopsie. Gaz Med (Paris) 4:127–129, 1875.
18. Cosgrove JL, Alexander MA, Kitts EL, et al: Late effects of poliomyelitis. Arch Phys Med Rehabil 68:4–7, 1987.
19. Dalakas MC: Why drugs fail in postpolio syndrome: Lessons from another clinical trial. Neurology 53:1166–1167, 1999.
20. Dalakas MC, Bartfeld H, Kurland LT (eds): The Post-Polio Syndrome: Advances in the Pathogenesis and Treatment. Ann NY Acad Sci 753, 1995.
21. Dalakas MC, Elder G, Cunningham G, Sever JC: Morphological changes in the muscles of patient with post-poliomyelitis muscular atrophy (PPMA): 38 biopsies [abstract]. Neurology 36(suppl 1):137, 1986.
22. Dalakas MC, Elder G, Hallet M, et al: A long-term follow-up study of patients with post-poliomyelitis neuromuscular symptoms. N Engl J Med 314:959–963, 1986.
23. Dalakas MC, Sever JL, Fletcher M, et al: Neuromuscular symptoms in patients with old poliomyelitis: Clinical, virological, and immunological studies. In Halstead LS, Wiechers DO (eds): Late Effects of Poliomyelitis. Miami, Symposia Foundation 1985, p 73.

24. Dauer C: The changing age distribution of paralytic poliomyelitis. Ann NY Acad Sci 61:943–955, 1955.
25. Dirard C, Ravaud JF, Held JP: French survey of postpolio sequelae. Am J Phys Med Rehabil 73:264–267, 1994.
26. Feinstein AR: Clinical Epidemiology: The Architecture of Clinical Research. Philadelphia, W.B. Saunders, 1985.
27. Frick NM: Demographic and psychological characteristics of the post-polio community. Paper presented at the First Annual Conference on the Late Effects of Poliomyelitis. Lansing, MI, 1985.
28. Gawne AC, Pham BT, Halstead LS: Electrodiagnostic finding in 108 consecutive patients referred to a post-polio clinic: The value of routine electrodiagnostic studies. Ann NY Acad Sci 25:383–385, 1995.
29. Halstead LS (ed): Managing Post-Polio: A Guide to Living Well with Post-Polio Syndrome. Washington, NRH Press, 1998.
30. Halstead LS, Rossi CD: New problems in old polio patients: Results of a survey of 539 polio surviviors. Orthopedics 8:845–850, 1985.
31. Halstead LS, Rossi DC: Post-polio syndrome: Clinical experience with 132 consecutive outpatients. In Halstead LS, Wiechers DO (eds): Research and Clinical Aspects of the Late Effects of Poliomyelitis. White Plains, NY, March of Dimes Birth Defects Foundation, 1987, pp 13–26.
32. Halstead LS, Silver JK: Nonparalytic polio and post-polio syndrome. Am J Phys Med Rehabil 79:13–18, 2000.
33. Halstead LS, Wiechers DO (eds): Late Effects of Poliomyelitis. Miami, Symposia Foundation, 1985.
34. Halstead LS, Wiechers DO, Rossi CD: Late effects of poliomyelitis: A national survey. In Halstead LS, Wiechers DO (eds): Late Effects of Poliomyelitis. Miami, Symposia Foundation, 1985, pp 11–31.
35. Hayward M, Seaton D: Late sequelae of paralytic polio in a clinical and EMG study. J Neurol Neurosurg Psychiatry 42:117–122, 1979.
36. Johnson EW, Alexander MA: Management of motor unit diseases. In Kotke FJ, Stillwell GK, Lehman JF (eds): Krusen's Handbook of Physical Medicine and Rehabilitation. Philadelphia, WB Saunders, 1982, pp 686–687.
37. Kayser-Gatchalian MC: Late muscular atrophy after poliomyelitis. Eur Neurol 10: 371–380, 1973.
38. Lonnberg F, Madsen M: Late onset polio sequelae in Denmark. Risk indicators of late onset polio sequelae. Results of a nation-wide survey of 3,607 polio survivors. Scand J Rehabil Med 28:17–23, 1993.
39. Maynard FM: Differential diagnosis of pain and weakness in post-polio patients. In Halstead LS, Wiechers DO (eds): Late Effects of Poliomyelitis. Miami, Symposia Foundation, 1985, pp 33–44.
40. McCain GA, Scudds RA: The concept of primary fibromyalgia (fibrositis): Clinical value, relation and significance to other chronic musculoskeletal pain syndromes. Pain 33: 273–287, 1988.
41. MacMahon B, Pugh TF: Epidemiology: Principles and Methods. Boston, Little, Brown, 1970.
42. Mulder DW, Rosenbaum RA, Layton DD: Late progression of poliomyelitis or forme fruste amyotrophic lateral sclerosis? Mayo Clin Proc 47:756–761, 1972.
43. Nathanson N, Martin JR: The epidemiology of poliomyelitis: Enigmas surrounding its appearance, epidemicity, and disappearance. Am J Epidemiol 110:672–692, 1979.

44. Nelson KR: Creatine kinase and fibrillation potentials in patients with late sequelae of polio. Muscle Nerve 13:722–755, 1990.
45. Parsons PE: National Center for Health Statistics: Letter to the editor. N Engl J Med 325:1108, 1991.
46. Paul JR: History of Poliomyelitis. New Haven, Yale University Press, 1971.
47. Plioplys AV, Plioplys S: Meeting the frustrations of chronic fatigue syndrome. Hospital Practice 147–166, 1997.
48. Postkanzer DC, Cantor HM, Kaplan GS: The frequency of preceding poliomyelitis in amyotrophic lateral sclerosis. In Norris Jr FH, Kurland LT (eds): Motor Neuron Disease: Research on Amyotrophic Lateral Sclerosis and Related Disorders. New York, Grune & Stratton, 1969.
49. Post-Polio Task Force: Post-Polio Syndrome. New York, BioScience Communications, 1999.
50. Ramlow J, Alexander M, Laporte R, Kaufman C, Kuller K: Epidemiology of the post-polio syndrome. Am J Epidemiol 136:769–784, 1992.
51. Raymond M (with contribution by Charcot JM): Paralysie essentiele de l'enfance: Atrophie musculaire consecutive. Gaz Med (Paris) 225, 1875.
52. Sabin AB, Steigman AJ: Poliomyelitis virus of low virulence in patients with epidemic summer grippe or sore throat. Am J Hygeine 49:176–193, 1949.
53. Silver JK: Post-Polio Syndrome: A Guide for Polio Survivors and Family Members. New Haven, Yale University Press, 2001.
54. Smith LK, McDermott K: Pain in post-poliomyelitis: Addressing causes versus treating effects. In Halstead LS, Weichers DO (eds): Research and Clinical Aspects of the Late Affects of Poliomyelitis. White Plains, NY, March of Dimes Birth Defects Foundation, 1987, pp 125–134.
55. Sonies BC, Dalakas MC: Dysphagia in patients with the post-polio syndrome. N Engl J Med 324:1162–1167, 1991.
56. Speier JL, Owen RR, Knapp M, Canine JK: Occurrence of post-polio sequelae in an epidemic population. In Halstead LS, Wiechers DO (eds): Research and Clinical Aspects of the Late Effects of Poliomyelitis. White Plains, NY, March of Dimes Birth Defects Foundation, 1987, pp 39–48.
57. Thompson JM: Subspecialty clinics: Physical medicine and rehabilitation. Tension myalgia as a diagnosis at the Mayo Clinic and its relationship to fibrositis, fibromyalgia, and myofascial pain syndrome. Mayo Clin Proc 65:1237–1248, 1990.
58. Tomlinson BE, Irving D: Changes in spinal cord motor neurons of possible relevance to the late effects of poliomyelitis. In Halstead LS, Wiechers DO (eds): Late effects of poliomyelitis. Miami, Symposia Foundation, 1985.
59. Trojan DA, Bernasconi A, Arnold DL: Brainstem neuronal injury in fatigued postpoliomyelitis syndrome patients [abstract]. Neurology 58(suppl 3):A197, 2002.
60. Trojan DA, Cashman NR: Current Trends in Post-Poliomyelitis Syndrome. New York, Milestone Medical Communications, 1996.
61. Trojan DA, Cashman NR, Jubelt B, et al: The response of post-poliomyelitis syndrome symptoms to pyridostigmine (Mestinon): A multi-centered, placebo-controlled trial. Arch Phys Med Rehabil 78:1027, 1997.
62. Trojan DA, Cashman NR, Shapiro S, et al: Predictive factors for post-poliomyelitis syndrome. Arch Phys Med Rehabil 75:770–777, 1994.
63. Vasiliadis HM, Collet JP, Shapiro S, et al: Predictive factors and correlates for pain in postpoliomyelitis syndrome patients. Arch Phys Med Rehabil 83:1109–1115, 2002.
64. Waring WP, Davidoff G, Werner RA: Serum creatine kinase in the post-polio population. Am J Phys Med Rehabil 72:923–931, 1989.

65. Weinstein L, Shelokov A, Seltser R et al: A comparison of the clinical features of polio-
    myelitis in adults and in children. N Engl J Med 246:296–302, 1952.
66. Weinstein L: Influence of age and sex on susceptibility and clinical manifestations in
    poliomyelitis. N Engl J Med 257:47–52, 1957.
67. Wiechers DO: Late effect of polio: Historical perspectives. In Halstead LS, Wiechers DO
    (eds): Research and Clinical Aspects of the Late Effects of Poliomyelitis. White Plains,
    NY, March of Dimes Birth Defects Foundation, 1987, pp 1–11.
68. Windebank AJ, Daube JR, Lichty WJ, et al: Late sequelae of paralytic poliomyelitis in
    Olmstead County, Minnesota. In Halstead LS, Wiechers DO (eds): Research and Clini-
    cal Aspects of the Late Effects of Poliomyelitis. White Plains, NY, March of Dimes Birth
    Defects Foundation, 1987, pp 27–38.
69. Wolfe F: Interrater reliability of the tender point criterion for fibromyalgia. J Rheumatol
    21:370–371, 1994.
70. Yunus MB: Primary fibromyalgia syndrome: A critical evaluation of recent criteria devel-
    opments. Zeitschrift fur Rheumatologic 48:217–222, 1989.

Evaluating and Treating Symptomatic Postpolio Patients

Daria A. Trojan, MD, MSc, Lois Finch, MSc, Deborah Da Costa, PhD, and Neil R. Cashman, MD

Patients with previous polio can present to their physician with a wide variety of complaints, which may or may not be related to polio or postpolio syndrome (PPS). Evaluation requires confirmation of previous polio and is usually followed by a search for other potential causes of new symptoms. Because there is no specific diagnostic test for PPS,[10] thorough evaluation is especially important before attributing new symptoms to PPS.

Management of polio-related difficulties should be symptom specific and typically requires an interdisciplinary team. This chapter discusses the evaluation of newly symptomatic postpolio patients and summarizes the development of a management program for polio-related difficulties. The management of the three primary symptoms of PPS—weakness, fatigue, and pain—is introduced. For further information on specific management options (e.g., exercise, bracing), and management of certain symptoms (e.g., pain, fatigue) the reader is referred to other chapters in this text. The same is true for management of patients with dysphagia, respiratory dysfunction, and psychological issues. Table 1 summarizes the evaluation and treatment of symptomatic postpolio patients.

EVALUATION

CONFIRMATION OF PREVIOUS PARALYTIC POLIO

When evaluating a newly symptomatic postpolio patient, the history of previous paralytic polio (or poliomyelitis producing motor neuron loss) should first be confirmed. In one study, approximately 10% of patients presenting consecutively to a postpolio clinic did not have previous paralytic polio.[61] However, the patient typically provides a (often childhood) history of an illness characterized by high fever, followed by paralysis, during a polio epidemic. On neurologic examination, signs of previous motor neuron loss are usually present (reduction or loss of deep tendon reflexes, muscular weakness, and atrophy). If the history of paralytic polio is unclear or un-

Table 1. SUMMARY OF EVALUATION AND TREATMENT OF SYMPTOMATIC POSTPOLIO PATIENTS

Evaluation
  Confirm previous paralytic polio
  Identify other medical, neurologic, and orthopedic causes of new symptoms
Treatment (interdisciplinary team)
  Management of weakness
    Judicious exercise (aerobic, strengthening, stretching)
    Avoidance of muscular overuse
    Weight loss
    Orthoses
    Use of assistive devices
  Management of fatigue
    Energy conservation techniques
    Lifestyle changes
    Regular rest periods or naps during the day
    Pacing (rest periods during activity)
    Improvement of sleep (e.g., relaxation techniques, medications such as
      amitriptyline, avoiding caffeine)
    Avoidance of excessive fatigue (with Borg Scale of Perceived Exertion)
  Management of pain
    Joint and soft tissue abnormalities
      Modification of extremity use
      Physiotherapy
      Strengthening exercise (when possible)
      Orthoses
      Assistive devices
      Medications (e.g., NSAIDs, acetaminophen)
      Steroid injections
      Surgery
    Postpolio muscular pain, muscular pain with activity, muscular cramps
      Activity reduction
      Pacing
      Moist heat, ice, stretching
      Use of assistive devices
      Lifestyle modifications
    Fibromyalgia
      Aerobic exercise
      Medications (e.g., amitriptyline, cyclobenzaprine, fluoxetine)
      Improvement of sleep
    Treatment of other superimposed neurologic disorders (e.g., carpal tunnel
      syndrome, ulnar neuropathy, spinal stenosis, radiculopathy)
Pharmacotherapy
  Avoidance of medications that can aggravate symptoms of PPS
  No well-proven, specific treatment currently available
Identification and treatment of other commonly associated conditions (e.g.,
  osteoporosis, sleep apnea, fibromyalgia, cardiovascular disease)

usual or if the examination is not suggestive of previous polio, electromyography (EMG) studies are recommended to document signs of previous motor neuron loss.[8] However, some investigators recommend EMG evaluation of all patients to identify the extent of motor neuron loss and to document signs of denervation.[27,40] The abnormalities seen on EMG studies in patients with previous paralytic polio are not specific for polio and may be found in other neurologic disorders characterized by motor neuron loss. Rarely, patients may present with no clear history of previous polio and little evidence for paralytic polio on examination but with complaints of progressive new weakness and fatigue and evidence of diffuse denervation on EMG studies.[32] These patients may have PPS, but the presence of other disorders such as spinal muscular atrophy should also be considered.

EXCLUSION OF OTHER CAUSES OF NEW SYMPTOMS

Postpolio patients are not immune to other disorders found in older adults, which could account for some or all of their new symptoms. In one study, the charts of 353 postpolio clinic patients were reviewed to identify PPS cases and stable postpolio control subjects. Forty-six percent of patients were excluded primarily because of the presence of other disorders that could account for new weakness and fatigue.[59,69] Fatigue is very common in the general adult population and may be caused by a variety of causes such as respiratory dysfunction, sleep apnea, depression, chronic pain, anemia, endocrinologic abnormalities (e.g., hypothyroidism), cardiac dysfunction, cancer, chronic infections, and rheumatologic disorders.[63] Sleep apnea is a common cause of fatigue in postpolio patients and may be obstructive and central. Obstructive sleep apnea has been reported in 7.3% of individuals with previous polio,[70] which is significantly higher than in the general adult population. Patients with current or previous bulbar involvement may have more frequent sleep apnea, especially central apnea.[14] Fibromyalgia may be the cause of diffuse muscular pain and fatigue and has been reported to occur in 10.5% of postpolio patients attending a postpolio clinic.[61] Other disorders such as polymyalgia rheumatica may also produce diffuse pain and fatigue. Spinal stenosis causes similar symptoms to PPS in ambulatory patients, and its diagnosis should be excluded.

A number of neurologic disorders can produce new weakness and abnormal muscle fatiguability, although with a disease course readily distinguishable from PPS. Neurologic disorders to consider include adult spinal muscular atrophy, amyotrophic lateral sclerosis, cauda equina syndrome, cervical and lumbosacral spinal stenosis, chronic inflammatory demyelinating polyneuropathy, diabetic neuropathy, entrapment neuropathy, heavy metal toxicity, inflammatory myopathy, multifocal motor conduction block, multiple sclerosis, myasthenia gravis, Parkinson's disease, peripheral neuropathy, radiculopathy, and spinal cord tumor.[63]

Exclusion of other potential causes of new symptoms requires a thorough evaluation. *Laboratory blood tests* should be done on most newly symptomatic postpolio patients, including complete blood count, chemistry (sodium, potassium, chloride, HCO_3, glucose, blood urea nitrogen, creatinine, calcium, phosphorus, total protein, albumin, magnesium, liver function studies, alkaline phosphatase, creatine kinase), thyroid function tests, erythrocyte sedimentation rate, and serum protein electrophoresis.[63] A mild elevation of creatine kinase is observed in a large proportion of postpolio patients[72] and may be related to activity.[45,73] In patients with higher elevations of creatine kinase, a myopathy should be considered. Essentially, all patients should undergo *pulmonary function tests,* including assessment of respiratory muscle strength, because postpolio patients who do not report current or previous respiratory symptoms may have respiratory abnormalities.[16] In patients with significant reductions in vital capacity (< 55% of predicted normal), a more thorough evaluation (including arterial blood gases, measurement of vital capacity sitting and supine, sleep studies) should be considered.[4,41] Hypercapnia is likely in patients with myopathy when vital capacity falls below 55%[7] and has been shown to be a predictor of "poor outcome" (defined as necessity of home ventilation or death from respiratory failure) in post-polio patients.[41] In patients with symptoms suggestive of sleep apnea, *sleep studies* should be performed. A *cardiac evaluation* may be necessary. Extensive *clinical electrophysiologic* evaluation may be indicated to exclude other neurologic disorders. *Radiologic studies* are frequently necessary to evaluate joint abnormalities. Baseline *scoliosis films* can be taken for patients with scoliosis to evaluate degree of scoliosis and previous spinal fusions. *Computed tomography (CT)* scans or *magnetic resonance imaging (MRI)* studies are frequently required to exclude other common conditions (e.g., spinal stenosis and cervical myelopathy) and to evaluate cervical or lumbar pathology. *Swallowing evaluation* with dynamic imaging including cine- and videofluoroscopy is recommended in postpolio patients with dysphagia.[34] Orapharyngeal dysfunction in patients with PPS may be quite common and unrelated to current or previous history of swallowing dysfunction. In a study of 32 patients with PPS (defined by new weakness in the limbs), Sonies and Dalakas reported some abnormality on detailed testing of oropharyngeal function in 31 patients.[56] This occurred regardless of whether or not the patient had new symptoms of dysphagia or gave a history of previous bulbar involvement.[56] Patients with dysphagia may also have concurrent laryngeal pathology. In one study, all nine postpolio patients with swallowing complaints had some degree of abnormality on videostroboscopic evaluation (including unilateral vocal cord paralysis in four patients with previous bulbar polio).[20]

MANAGEMENT

Many newly symptomatic postpolio patients appear to benefit from a management program, although no controlled studies of management programs have been completed to date. Uncontrolled studies of management programs in postpolio patients have reported that patients who adhere to treatment recommendations can experience an improvement of symptoms. In one study, 77 PPS patients were followed for a mean of 2.2 years.[46] Patients who complied with treatment recommendations ($n =$ 30) experienced improvement or resolution of PPS symptoms and a mean improvement in strength on manual muscle testing of 0.6% per year. In contrast, patients who partially complied with recommendations ($n = $ 32) experienced no improvement or improvement in PPS symptoms with a mean annual reduction in strength of -1.3%, and patients who did not comply ($n = $ 15) experienced no change or a worsening of symptoms with an annual mean decline in strength of -2.0%.[46] In a retrospective chart review of 79 postpolio patients, recommendations were helpful in 25 of 32 (78%) of patients seen at follow-up. Of the seven patients who did not note improvement, six had not followed recommendations.[3]

Based on the results of these studies, the health benefits of a PPS management program depend on patient adherence; however, the factors determining adherence to treatment recommendations in PPS have received limited attention.[11,12] Studies completed in other disorders suggest that potentially modifiable psychosocial variables (e.g., coping, depression, social support, stress) are important predictors of adherence.[21,36,52] This area requires further study.

Because most postpolio patients present with such a wide variety of difficulties, an interdisciplinary approach to management with a team of physicians and health care personnel is usually most effective. Team members can include a primary care physician, physiatrist, neurologist, pulmonary specialist, psychiatrist, orthopedist, rheumatologist, physical and occupational therapists, orthotist, psychologist, social worker, dietitian, nurse, and respiratory therapist.[67] The team is usually headed by a specialist such as a physiatrist or neurologist.

Management should be symptom specific and may need to change over time because of the evolution of PPS and normal aging.[40] In most cases, patients should first concentrate on learning to avoid overuse with a reduction in activities, pacing, and education on energy conservation techniques. Difficulties with mobility and pain should also be addressed. After the patient has learned to monitor and manage his or her weakness and fatigue, an individualized exercise program can be introduced. However, additional exercise should not be recommended in patients with severe weakness and fatigue who are already spending most of their energy completing activities of daily living.

Management should also address treatment of other conditions such as osteoporosis and peripheral neuropathies (which are generally associated with repetitive use of an extremity or pressure on a nerve), which may occur more commonly in individuals with previous paralytic polio. The exact prevalence of osteoporosis in postpolio individuals is unknown, but it is likely related to weakness severity. One study found a strong association between bone mineral content and lean tissue in limbs of 38 postpolio subjects, suggesting that the weakest patients are at greatest risk for developing osteoporosis.[17] In a study of 6 male postpolio patients, an association between hip bone density and hip muscular strength was reported.[53] In addition, postpolio patients may have a higher prevalence for various cardiovascular risk ractors such as hyperlipidemia and diabetes because of their reduced levels of physical activity.[29] These conditions should be identified and treated.

MANAGEMENT OF WEAKNESS

Management of patients with weakness can include various strategies such as exercise, avoidance of muscular overuse, weight loss, orthoses, and use of assistive devices.[67] Exercise is discussed in detail in Chapter 9. Aerobic exercise is the only treatment that has been shown to be useful in controlled studies,[15,35,37,48] but other forms of exercise (e.g., isotonic) are also likely useful.[2,22–25] The recommended exercise program for a patient is dependent on a number of factors. Isotonic or isokinetic strengthening can be used to strengthen muscles that are ≥ 3 on the Medical Research Council (MRC) scale. Isometric exercise can be used to strengthen muscles over a painful joint. Aerobic exercise (e.g., bicycle ergometry, swimming, walking) can be recommended and preferably should be an activity that the patient enjoys. The concept of cross-training, which is so effectively used in sports medicine, can be introduced in order to have patients alternate exercises and thus not overuse any particular muscle group. Stretching exercises can be useful to maintain or improve range of motion and may improve function. For example, stretching of a knee flexion contracture may improve gait and stability. However, certain contractures may be useful for a patient and should not be stretched (e.g., ankle plantar flexion contracture in the presence of severe weakness of the quadriceps). The exercise program should include warm-up and cool-down periods. Initially, the patient should be monitored frequently to ensure that the exercises are being performed correctly and that no adverse effects are present. Muscular overuse (i.e., exercising to the point of muscle pain and fatigue) should be avoided during physical activity because overuse in postpolio patients has been reported to produce permanent increased weakness.[5,63,67] Orthoses and assistive devices (e.g., canes, crutches, manual wheelchairs, electric wheelchairs, motorized scooters) can be very useful in the management of weakness and resultant gait difficulties, as well as pain and joint deformities. In a retrospective study of 104 postpolio patients, the new lower extremity orthoses recommended to 37 patients improved patients' subjective ability to walk, perceived walking safety, and pain.[74] The reader is referred to other chapters in this volume for further details on orthoses and mobility aids.

MANAGEMENT OF FATIGUE

Recommendations for management of patients with excessive fatigue can include use of energy-conservation techniques, lifestyle changes, regular rest periods or naps during the day, pacing, and improvement of sleep. Examples of energy conservation techniques are discontinuing certain unnecessary and energy-consuming activities, making seating and work station corrections, using a handicapped license plate, sitting instead of standing, and using an electric scooter or wheelchair for longer distances. Lifestyle changes can include changing to a more sedentary employment, working at home, working part time, and discontinuing or modifying certain activities (e.g., ordering groceries online versus going to the store). Regular naps or rest periods during the day, especially in the early afternoon, can be beneficial, and, if possible, can be used even by working patients with significant fatigue.[67] Pacing (i.e., regular rest periods during activity) can be useful in managing local muscle fatigue. Agre and Rodriquez studied 7 PPS patients with three different exercise protocols, on three separate occasions, at least one week apart.[1] With regular rest periods during an isometric endurance test of the quadriceps at 40% maximum voluntary contraction (MVC), patients had less local muscle fatigue, increased work capacity, and improved ability to recover strength after activity. Improvement of sleep can occur with measures such as use of relaxation techniques and medications such as amitriptyline, L-tryptophan, and gabapentin.

To help patients avoid excessive muscular and general fatigue, they can be taught to attend to their perception of fatigue by using the Borg Rating Scale of Perceived Exertion (RPE; Fig. 1).[6,49,67] The RPE is a 15-point scale, from 6 to 20, with verbal anchors from a level of 6 (light) to 20 (very, very hard). The RPE is used as a limit of exercise capacity in PPS as well as other conditions.[15,26,38] Patients with previous polio can use the RPE reliably ($r = 0.83$) to monitor their effort after only one training session.[26] We recommend teaching patients to end their daily activities at an RPE level of 14 (or lower), with an anchor word of *hard*.[67] Even though we have found this technique useful in fatigue management, the potential benefits have not yet been well evaluated.

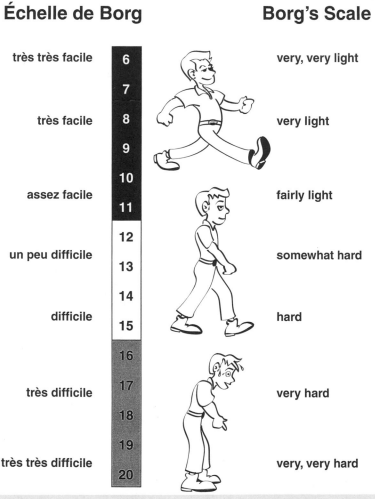

Échelle de Borg   **Borg's Scale**

très très facile	6	very, very light
	7	
très facile	8	very light
	9	
	10	
assez facile	11	fairly light
	12	
un peu difficile	13	somewhat hard
	14	
difficile	15	hard
	16	
très difficile	17	very hard
	18	
	19	
très très difficile	20	very, very hard

Figure 1. The Borg scale of perceived exertion. The original Borg scale has been modified. The numbers from 6 to 11 are in green, the numbers from 12 to 15 are in yellow, and the numbers from 16 to 20 are in red, similar in concept to traffic lights. A figure has been added for each colored area to depict the amount of effort represented by the numbers and anchor words. (Reprinted with permission from the Scandinavian University Press (Borg GV: Scand J Rehab Med 21:82–89, 1970) and from IOS Press B.V. (Trojan DA, Finch L: NeuroRehabil 8:93–105, 1997).)

MANAGEMENT OF PAIN

Pain in postpolio patients may be localized to the joints and soft tissues or to muscles, or it may be caused by superimposed neurologic disorders. Overuse or chronic abnormal use (caused by weakness) may lead to many of the pain syndromes experienced by postpolio patients. Pain is dependent upon the method of locomotion; pain occurs more frequently in the lower extremities and lower back in ambulatory patients and more often in the upper extremities in patients who use wheelchairs or crutches.[55] Pain in postpolio patients is also associated with physical exertion and spontaneous walking speed.[78] However, weakness (at acute polio and current) is associated with joint pain but not muscle pain.[69,71]

Joint and soft tissue abnormalities may be caused by osteoarthritis, tendonitis, bursitis, ligamentous strain secondary to joint deformities and weakness, and previous arthrodeses. Osteoarthritis of the hand and wrist is common in postpolio patients. In a cross-sectional study of 61 postpolio patients, 13% had moderate or severe osteoarthritis and 68% had mild osteoarthritis of the hand and wrist. Associated factors were age > 50 years, increased lower extremity weakness, a greater locomotor disability, and a greater usage of assistive devices.[77] Many patients underwent joint arthrodeses during childhood after acute paralytic polio. In one study of 57 patients with triple arthrodeses of the hindfoot and various neuromuscular disorders (most commonly poliomyelitis), 55% of feet and ankles were painful, and all ankles had some degenerative changes at the time of a follow-up evaluation performed an average of 45 years after the surgery.[50] Recommendations for management of joint and tissue abnormalities are modification of extremity use, physiotherapy, strengthening (when possible), orthoses to control joint deformities and difficulties with previous joint fusions, assistive devices, nonsteroidal anti-inflammatory drugs, acetaminophen, and rarely, corticosteroid injection or surgery.[67]

Muscular pain can include a postpolio muscular pain (i.e., a deep aching muscular sensation similar to that experienced during acute paralytic polio, usually occuring late in the day), muscular pain with activity, muscular cramps, fasciculations, and fibromyalgia. Muscular cramps and muscular pain with activity are usually signs of overuse and should be avoided. Management options can include reduction of activity, pacing, use of physical modalities (e.g., moist heat, ice), stretching, use of assistive devices, and lifestyle modifications.[27,67] In a few postpolio patients with severe cramps, we have found the medications gabapentin and lioresal useful. Fasciculations are commonly found in postpolio patients. Although painless, fasciculations may prompt anxiety in some patients because of their presumed association with motor neuron diseases. Aside from reassurance, they are untreatable. Fibromylagia can be treated with a number of interventions, including amitriptyline, cyclobenzaprine, fluoxetine, aerobic exercise, and other measures.[61]

Superimposed peripheral neurologic disorders can be another cause of pain and are common in postpolio patients. In a study of electrodiagnostic findings in 100 postpolio patients, carpal tunnel syndrome was found in 35% of patients, ulnar neuropathy at the wrist in 2%, peripheral neuropathy in 3%, combined carpal tunnel syndrome and ulnar neuropathy in 3%, and radiculopathy in 4%.[28] Ulnar neuropathy at the elbow has been reported in > 50% of 48 postpolio patients.[54] Use of assistive devices is a major risk factor for carpal tunnel syndrome in postpolio patients,[76] and for ulnar neuropathy at the elbow.[54] Spinal stenosis can produce similar symptoms as PPS in ambulatory patients and is another cause of lower back and lower extremity pain. Treatment options for carpal tunnel syndrome include splinting, use of special pads or grips on canes or crutches (which place the wrist in a more neutral position and increase the weight-bearing surface of the hand), corticosteroid injection, and carpal tunnel release.[27,67] However, surgery for carpal tunnel syndrome should be recommended with caution.[75] For patients with spinal stenosis, treatment options include medications, spinal injections, physiotherapy, use of an assistive device (e.g., a cane), transcutaneous electrical nerve stimulation (TENS), lumbosacral orthosis, and (in some cases) surgery.

PHARMACOTHERAPY

Some medications may produce or aggravate the symptoms of PPS and may interfere with the function of the neuromuscular junction. Therefore, medications should be considered as a possible cause of symptoms, and some medications should be avoided, if possible. Such medications include beta-blockers, benzodiazepines, certain anesthetics (e.g., succinylcholine[39]), some antibiotics (e.g., tetracycline and aminoglycosides), certain anticonvulsants (e.g., phenytoin), some antipsychotics (e.g., lithium, phenothiazines), and barbiturates.[47]

Currently, there is no well-proven pharmacologic treatment for patients with PPS, but relatively few studies have been conducted on a small number of agents. Potential treatments evaluated include pyridostigmine, carnitine, amantadine, prednisone, insulin-like growth factor (IGF) I, growth hormone, and bromocriptine. Only two multicenter, randomized, double-blinded trials and several small clinical trials of pharmacologic treatments have been completed in PPS.[9,18,31,33,42,44,51,57,57a,60,62,68]

Several studies have evaluated the anticholinesterase pyridostigmine in PPS. Many patients with previous paralytic polio have neuromuscular junction transmission defects, which have been hypothesized to be a cause of muscular—and, consequently, general—fatigue. Pyridostigmine may improve fatigue by repairing defective neuromuscular junction transmission in PPS. Chronic, trophic effects of pyridostigmine are also possible and may be mediated through growth hormone and IGF-I,[30,43] an acetylcholine trophic effect on partially denervated muscle,[19] and induction of calcitonin gene related peptide (CGRP) secretion.[58] Neuromuscular junction transmission has been reported to improve with anticholinesterases in postpolio patients.[33,68] In an open trial in 17 PPS patients, we found a significant association of improvement of subjective fatigue with pyridostigmine and edrophonium-responsive neuromuscular junction transmission defects on stimulation single fiber electromyography.[60,68] This finding suggested that fatigue in PPS may be caused partly by anticholinesterase-responsive neuromuscular junction transmission defects.

In another open trial, we found that approximately 60% of 27 PPS patients reported improvement of subjective fatigue with pyridostigmine.[62] In a placebo-controlled, crossover trial in 27 PPS patients, another group of investigators[51] reported improved subjective fatigue and strength in the upper extremities with pyridostigmine. After these encouraging results, a six-center, randomized, placebo-controlled, double-blind trial was completed to evaluate the effect of pyridostigmine on health-related quality of life, isometric muscle strength in 12 muscle groups, subjective fatigue, and serum IGF I levels in 126 PPS patients.[65] The study showed no significant differences between pyridostigmine and placebo-treated patients at 6 months of treatment. There were no differences between patient groups at 6 and 10 weeks of treatment. However, the very weak muscles (1–25% predicted normal at baseline) were somewhat stronger ($P = 0.10$), and in compliant patients, IGF-I was somewhat increased ($P = 0.15$) at 6 months of treatment with pyridostigmine.[65]

A single-center, randomized, placebo-controlled, double-blind trial of pyridostigmine in 67 PPS patients over 14 weeks was also done.[44] Preliminary results showed no significant differences between pyridostigmine and placebo-treated patients with regard to changes in subjective fatigue, isometric strength (quadriceps), and neuromuscular junction transmission defects (as assessed by jitter on single fiber electromyography). However, there was a small significant improvement on walking performance (timed walking test) in pyridostigmine-treated patients at 14 weeks.[44] Thus, despite encouraging preliminary results from smaller trials, the more comprehensive trials completed to date have not shown a definitive benefit of pyridostigmine in patients with PPS.

Other agents have been evaluated in PPS in smaller trials. A multicenter, randomized, placebo-controlled trial of the vitamin carnitine has been completed in 60 PPS patients, but the results have not yet been published. Preliminary reports did not show a beneficial effect of the medication.[57a] Amantadine (an antiviral agent used for the treatment of fatigue in several neurologic disorders) has been evaluated in a randomized, placebo-controlled trial in 25 PPS patients treated for 6 weeks. No significant improvement of subjective fatigue was reported; however, patients treated with amantadine were more likely to note an overall improvement of fatigue compared with placebo.[57]

High-dose prednisone has been evaluated in a randomized, placebo-controlled trial in 17 PPS patients treated for 25 weeks. Prednisone has been proposed as a possible treatment because of the presence of various immunologic abnormalities reported in PPS by some investigators. Patients in the treatment group received prednisone 80 mg/day for the first 4 weeks, followed by a gradual reduction for the remainder of the study. The investigators reported no significant improvement in muscular strength (assessed by electronic strain gauge tensiometer and manual muscle testing) or subjective fatigue; however, a trend to an increase in isometric strength with prednisone was observed.[18]

Recombinant human IGF-I (rhIGF-I), a neurotrophic factor, has been evaluated in a randomized, placebo-controlled trial in 22 PPS patients treated for 3 months. In rhIGF-I–treated patients, an improvement in recovery after fatiguing exercise—but no change in strength and fatiguability—was reported.[42] Human growth hormone (which stimulates IGF-I secretion) has been evaluated in an open trial in six PPS patients for a period of 3 months. Little or no improvement in muscle strength, endurance, or recovery after fatigue was found.[31]

Bromocriptine mesylate, a postsynaptic, dopamine 2 receptor agonist used in the treatment of patients with Parkinson's disease, has been evaluated in a placebo-controlled, crossover trial in five patients. This medication has been proposed as a possible treatment for PPS general fatigue, which may be caused by poliovirus-induced damage to the brain's reticular activating system, including dopaminergic neurons in the substania nigra. Subjective fatigue symptoms were noted to improve in three patients in this study.[9]

In summary, even though some of the agents evaluated show promise as potential treatments, the trials completed thus far have not shown conclusive evidence for a benefit in PPS. However, the majority of these trials have been limited in power because of small sample size and other factors such as trial duration. The two larger trials may have been limited by inadequate outcome measures and other factors.[13,65,66]

CONCLUSION

Postpolio patients with new symptoms require confirmation of previous polio and exclusion of other medical, neurologic, and orthopedic causes of new symptoms. Many patients appear to benefit from an individualized management program developed by a team of physicians and health care personnel. Further research on the effects of management programs and specific treatments (including pharmacologic agents) is necessary in clinical trials using adequate sample sizes and disease-specific, responsive outcome measures.

ACKNOWLEDGMENTS

This work was supported in part by the Fonds de la recherche en santé du Québec, the Montreal Neurological Institute, and the Association Polio Quebec.

References
1. Agre JC, Rodriquez AA: Intermittent isometric activity: Its effect on muscle fatigue in postpolio subjects. Arch Phys Med Rehabil 72:971–975, 1991.
2. Agre JC, Rodriquez AA, Franke TM, et al: Low-intensity, alternate-day exercise improves muscle performance without apparent adverse affect in postpolio patients. Am J Phys Med Rehabil 75:50–58, 1996.
3. Agre JC, Rodriquez AA, Sperling KB: Symptoms and clinical impressions of patients seen in a post-polio clinic. Arch Phys Med Rehabil 70:367–370, 1989.
4. Bach JR, Alba A: Pulmonary dysfunction and sleep-disordered breathing as postpolio sequelae: Evaluation and management. Orthopedics 14:1329–1337, 1991.
5. Bennett RL, Knowlton GC: Overwork weakness in partially denervated skeletal muscle. Clin Orthop 12:22–29, 1958.
6. Borg GV: Perceived exertion as an indicator of somatic stress. Scand J Rehab Med 21:82–98, 1970.
7. Braun NMT, Arora MS, Rochester DF: Respiratory muscle and pulmonary function in polymyositis and other proximal myopathies. Thorax 38:616–623, 1983.
8. Bromberg MB, Waring WP: Neurologically normal patients with suspected postpo-

liomyelitis syndrome: Electromyographic assessment of past denervation. Arch Phys Med Rehabil 72:493–497, 1991.

9. Bruno RL, Zimmerman J, Creange SJ, et al: Bromocriptine in the treatment of post-polio fatigue. Am J Phys Med Rehabil 75:340–347, 1996.

10. Cashman NR, Maselli R, Wollman RL, et al: Late denervation in patients with antecedent paralytic poliomyelitis. N Engl J Med 317:7–12, 1987.

11. Creange SJ, Bruno RL: Family support as a predictor of participation in rehabilitation for post-polio sequelae. N J Rehabil 8:8–11, 1994.

12. Creange SJ, Bruno RL: Compliance with treatment for post-polio sequelae. Am J Phys Med Rehabil 76:378–382, 1997.

13. Dalakas MC: Why drugs fail in postpolio syndrome: lessons from another clinical trial. Neurology 53:1166–1167, 1999.

14. Dean AC, Graham BA, Dalakas M: Sleep apnea in patients with postpolio syndrome. Ann Neurol 43:661–664, 1998.

15. Dean E, Ross J: Effect of modified aerobic training on movement energetics in polio survivors. Orthopedics 14:1243–1246, 1991.

16. Dean E, Ross J, Road JD, et al: Pulmonary function in individuals with a history of poliomyelitis. Chest 100:118–128, 1991.

17. Delahunt JW, Falkner ME, Krebs J, et al: Correlations between bone mineral content, bone area, and lean tissue in individual limbs of subjects with limb weakness after acute poliomyelitis in the past [abstract]. In Proceedings of the Endocrine Society of Australia, 1999, p NZ18.

18. Dinsmore S, Dambrosia J, Dalakas MC: A double-blind, placebo-controlled trial of high-dose prednisone for the treatment of post-poliomyelitis syndrome. Ann NY Acad Sci 753:303–313, 1995.

19. Drachman DB: The role of acetylcholine as a neurotrophic transmitter. Ann NY Acad Sci 228:160–175, 1974.

20. Driscoll BP, Gracco C, Coelho C, et al: Laryngeal function in postpolio patients. Laryngoscope 105:35–41, 1995.

21. Dunbar-Jacob JM, Schlenk EA, Burke LE, Matthews JT: Predictors of patient adherence: Patient characteristics. In Shumaker SA, Schron EB (eds): The Handbook of Health Behavior Change, 2nd ed. New York, Springer, 1998, pp 491–511.

22. Einarsson G: Muscle conditioning in late poliomyelitis. Arch Phys Med Rehabil. 72: 11–14, 1991.

23. Einarsson G, Grimby G: Strengthening exercise program in post-polio subjects. In Halstead LS, Weichers DO (eds): Research and Clinical Aspects of the Late Effects of Poliomyelitis. White Plains, NY, March of Dimes Birth Defects Foundation, 1987, pp 275–283.

24. Feldman RM, Soskolne CL: The use of non-fatiguing strengthening exercises in post-polio syndrome. In Halstead LS, Weichers DO (eds): Research and Clinical Aspects of the Late Effects of Poliomyelitis. White Plains, NY, March of Dimes Birth Defects Foundation, 1987, pp 335–341.

25. Fillyaw MJ, Badger GJ, Goodwin GD, et al: The effects of long-term non-fatiguing resistance exercise in subjects with post-polio syndrome. Orthopedics 14:1253–1256, 1991.

26. Finch L, Trojan D, Wilford C, Venturini A: A treadmill walking test in post-polio syndrome patients: Preliminary results [abstract]. Physiother Canada 46:117, 1994.

27. Gawne AC, Halstead LS: Post-polio syndrome: Pathophysiology and clinical management. Crit Rev Phys Rehabil Med 7:147–188, 1995.

28. Gawne AC, Pham BT, Halstead LS: Electrodiagnostic findings in 108 consecutive patients referred to a post-polio clinic. Ann NY Acad Sci 753:383–385, 1995.

29. Gawne AC, Wells KD, Wilson KS: Cardiac risk factors in polio survivors [abstract]. Arch Phys Med Rehabil 82:1306, 2001.
30. Ghigo E, Goffi S, Arvat E, et al: Pyridostigmine partially restores the GH responsiveness to GHRH in normal aging. Acta Endocrinologica (Copenh) 123:169–174, 1990.
31. Gupta KL, Shetty KR, Agre JC, et al: Human growth hormone effect on serum IGF-I and muscle function in poliomyelitis survivors. Arch Phys Med Rehabil 75:889–894, 1994.
32. Halstead LS, Silver JK: Nonparalytic polio and post-polio syndrome. Am J Phys Med Rehabil 79:13–18, 2000.
33. Hodes R: Electromyographic study of defects of neuromuscular transmission in human poliomyelitis. Arch Neurol Psychiatry 60:457–473, 1948.
34. Jones B, Buchholz DW, Ravich WJ, Donner MW: Swallowing dysfunction in the post-polio syndrome: a cinefluorographic study. AJR 158:283–286, 1992.
35. Jones DR, Speier J, Canine K, et al: Cardiorespiratory responses to aerobic training by patients with postpoliomyelitis sequelae. JAMA 261:3255–3258, 1989.
36. Kravitz RL, Hays RD, Sherbourne CD, et al: Recall of recommendations and adherence to advice among patients with chronic medical conditions. Arch Intern Med 153:1869–1878, 1993.
37. Kriz JL, Jones DR, Speier JL, et al: Cardiorespiratory responses to upper extremity aerobic training by postpolio subjects. Arch Phys Med Rehabil 73:49–54, 1992.
38. Levine GN, Balady GJ: The benefits and risks of exercise training: The exercise prescription. Adv Intern Med 38:57–79, 1993.
39. Liu S, Modell JH: Anesthetic management for patients with postpolio syndrome receiving electroconvulsive therapy. Anesthesiology 95:799–801, 2001.
40. March of Dimes: Post-polio Syndrome: Identifying Best Practices in Diagnosis and Care. White Plains, NY, March of Dimes Birth Defects Foundation, 2001. Available at www.modimes.org.
41. Midgren B: Lung function and clinical outcome in postpolio patients: A prospective cohort study during 11 years. Eur Respir J 10:146–149, 1997.
42. Miller RG, Gelinas DF, Kent-Braun J, et al: The effect of recombinant insulin-like growth factor I (rhIGF-I) on exercise-induced fatigue and recovery in patients with postpolio syndrome [abstract]. Neurology 48(suppl A):217, 1997.
43. Muller EE, Locatelli V, Ghigo E, et al: Involvement of brain catecholamines and acetylcholine in growth hormone deficiency states: Pathophysiological, diagnostic, and therapeutic implications. Drugs 41:161–177, 1991.
44. Nollet F, Horemans HLD, Beelen A, et al: Pyridostigmine in postpolio syndrome: A randomized double-blinded trial [abstract]. Neurology 58(suppl 2):199–200, 2002.
45. Peach PE: Overwork weakness with evidence of muscle damage in a patient with residual paralysis from polio. Arch Phys Med Rehabil 71:248–250, 1990.
46. Peach PE, Olejnik S: Post-polio sequelae: Effect of treatment and noncompliance on post-polio sequelae. Orthopedics 14:1199–1203, 1991.
47. Post-Polio Task Force: Post-polio syndrome update. Bioscience Rep 5:1997.
48. Prins JH, Hartung H, Merritt DJ, et al: Effect of aquatic exercise training in persons with poliomyelitis disability. Sports Med Training Rehab 5:29–39, 1994.
49. Rodriquez AA, Agre JC: Physiologic parameters and perceived exertion with local muscle fatigue in postpolio subjects. Arch Phys Med Rehabil 72:305–308, 1991.
50. Saltzman CL, Fehrle MJ, Cooper RR, et al: Triple arthrodesis: twenty-five and forty-four-year average follow-up of the same patients. J Bone Joint Surg 81A:1391–1402, 1999.
51. Seizert BP, Speier JL, Canine JK: Pyridostigmine effect on strength, endurance, and fatigue in post-polio patients [abstract]. Arch Phys Med Rehabil 75:1049, 1994.

52. Sherbourne CD, Hays RD, Ordway L, et al: Antecedents of adherence to medical recommendations: results from the Medical Outcomes Study. J Behav Med 15:447–468, 1992.
53. Silver JK, Aiello DD: Bone density and fracture risk in male polio survivors [abstract]. Arch Phys Med Rehabil 82:1329, 2001.
54. Slowman LS, Silver JK: Prevalence of median and ulnar neuropathy in postpolio patients [abstract]. Arch Phys Med Rehabil 82:1312–1313, 2001.
55. Smith LK, McDermott K: Pain in post-poliomyelitis: Addressing causes versus treating effects. In Halstead LS, Wiechers DO (eds): Research and Clinical Aspects of the Late Effects of Poliomyelitis. White Plains, NY, March of Dimes Birth Defects Foundation, 1987, pp 121–134.
56. Sonies BC, Dalakas MC: Dysphagia in patients with the post-polio syndrome. N Engl J Med 324:1162–1167, 1991.
57. Stein DP, Dambrosia J, Dalakas MC: A double-blind, placebo-controlled trial of high-dose prednisone for the treatment of post-poliomyelitis syndrome. Ann NY Acad Sci 753:296–302, 1995.
57a. Tesch, et al: Medikamentöse therapie bei PPS. Presented at the International Polio Conference, Jena, Germany, October 30–31, 1998.
58. Trasforini G, Margutti A, Vergani L, et al: Evidence that enhancement of cholinergic tone increases basal levels of calcitonin gene-related peptide in normal man. J Clin Endocrinol Metab 78:763–766, 1994.
59. Trojan DA: A case-control study of risk factors for post-poliomyelitis syndrome. Master of Science thesis submitted to the Department of Epidemiology and Biostatistics, McGill University, Montreal, 1992.
60. Trojan DA, Cashman NR: Anticholinesterases in post-poliomyelitis syndrome. Ann NY Acad Sci 753:285–295, 1995.
61. Trojan DA, Cashman NR: Fibromyalgia is common in a postpoliomyelitis clinic. Arch Neurol 52:620–624, 1995.
62. Trojan DA, Cashman NR: An open trial of pyridostigmine in a post-poliomyelitis clinic. Can J Neurol Sci 22:223–227, 1995.
63. Trojan DA, Cashman NR: Current Trends in Post-Poliomyelitis Syndrome. New York, Milestone Medical Communications (a division of Ruder-Finn), 1996.
64. Trojan DA, Cashman NR, Shapiro S, et al: Predictive factors for post-poliomyelitis syndrome. Arch Phys Med Rehabil 75:770–777, 1994.
65. Trojan DA, Collet J-P, Shapiro S, et al: A multicenter, randomized, double-blinded trial of pyridostigmine in postpolio syndrome. Neurology 53:1225–1233, 1999.
66. Trojan DA, Collet J-P, Shapiro S, et al: Letter. Neurology 55:900–901, 2000.
67. Trojan DA, Finch L: Management of post-polio syndrome. Neurol Rehabil 8:93–105, 1997.
68. Trojan DA, Gendron D, Cashman NR: Anticholinesterase-responsive neuromuscular junction transmission defects in post-poliomyelitis fatigue. J Neurol Sci 114:170–177, 1993.
69. Trojan DA, Vasiliadis H-M, Shapiro S, et al: Predictive factors and correlates of joint and muscle pain in post-poliomyelitis syndrome [abstract]. Arch Phys Med Rehabil 81:1292, 2000.
70. Ulfberg J, Jonsson R, Ekeroth G: Sleep apnea syndrome among poliomyelitis survivors [letter]. Neurology 49:1189, 1997.
71. Vasiliadis H-M, Collet J-P, Shapiro S, et al: Predictive factors and correlates for pain in post-poliomyelitis syndrome. Arch Phys Med Rehabil 83:1109–1115, 2002.
72. Waring WP, Davidoff G, Werner RA: Serum creatine kinase in the post-polio population. Am J Phys Med Rehab 68:86–90, 1988.

73. Waring WP, McLaurin TM. Correlation of creatine kinase and gait measurement in the postpolio population: a corrected version. Arch Phys Med Rehabil 73:447–450, 1992.
74. Waring WP, Maynard F, et al: Influence of appropriate lower extremity orthotic management on ambulation, pain, and fatigue in a postpolio population. Arch Phys Med Rehabil 70:371–375, 1989.
75. Waring WP, Werner RA: Clinical management of carpal tunnel syndrome in patients with long-term sequelae of poliomyelitis. J Hand Surg 14A:865–869, 1989.
76. Werner RA, Waring W, Davidoff G: Risk factors for median mononeuropathy of the wrist in postpoliomyelitis patients. Arch Phys Med Rehabil 70:464–467, 1989.
77. Werner RA, Waring W, Maynard F: Osteoarthritis of the hand and wrist in the post poliomyelitis population. Arch Phys Med Rehabil 73:1069–1072, 1992.
78. Willen C, Grimby G: Pain, physical activity, and disability in individuals with late effects of polio. Arch Phys Med Rehabil 79:915–919, 1998.

The Interdisciplinary Team Assessment

Anne C. Gawne, MD

Assessment of polio survivors can be difficult because of the diversity and the persistent nature of their complaints. The most frequent symptoms experienced by polio survivors in five separate studies are summarized in Table 1.[1–4,6] The most common new functional problems in four studies are summarized in Table 2.[2,3,5,6] The most common problems reported are pain, fatigue, and difficulty with walking. Appropriate treatment is a challenge because of the heterogeneity of the symptoms and the lack of curative therapeutic interventions. However, using the traditional rehabilitative model of an interdisciplinary team approach can be tremendously helpful to polio survivors who are suffering from new problems. This chapter is based on the author's polio clinic. Obviously, clinics can be set up in a variety of ways, and this model is simply an example of what we have found to be successful.

Our patients often travel great distances, and the trip to our clinic can be arduous for them. Because they may have decreased stamina, the usual evaluation is completed in 1 or 2 days. This is achieved by having team members come to the patient in a central location, rather than having the patient go for a series of single-service outpatient evaluations. All laboratory, radiologic and electrodiagnostic procedures are performed on location the same day as the evaluations. A typical interdisciplinary evaluation includes assessments by a nurse, physician, physical therapist (PT), occupational therapist (OT), orthotist, and social worker. When necessary, referrals are made to other health care providers, including a psychologist, pharmacist, podiatrist, dietitian, speech language pathologist (SLP), or respiratory therapist. The team attempts to set realistic goals for patients to help them to feel better physically and emotionally. These goals often center around improving the ease in performing activities of daily living (ADLs) and mobility. This chapter focuses on how the roles of the team members assist in the development of a comprehensive treatment plan.

Table 1. MOST COMMON NEW COMPLAINTS IN POLIO SURVIVORS IN FIVE STUDIES					
SYMPTOM	HALSTEAD AND ROSSI[1] (N = 539)	HALSTEAD AND ROSSI[2] (N = 132)	CHETWYND AND HOGAN[3] (N = 694)	AGRE ET AL.[4] (N = 79)	RAMLOW (N = 474)
Fatigue	87%*	89%*	48%	86%*	34%
Joint pain	80%	71%	60%*	77%	42%*
Muscle pain	79%	71%	52%	86%	38%
New weakness in affected muscle	87%	69%	47%	80%	38%
Cold sensitivity	N/A	29%	N/A	N/A	26%

*Most common new problem.

CLINIC COORDINATOR

The initial contact begins with the clinic coordinator. This person can be one of the core team members or may be a case manager, nurse, or physician's secretary. The clinic coordinator can supply the patient with appropriate articles and pamphlets about postpolio syndrome (PPS) and about the clinic. The clinic coordinator may send prospective patients a packet that includes the clinic's brochure, directions, and a health questionnaire. By using the questionnaire, patients tell their history only once. This practice also allows time for a discussion of items identified as important by the patient and the team. For instance, if a patients needs specific equipment such as a wheeled mobility system or a custom-made orthosis, the coordinator can usually able to determine this in advance based on the initial questionnaire and then schedule the appropriate appointments. The clinic coordinator is responsible for setting up the appointments and ensuring that all necessary team members will be present during the evaluation. Also in this initial encounter, inquiries can be made regarding insurance coverage, the need for precertification, and

Table 2. NEW FUNCTIONAL PROBLEMS IN POLIO SURVIVORS IN FOUR STUDIES				
FUNCTIONAL PROBLEM	CODD ET AL.[5] (N = 28)	HALSTEAD AND ROSSI[2] (N = 132)	AGRE ET AL.[4] (N = 79)	HALSTEAD AND ROSSI[1] (N = 539)
Difficulty walking	25%*	63%*	N/A	85%*
Difficulty climbing stairs	N/A	61%	67%*	82%
Difficulty with ADLs	14%	17%	16%	62%

*Most common new problem.

other administrative issues. The coordinator also provides information concerning local accommodations and other arrangements that patients may need when they are traveling. This way, they can stay for a complete evaluation and have ample time to get all equipment made, repaired, or fitted.

THE REHABILITATION NURSE

The evaluation begins with a rehabilitation nurse, who assesses the patient's health status by reviewing the medical history, medications, and functional status and takes vital signs, including weight and blood pressure. The nurse then helps coordinate the remaining evaluations and tests. The "nursing model of case collaboration" is based on principles of collaborative management of chronic illness developed by Van Korff et al.[6] The essential elements of nursing care that can enhance this process are (1) collaborative definition of the problems experienced by the person with PPS; (2) focus on a specific problem (after it is mutually identified and defined), set goals, and plan for the future; (3) create a continuum of self-management training and support services for the polio survivor; and (4) provide active and sustained follow-up at regular intervals, not just at times of crisis. The rehabilitation nurse also assists in identifying additional medical problems such as hypertension and obesity. Moreover, a good nurse can provide extremely important preventive medicine information and help reinforce wellness behaviors, such as patient education about weight loss and smoking cessation. The nurse can also promote compliance with medications, the team's recommendations, and regular follow-up appointments.

PHYSICIAN

The physician's role is obviously extremely important. He or she obtains a comprehensive history and performs a physical examination with attention to present complaints, polio history, and musculoskeletal and neurological examinations, taking into account the medical history and review of systems. The physician should ideally be a physiatrist, neurologist, or orthopedist with a background in the treatment of patients with PPS. It is wise for polio survivors to start with postpolio physicians whom they trust. In a recent study of 659 polio survivors, only 36% said their primary care physician (PCP) was knowledgeable about PPS, and 47% said they thought they should be referred to a polio specialist because they believed their PCPs were unlikely to take time to educate themselves about PPS.[7] It was noted that many times the PCP would prescribe strenuous exercise, doing more harm than good. Roller and Maynard suggest that polio survivors need to establish an "exercise coaching team," which includes the patient, the physician, and a therapist.[8] They state that: "If you need to first find these professionals, the journey will be longer since knowledgeable post-polio helping professionals can be difficult to find or cultivate. If you sense that a professional is not interested in post-polio issues, move on quickly to find someone who will work with you and is willing to learn and help." The International Polio Network in St. Louis (www.post-polio.org) is a good resource that publishes a national and international directory of self-identified postpolio health professionals and support groups whose members know about the best specialists in their geographic area.

The physician determines the need for diagnostic tests, including laboratory tests, imaging studies, pulmonary function tests, and electrodiagnostic studies (e.g., electromyography [EMG], nerve conduction studies [NCS]).[9] Physicians can also make referrals to other specialists. The need for referrals and tests depend on the patient's symptoms and functional problems. The differential diagnosis for PPS is difficult because the symptoms experienced by postpolio patients are common and nonspecific. The physician's job is to determine whether the patient has PPS or other diagnoses related to the late effects of polio by ruling specific diagnoses in or out. Even if the patient does not meet all criteria for PPS, the patient needs to be treated for the chief complaints, reassured, and given education regarding how to help prevent or lessen the effects of PPS in the future.

The most common and often most debilitating symptom that polio surivors complain of is a sense of fatigue. This can be described as focal, such as the legs only, but is usually more generalized and is described as an overwhelming exhaustion that typically occurs at the end of the day when patients "hit the polio wall."[9] It is typically brought on by an accumulation of activities, such as an occupation, that was previously carried on without special effort or noticeable sequelae. The differential diagnosis for fatigue is extensive but includes common problems such as thyroid dysfunction, diabetes mellitus, depression, and the side effects of medications. Therefore, routine baseline laboratory values should be done to rule out various causes of fatigue. These include thyroid studies, a serum fasting glucose, and a screening test for anemia. The physician also needs to perform a careful review of all drugs, including over-the-counter medications and herbal remedies.

Recent studies have shown that polio patients are at high risk for risk factors for hyperlipidemia and coronary heart disease (CHD). In a study of 64 postpolio patients, Agre et al.[10] found hyperlipidemia in 66% of all men evaluated and 25% of all women.[10] In a study of 50 women and 38 men, Gawne et al. found that a total of 61.3% had dyspidemia and 46.5% had more than one risk factor for CHD.[11] Therefore, a lipid profile should be performed during the initial evaluation to determine the patient's risk for CHD.

The use of certain tests such as creatine kinase (CK) is uncertain but needs to be studied further. Muscle pain may be a sign of overuse because some studies have found elevated CK levels in PPS patients. Windebank et al. found that 10 of 32 symptomatic patients had elevated CK levels, but none of the 18 asymptomatic patients did,[12] although other studies failed to demonstrate this relationship. Nelson found that the incidence of an elevated CK in a group of polio patients with delayed weakness (15 of 29 patients) did not differ from polio patients without delayed weakness.[13] Trojan et al. also failed to demonstrate a relationship between muscle pain and elevated CK levels.[14]

New weakness is the hallmark of PPS and can be partly evaluated by electrodiagnostic studies (i.e., EMG, NCS). These tests can detect the presence of other conditions such as carpal tunnel syndrome (CTS) and rule out alternative causes of weakness such as a radiculopathy. In a prospective study of 100 consecutive patients, 35% were found to have CTS, 2% ulnar neuropathy at the wrist, 3% ulnar neuropathy and CTS, 3% peripheral neuropathy, 4% radiculopathy, and 2% other neuropathies, as shown in Table 3.[15] In addition, EMG can be useful in identifying previous injury from polio in "unaffected limbs." This is important when recommending specific exercise programs.[15] The frequency of this finding of "subclinical polio" can be significant (see Table 3).[16]

Pain is another very common complaint; it has many possible causes. Three types of pain seen in polio survivors are postpolio muscle pain, overuse pain, and biomechanical pain.[17] Fibromyalgia may also be identified in some patients who complain of pain.[18] Proper treatment of patients with these pain problems leads to improved comfort as well as functional gains. Treatment options may include medications, injections, surgery, assistive devices, modalities and therapeutic exercise provided by either an OT or PT, and bracing.

Physicians must also address a number of other issues; these are best done on a patient-by-patient basis. Physician play a pivotal role in the care of patients and in the coordination of the other team members as well as other specialists who may become involved in the care of patients.

PHYSICAL THERAPIST

The PT's role in the evaluation includes a baseline manual muscle test; range of motion (ROM) of major joints; and evaluation of posture, gait, and mobility. The PT evaluates the patient's posture in sitting, sleeping, and standing (if appropriate) and analyzes activities and positions that provoke or relieve muscle and joint pains. Gait patterns are evaluated, with modifications made as needed with appropriate assistive devices. Smith et al. evaluated 111 postpolio patients, noting any significant postural or gait deviations.[19] In the 111 persons evaluated in a sitting position, 64% had an absent lumbar curve, 38% had structural scoliosis, and 50% had a forward head. In addition, it was found that 100% of the 76 patients who were ambulatory demonstrated gait deviations such as lateral trunk oscillations and forward lean.

Table 3. ABNORMAL ELECTRODIAGNOSTIC FINDINGS IN 100 CONSECUTIVE POSTPOLIO PATIENTS		
FINDING	**NUMBER OF PATIENTS**	**PERCENT OF PATIENTS**
Carpal tunnel syndrome (CTS)	35	35%
Ulnar neuropathy at the wrist	2	2%
CTS and ulnar neuropathy	3	3%
Peripheral neuropathy	3	3%
Brachial plexopathy	1	1%
Tibial neuropathy	1	1%
Radiculopathy	4	4%
Total abnormal studies	49	49%
Subclinical polio	49	49%

While standing, they had an uneven pelvic base 40% of the time and an absent lumbar curve in 52%, with a tendency to bear weight on the stronger leg.

A baseline manual muscle test is performed of major muscle groups, noting any history of muscle transfers, stabilization, or surgical interventions. Many times, polio survivors have found ways of "cheating" with manual muscle testing. They substitute one group of muscles to perform the joint motion normally performed by another such as using wrist flexors to flex the elbow. For this reason, it is sometimes wise to test individual muscle groups rather than a joint action such as elbow flexion. ROM and leg length discrepancy measurements are also important and should be followed over time along with manual muscle testing. It is well known that there are changes in muscle strength in different muscles over time. Klein et al. evaluated 120 polio patients initially and then at 3 and 5 months later.[20] They found that upper extremity strength decreased 1.39 lbs each visit, with more severe weakness in the wrist flexors, elbow extensors, shoulder external rotators, abductors, and extensors. In the lower extremity, strength dropped 0.8 lbs per visit, a less significant effect than was observed in the upper extremity. The greatest loss was in the dorsiflexors of the ankle, followed by the knee flexors, knee extensors, and finally the ankle plantar flexors. It was observed that there was greater loss in flexor rather than extensor muscles, implying that persons can use "tricks" to rest the extensors while ambulating by doing things such as going into genu recurvatum. This relative rest would helps preserve strength by avoiding muscle overuse. It should be noted that this study uses muscle strength measured in pounds obtained with the use of hand-held dynamometer. This is in contrast to the standard way most therapists use to measure strength, which is using the Medical Research Council (MRC) scale in which 5/5 is considered normal, 4/5 greater than antigravity, 3/5 antigravity, 2/5 less than antigravity, and 1/5 a "flicker" or trace. Although this method is well known to all, studies have shown that inter- and intrarater reliability are poor. In a study of polio subjects compared with a hand-held dynamometer, there was found to be good interexaminer correlation with experienced examiners, especially for weaker muscles.[21] Therefore, for research purposes, the more valid method is encouraged.

The PT addresses mobility issues in the Seating and Wheeled Mobility Clinic. There, patients have the opportunity to try manual wheelchairs, power-operated vehicles (POV), or scooters and power wheelchairs. Seating systems are also used to provide pelvic and trunk support in order to decrease pain and prevent deformity. Studies have found that the use of a wheelchair can conserve energy as well as decrease stress on the lower extremities. Hildebrandt et al. studied the energy cost of wheelchair mobility and found that at speeds ranging from 16 to 50 m/min, the energy expenditure in kcal/min kg was nearly half that of normal ambulation and compared with ambulation with an assistive device, it was almost one tenth the energy expenditure.[22] However, use of a manual wheelchair is rarely indicated because of the problems with overuse of the arm muscles and injuries to such structures as the rotator cuff. Occasionally, patients want a lightweight wheelchair that is easily transportable. This is particularly useful for patients who travel with a partner who can push them when they are in the chair. For most polio survivors, the appropriate mobility device is one that is powered, either a POV or a power wheelchair. These, however, are usually larger and more difficult to drive and transport. It is the duty of the PT to discuss the different options with the patient and to determine which device is most appropriate. The PT can also generate an appropriate letter and certificate of medical necessity in order for the item to be covered by third-party payers.

Finally, the PT provides patient education. Patient education includes information on appropriate exercise protocols, known as nonfatiguing paced exercises using the less affected extremities.[16] The PT can also work with the patient in a swimming pool. The benefits of aquatic therapy include increasing strength, flexibility, and endurance. It can also help to normalize movement and provide muscle re-education, relaxation of muscles, and tone reduction. It may offer improvements in the functional abilities, trunk stability, quality of gait, balance, and posture as well as pain reduction and enhanced psychological well-being.

OCCUPATIONAL THERAPIST

The occupational therapist assesses patients' independence with ADLs such as dressing, bathing, cooking, and driving. The OT is also an expert in upper extremity related problems (e.g., overuse injuries, CTS). In addition to the polio history and an assessment of the present problems, the OT evaluates the equipment patients have been using, including upper extremity orthoses and adaptive equipment such as built-up utensils and bathroom equipment. The OT is an expert at examining how an individual moves about in his or her world, both at work and at home. The OT analyzes daily activities to determine the amount of energy required and the amount of stress placed on each specific muscle group. The OT is particularly interested in activities that cause pain, fatigue, or weakness or place the patient at risk for falls. Special attention is paid to the frequency of these symptoms in the home, at work, and in the community and the need for adaptive equipment.

The focus of occupational therapy is an appropriate exercise program that involves the upper extremities, prevention of overuse injuries, treatment of any existing arm problems, and education about the principles of energy conservation. In terms of pacing and energy conservation, it is important to keep in mind that people do things very differently. For example, for some people, going to the store may involve a long walk, a lot of shopping, carrying heavy bags home, and putting away the purchased goods. Another person may drive to the store, use a scooter provided in the store, and purchase only a few light items. It is also important to remember that people value tasks in a variety of ways. Some people would love to order their groceries online and have them delivered, but others cannot bear the thought of someone else choosing their produce. A good OT understands the subtleties involved in making recommendations about lifestyle changes to improve patient's energy level and quality of life.

As the overuse theory suggests, people with PPS have a limited amount of energy with which to power their muscles; therefore, it should be carefully managed, just as money has to be budgeted. Energy conservation is a method of organizing daily activities so that the least amount of energy is used to complete a task. It is based on five principles; the "five P's" are *p*lanning, *p*rioritizing, *p*acing, *p*ositioning, and *p*ower-saving devices.[23] **Planning** involves making a schedule of the day's or week's tasks. The patient is encouraged to alternate heavy tasks with lighter ones and organize proper rest periods into the day. Errands should be spread throughout the week. **Prioritizing** consists of deciding which activities have to be done and which can wait, as well as delegating tasks to others. **Pacing** involves interdispersing activity and rest periods, even when exercising. It is important to remember not to do too many things at once. **Positioning** involves placing one's self in the most comfortable position to perform a task (e.g., sitting or leaning on a high stool). Occupational therapists are trained how to evaluate patients for and prescribe not only power-saving devices but also other equipment such as tub lifts or shower benches, handheld showers, and reachers. For people with weak arms, computer or desk work is made easier with mobile arm supports attached to the desk or power chair. It is important that the chair or work area is the correct height. Finally, **power-saving devices** such as an electric can or jar opener makes the job easier and other bathroom equipment. The evaluation helps determine which activities, responsibilities, and environmental surroundings need to be changed to help decrease symptoms such as pain and fatigue. Energy conservation is a lifelong process. OT evaluation and treatment are designed to help individuals on a course of awareness of themselves, their surroundings, and their activities to decrease the symptoms of PPS.[24]

Additional OT treatment can also include upper extremity stretching, gentle strengthening (if indicated), and cardiovascular exercises that involve the arms. OTs also provide information about adaptive equipment to compensate for weak or atrophied muscles and provide hand splints to improve hand function or protect weak muscles.

ORTHOTIST

Orthotists evaluate the gait and bracing needs, usually along with a physician and a physical therapist. Orthotists also make necessary adjustments and repairs to existing braces and crutches. They can help determine whether someone who has never worn a brace or has not worn one since childhood might benefit from using one now. Orthotists who are skilled at treating polio survivors are sensitive to the fact that for many people who gave up their braces years ago, resorting to wearing a brace again may be a difficult experience. However, many times the brace may be necessary to improve gait, decrease pain, or prevent further joint deformity such as knee hyperextension (genu recurvatum). Examples of bracing options include a posterior leaf spring ankle foot orthosis (AFO) for flaccid dorsiflexors weakness and a solid AFO for those with both plantar and dorsiflexor weakness. Equinovarus can be treated with a solid AFO or a short leg brace with a lateral T strap.[25] Plastic molded AFOs made of polyethylene, polypropylene, Orthoplast, or other materials permits custom design of lightweight flexible to rigid orthoses, depending on the ratio of flexible monomer.[26] The materials used and the type of brace required depend on the patient's strength, lifestyle, and what he or she has worn in the past. A double metal upright brace should be used when there is loss of sensation, skin breakdown such as foot ulcers, or fluctuating edema. Some patients prefer these braces because they have worn them in the past despite the decreased weight and convenience of slipping the brace into many different shoes that plastic braces offer.

Objectives for nonsurgical treatment of foot and leg disorders in poliomyelitis patients include:

- Accommodation of rigid conditions and toe deformities
- Offweighting, which provides shock absorption and cushioning of bony prominences and contracted digits
- Control of flexible conditions and rigid deformities to allow a stable plantigrade foot that will help prevent strain on soft tissues and joints and allow better fit of shoe wear
- Patient education on shoe wear, proper orthotic use, skin care, and temperature regulation
- Improvement of gait
- Prevention of falls[27]

In a study of 104 postpolio patients, Waring et al. prescribed lower extremity orthoses for 36 patients.[28] Orthotics were recommended to improve safety by reducing the risk of falls, reduce pain, and decrease fatigue by improving gait speed and symmetry. Subjects who used orthoses reported significant improvements in pain relief, especially at the knee.

Table 4 shows the numbers and types of braces or assistive devices that were used in a survey of 83 polio survivors.[29]

SOCIAL WORKER OR PSYCHOLOGIST

A clinical social worker or psychologist evaluates the psychological impact of new health problems and functional loss on the patient and the family. Typically, there is also an effort to identify coping strategies used by, and available to, the individual and

Table 4. ASSISTIVE DEVICES IN 83 POLIO SURVIVORS		
ORTHOTICS OR ASSISTIVE DEVICES	**NUMBER OF PATIENTS**	**PERCENTAGE OF PATIENTS**
Prescription shoes	12	14%
Molded AFO	14	17%
Cane	40	48%
Crutches	7	8%
Wheelchair or scooter	35	42%
Metal upright AFO	28	33%
Inserts or lifts	20	24%
Orthodigita or padding	6	7%
Knee brace or KAFO	6	7%
Walker	5	6%
Prescription hose	1	1%
Magnet therapy	2	2%

assess the emotional impact of the original polio experience and how it relates to current feelings of having a second disability. Social workers can also help to facilitate referrals and access to community resources and services, including local postpolio support groups and polio resources within the United States and abroad.

The adjustments and changes in lifestyle required to live with both polio and PPS represent a lifelong process. Maynard and Roller surveyed 100 polio survivors to identify their coping strategies and identified three distinct patterns of emotional reaction to the need for re-rehabilitation.[30] Their model designates polio survivors as *passers, minimizers,* and *identifiers,* which are labels that characterize typical attitudes and behaviors that were adopted in order to cope with long-term mild, moderate, or severe disability. Passers had a disability that was so mild it could be hidden easily in casual social interactions. Minimizers had a moderate disability that was readily recognized by other people, and they often used visible adaptive equipment to function optimally. They typically minimized the importance of their physical differences. Identifiers were severely disabled by acute polio and generally needed wheelchairs for independent mobility. A closer look at each group's coping style is presented in order to clarify the typical patterns of emotional reaction that occur when polio survivors experience disabling late effects of the disease.

Passers work directly to hide their long-term disabilities. By using denial, they have been able to put their disability out of existence mentally and physically by hiding any physical impairment. Passing is a coping style that requires constant vigilance or one might become stigmatized as part of society's disabled minority. Maynard and Roller administered an attitudes survey and discovered that passers were the group that was most distressed in having to adjust to the late effects of polio. Passers were more likely to be emotionally overwhelmed by the physical changes from the late effects than any of their postpolio counterparts. It is important for health professionals to know that among postpolio patients, the passers have the greatest resistance to making—and the most emotional difficulty in accepting—some of the relatively minor lifestyle adaptations that are needed to cope with the late effects of polio. Passers who are confronted with postpolio sequelae often have their self-image threatened when they can no longer pass as someone who does not have a disability. They may become frightened because they do not know how far their disabilities will progress. When confronted with PPS, passers must often alter their self-perceptions and lifestyles to continue successful coping. Their former coping styles may no longer be effective, and they must learn new attitudes and behaviors. Ironically, in clinical terms, passers can often be fully rehabilitated because their new disabilities are less severe than those in the other groups. They can be reassured that modern orthotics, such as plastic braces, can be nicely worn under clothing and completely hidden under shoes. Passers may require an unexpected amount of understanding, patience, and empathetic support from health care professionals because of strong emotional reactions that are not only triggered by the impending public nature of their new disability but also by memories of past polio-related experiences.[31] When their disability progresses from mild to moderate, they become undeniably disabled for the first time. This can be a harsh reality for them to finally face, accept, and adapt to.

Minimizers are postpolio patients who have had a moderate disability that was always apparent to themselves and to others. They have coped with polio's first effects by minimizing the negative; adapted by de-emphasizing physical pain, deformity, and functional shortcomings; and accentuated the positive by pursuing intellectual vocations and avocations in place of more physical activities. However, minimizers are often so adept at their ability to deny pain and other physical challenges that they often recognize polio's late effects only when physical symptoms become unbearable and sometimes insurmountable. In order to survive and function at peak capacity, they use minimizing as a defense mechanism to such an extent that they are quite insensitive to their own pain, weakness, and frustration. Minimizers tend to have negative attitudes about severely disabled individuals. Frequently, they admit to difficulty being socially linked with someone in a wheelchair because the very association might somehow generate their own need to use one. Not surprisingly, these patients are the most likely to physically benefit from beginning to use a wheelchair. It is useful for professionals to recognize these phobic-like reactions when they occur and to use techniques for helping minimizers change their perceptions of wheelchairs and wheelchair users. It is important to recognize that they may have difficulty verbally describing new physical symptoms because they are skilled at ignoring or denying such problems. They need coaching and encouragement to fully focus on their body's sensations and reactions and to become what might be called "wise hypochondriacs." Health care providers must listen closely to minimizers for the slightest mention of new medical problems and give them permission to elaborate.[32] Despite many negative emotional reactions, minimizers know how to set goals and achieve them with persistence and determination. Astute health care professionals encourage and help empower minimizers to use these qualities to refocus on what is important in life, to take another look at how to be successful, and to set new goals and achieve them in new ways. Health care professionals must be patient in helping minimizers work through understandable resistance, fears, and anger with re-rehabilitation. They must respect, remember, and sometimes remind minimizers that they are experienced copers who have a well-proven capacity to adapt effectively.

Identifiers are polio survivors who have been sufficiently disabled since their acute polio to require wheelchairs for mobility. They have needed to more fully integrate their disability into their self-image in order to create successful and meaningful lives. They have gained the strength to tolerate social prejudices and architectural barriers, and many have become disabled rights activists and helped start the independent living movement. Among the three groups sampled through the attitudes survey, identifiers most strongly endorsed the statement "high achievement is a requirement for survival as a disabled person." With the onset of PPS, many identifiers confront the loss of their independence. The smallest functional forfeiture can be extremely distressing to a person who has been chronically severely disabled. If breathing function becomes significantly impaired, death may be a realistic threat. For identifiers who have had to work diligently to learn to feed themselves and perform other simple self-care activities, independence in ADLs may be one of the most important accomplishments of their lives. Therefore, if postpolio sequelae threaten a decline in strength, they can be expected to appear extremely distressed. Effective, helping professionals need to anticipate identifiers' concerns and recognize that their intense interest in autonomy and control of their environments are not pathologic. Identifiers have needed to develop a heightened concern about physical independence and about personal choice with how required help is given in order to attain high self-esteem and survive with their severe disability. When their freedom to control their life activities is threatened by new physical limitations or even by temporary dependency imposed by a hospital setting, identifiers may experience a threat to their whole lives and purpose for living. This reaction often leaves identifiers vulnerable to others' false perceptions of them as being overly controlling, difficult, and demanding people. In reality, they simply know what they need and are not too timid to ask for it. Informed health care professionals accept this and do everything possible to let identifiers continue to feel—and actually be—in charge of what happens to them.

Health care professionals need to be aware of polio survivors' typical past coping styles and of their need to use different tactics for coping during the re-rehabilitation process. They can point out to polio survivors that it is possible to find opportunity in their time of change. Passers can "come out of the closet," relax, and enjoy a little more freedom with their very acceptable natural physiques and identities. Minimizers can also be empowered to live life with a greater sense of wholeness through more fully recognizing, accepting, and integrating all aspects of their bodies. By relinquishing their struggle for physical independence and accepting new personal and technological assistance, identifiers can gain the time and energy to develop new pursuits and cultivate other realms of interest. In this honest and supportive spirit of healthy transition, successful rehabilitation can occur for the ever-adapting group of polio survivors.

Many times, a mental health professional can be extremely beneficial to polio survivors who are coping with new health problems. Bruno and colleagues describe an evaluation process in their postpolio clinic.[33] Initially, all patients who present for treatment by the Post-Polio Service undergo complete physiatry and psychological evaluations. They are administered the Reinforcement Motivation Survey (RMS)[34] and Beck Depression Inventory (BDI).[35] Bruno has found that the majority of patients have elevated type A scores compared with control subjects and sensitivity to both criticism and failure scores on the RMS but had insignificantly elevated BDI scores. This indicates no serious depression; although 57% of patients reported "low mood," only 31% met *Diagnostic and Statistical Manual of Mental Disorders,* Third Edition, Revised, (DSM-IIIR) criteria for a major depressive episode (MDE). This is similar to the 32% reported by Freidenberg et al.[36] but higher than the prevalence of MDE in the general population (i.e., 3–7%)[37,38] and in those with medical illness (20%).[39]

The presence of major depression in polio patients is important, not only because it requires treatment, but also because MDE is significantly correlated with treatment noncompliance. MDE was diagnosed in 63% of patients who refused further treatment after the initial evaluation and in 50% of those who were discharged for therapeutic noncompliance. Only 11% of patients who were fully compliant and 29% of those who were partially compliant with therapy were diagnosed as having a MDE. Patients with MDE are always treated with psychotherapy, although depression was sufficiently severe in 70% of patients that an antidepressant was recommended. Mental health professionals can provide individual counseling and assist physicians with suggestions regarding medication management in cases of depression or anxiety.

RESPIRATORY THERAPIST

Another health professional who participates in the interdisciplinary clinic is a respiratory therapist. The respiratory therapist performs a screening pulmonary function test (PFT), including vital capacity (VC), and forced expiratory volume in 1 second (FEV_1), and peak expiratory flow in both a sitting and supine position. For individuals with evidence of chronic obstructive pulmonary disease (COPD), PFTs with a bronchodilator can be done. At times, it is necessary to obtain an arterial blood gas (ABG) to measure O_2, CO_2 saturation, and pH.

In a national study of 539 polio survivors, Halstead reported that 42% of respondents reported new problems with breathing.[40] These typically are restrictive pulmonary disease caused by weak muscles, including the diaphragm, but in some patients, especially those with a history of smoking, COPD can develop as well. Sleep-disordered breathing, including central or obstructive apnea, occurs in the postpolio population to a greater degree than in the general population. Sleep-disordered breathing can result in chronic alveolar hypoventilation (CAH); hypoxia; right ventricular strain; and, finally, cardiopulmonary failure. When not corrected, insidiously progressive hypercapnia leads to a compensatory metabolic alkalosis. The resulting central nervous system bicarbonate levels can lead to depression of the ventilatory response to the hypercapnia and hypoxia and worsening of the CAH.

When a nocturnal sleep disorder is suspected, polysomnography may be needed.[41] A CO_2 level > 50 mmHg or an O_2 saturation level < 95% for 1 hour or more in a patient with a VC < 50% of predicted is diagnostic of CAH. For symptomatic patients with VC > 50% of predicted and inconclusive sleep studies, sleep-disordered breathing and inspiratory muscle weakness may be responsible for symptoms.[42]

Both sleep-disordered breathing and CAH can be reversed and their symptoms improved with the initiation of ventilatory assistance. Inspiratory positive pressure ventilation (IPPV) can be delivered in many ways. Continuous positive airway pressure (CPAP) or bilevel positive pressure airway pressure (BiPAP), which independently varies the inspiratory and expiratory pressures, are both suitable alternatives. These can be delivered via an oral, nasal, or oral-nasal ventilator hose.[43] Inspiratory muscle training has been found to be of help in some patients with restrictive pulmonary disease. In a study of 10 polio patients with restrictive lung disease using part-time assisted ventilation, Kleback et al. performed inspiratory muscle training using a threshold inspiratory muscle trainer, monitoring the rating of perceived exertion (RPE).[44] They found significant ($P < 0.05$) improvements in endurance in the training group at RPEs of 15 (hard) and 17 (very hard).

PODIATRIST

The polio virus destroys the anterior horn cells of the spinal cord, leaving muscles weak and flaccid. With time, there is reinnervation and improvement of strength in many muscle groups, but sometimes this can lead to muscle imbalance, such as weak dorsiflexors and stronger plantar flexors. Also, there may also be asymmetry in the pattern of involvement with one lower extremity affected more than the other, leading to a leg length discrepancy. Extensive rehabilitation is done to strengthen the extremities and prevent deformity, and a number of surgical procedures were performed on the lower extremities to make the limbs functional once again. Chronically, as the polio survivor ages, residual deformities slowly become established and rigid and osteoarthritis becomes common. This leads to pain and further problems.

A podiatrist can evaluate patients for the presence of foot pain, deformity, past surgeries, and use of an assistive device. He or she can obtain radiographs and perform a gait analysis and evaluation of plantar pressures with the use of a pedobaragraph. A questionnaire was sent to 150 members of a polio support group; 83 polio survivors completed the questionnaire, 45 women and 38 men, ages 46 to 82 years (mean age, 60 years). A total of 54.3% of responders reported that they had foot pain, and 89% reported that they had foot deformity, ranging from limb length discrepancies to hammertoes, cavus feet, and equinus deformity (Table 5). Seventy percent of the patients reported some type of lower extremity surgery (Table 6). All of the patients reported using some type of appliance, assistive device, special shoe, or brace for ambulation. Only 8.4% reported currently seeing a podiatrist, and 37% saw a physiatrist.[29]

In another study of 39 consecutive patients evaluated in the foot clinic, 22 female and 17 male polio survivors ages 44–84 years (mean age, 64 years) were identified as having foot problems.[45] All had complaints of foot pain, and 89% had foot de-

Table 5. FOOT PROBLEMS IN 83 POLIO SURVIVORS

CHIEF COMPLAINT OR DEFORMITY	NUMBER OF PATIENTS, N	PERCENT OF PATIENTS
Equinus	26	31%
Osteoarthritis	27	32%
Limb length discrepancy	40	48%
Pes cavus	18	21%
Pes planus	11	13%
Digital deformities	10	12%
Scar complaints	21	25%
Bunion	11	13%
Keratosis	2	2.4%
Autonomic dysreflexia	61	73%
Swelling	1	1%
Dropfoot	3	4%

Table 6. SURGICAL HISTORY IN 83 POLIO SURVIVORS		
SURGICAL HISTORY	**NUMBER OF PATIENTS, N**	**PERCENT OF PATIENTS**
Achilles lengthening	17	20%
Ankle fusion	18	22%
Bunion surgery	3	4%
Digital surgery	7	8%
Tendon or muscle surgery	25	30%
Triple arthrodesis	14	17%
Epiphysiodesis	13	16%
Limb lengthening	1	1%
Calcaneal osteotomy	3	4%
Neuroma excision	2	2%
Ankle stabilization	1	1%
Hip fusion	1	1%
Tibial osteotomy	1	1%
Femoral osteotomy	1	1%

formity, including degenerative joint disease (28%), equinus or equinovarus deformities (25%), toe deformities (18%), cavus feet (15%), limb length discrepancies (10%), dropfoot (10%) and pes planus (5%), and calcaneus (5%) deformity. Twenty percent of the patients reported a history of lower extremity surgery. Treatments offered included orthoses, adjustment of a brace, watchful waiting, injections, and surgery.

PHARMACOLOGIST AND DIETITIAN

The dietitian and pharmacist can advise patients on diet and medications respectively. A low cholesterol level or weight loss diet is essential for many individuals because dyslipidemia is prevalent in polio survivors and management of obesity has been found to have a significant effect on patients' symptoms. In addition, counseling can be done about the other risk factors for heart disease such as smoking cessation and treatment of hypertension. Because osteoporosis is a problem in polio survivors, pharmacologists and dietitians can make recommendations about vitamin supplements and diets that contain enough vitamin D and calcium. The author's clinic provides counseling regarding heart disease risk factors. Over the first year, 46 consecutive postpolio patients (33 women, ages 44–75 [mean, 63.0 years] and 13 men, ages 44–80 [mean 57.5 years]) were evaluated in the Lipid Care Clinic. The mean cholesterol and high-density lipoprotein (HDL) levels were 233 and 61 for women and 221 and 39 for men, respectively. The mean Framingham score was 15.7 in women and 13.6 in men. A total of 21 patients had hypertension and 9 had diabetes. The results of the interventions with six patients showed that their mean cholesterol level dropped 40.3 points, mean HDL increased 19 points, non-HDL decreased 79 points, and triglyceride level decreased 37 points; the Framingham score decreased in three patients.[46]

SPEECH LANGUAGE PATHOLOGIST

In addition to damaging centers of respiration, the polio virus can also damage bulbar areas involved with the swallowing process. In some cases, bulbar involvement may be mild, with complaints of difficulty swallowing large pieces of food; however, in more severe cases, it can lead to aspiration pneumonia. Difficulty with swallowing has been reported to be a significant complaint in 10–15% of all patients with acute poliomyelitis[47] and 10–22% of all patients with PPS.[48]

Sonies and Dalakas studied 32 postpolio patients and found that 44% had complaints of new swallowing difficulties.[49] New swallowing difficulties were noted by nine of the 12 patients with a history bulbar involvement and five patients with no history of bulbar involvement. Detailed evaluation of these 32 patients, including ultrasonography and a modified barium swallow (MBS), revealed abnormalities in 31 patients, regardless of whether they were symptomatic or had a history of previous bulbar involvement. Trace aspiration was noted in only two subjects.

In another study of 109 postpolio patients, Coelho and Ferranti evaluated 21 patients who had complaints of difficulty swallowing.[50] Of the patients, 12 complained that foods got stuck, five had difficulty swallowing pills or dry foods, two complained of frequent choking, and two had complaints of coughing or tightness in the throat. These patients were evaluated using an MBS, which used video fluoroscopy to examine swallowing of liquids, paste, and crackers coated with barium. Twenty of these 21 patients had abnormal results. Twelve patients (57%) had mild involvement, six (29%) had moderate involvement, and two (10%) had severe involvement. Pulmonary function tests demonstrated abnormalities, including decreased peak expiratory flow and maximum expiratory pressure in all but three subjects; therefore, it was concluded that this combination put patients at risk for aspiration.

For patients who present with dysphagia, evaluation and treatment recommendations can be done by a speech language pathologist (SLP). The SLP should evaluate the patient clinically with attention to the cranial nerves and observe the patient swallowing, if possible. The SLP can perform an MBS, PFTs, or ultrasonography as indicated.

If abnormalities indicate that the patient is at risk for aspiration, recommendations for compensatory techniques include changing the consistency of the food or liquid, turning the head to one side, tucking the chin, alternating food and liquid, and avoiding eating when fatigued.[50] This subject is discussed in greater detail in Chapter 8.

THE INTERDISCIPLINARY TEAM

After the patient has been seen by the team members and all tests have been completed, it is imperative that the team members meet to discuss their findings with each other, the patient, and the patient's loved ones. A team conference can be conducted with the patient and significant others on the second day of the evaluation. This conference is used to review the results of diagnostic tests and discuss impressions and recommendations for interventions. At that time, prescriptions for medication and equipment are written and a follow-up appointment can be scheduled. Every patient and referring physician should receive a copy of the physician's summary as well as a copy of the team's recommendations.

It may be worthwhile to provide patients with a list of polio support groups in their geographic region (available from the International Polio Network). Polio survivors tend to be information seekers who appreciate reading materials. Books that we typically recommend to patients and their loved ones include *Post-Polio Syndrome: A Guide for Polio Surivors and Their Families* (Yale University Press) by Julie Silver, M.D., and *Managing Post-Polio: A Guide to Living Well with Post-Polio Syndrome* (Vandamere Press) edited by Lauro S. Halstead, M.D.

Follow-up appointments are scheduled according to the patient's needs and proximity to the clinic; the author's institution generally does a reassessment in person or by phone in 6 weeks and then on a yearly basis. For those with medication changes that need to be monitored, more frequent follow-ups may be needed. This helps the patients and also gives the team members an opportunity to see how patients have done with recommendations that were made. Peach and Olejnik studied 77 polio survivors, dividing them into compliers (i.e., complied with all recommendations) partial compliers (i.e., accepted some recommendations), and noncompliers.[51] At the time of follow up (mean, 2.1 years), the complier group reported either resolution or improvement in symptoms such as pain and fatigue; the noncompliers showed worsening or progression of symptoms; and the partial compliers demonstrated a wider range or responses, either no change or some improvement. Muscle strength increased in compliers but decreased in the other groups. Reasons for noncompliance included resistance to orthotics and other assistive devices as well as lifestyle. Thus, follow-up can be a way of both monitoring symptoms as well as compliance, giving providers an opportunity to suggest changes that patients can accept more readily.

In summary, an interdisciplinary clinic provides a thorough evaluation for all patients who present to a postpolio clinic. Because a polio survivors' needs are so diverse, it is highly unlikely that one health professional, regardless of how skilled he or she is, can meet them all. Ideally, team members should share physical workspace in order to communicate ideas and deliver a consistent message. When services are provided over a 2- or 3-day period, polio survivors are given a more energy efficient evaluation, yet there is adequate time for questions to be answered, education to be done, brace work to be completed, and laboratory work to be received while patients are still in the clinic. This interdisciplinary model can serve as an example for other postpolio clinics to follow in order to provide the best care possible for postpolio patients.

References

1. Halstead LS, Rossi CD: Post-polio syndrome: Results of a survey of 539 survivors. Orthopedics 8:845–850, 1985.
2. Halstead LS, Rossi CD: Post-polio syndrome: Clinical experience with 132 consecutive outpatients. In Halstead LS, Weichers DO (eds): Research and Clinical Aspects of the

Late Effects of Poliomyelitis. White Plains, NY, March of Dimes Birth Defects Foundation, 1987, pp 13–26.

3. Chetwynd J, Hogan D: Post-polio syndrome in New Zealand: A survey of 700 polio survivors. N Z Med J 106:406–408, 1993.

4. Agre JC, Rodriquez AA, Sperling KB: Symptoms and clinical impressions of patients seen in a post-polio clinic. Arch Phys Med Rehabil 70:367–370, 1989.

5. Codd MP, Mulder DW, Kurland LT, et al: Poliomyelitis in Rochester, MN, 1935 to 1955. Epidemiology and long-term sequelae: A preliminary report. In Halstead LS, Weicher DO (eds): Late Effects of Poliomyelitis. Miami, Symposium Foundation, 1985, pp 121–133.

6. Stuifbergen AK, Harrison T: Nursing interventions for persons with post-polio syndrome. Presented at the International Conference on Post-polio Syndrome: Identifying Best Practices in Diagnosis and Care. March of Dimes Birth Defects Foundation, Warm Springs, GA, May 19–20, 2000.

7. Zink J: Research report: How aging polio survivors perceive their primary care physician's knowledge of PPS. Options Polio Soc Newslett (Feb):4–5, 2001.

8. Roller S, Maynard FM: To Reap the Rewards of Post-Polio Exercise. Chicago, The National Center on Physical Activity and Disability, 2002.

9. Halstead LS: Assessment and differential diagnosis for post-polio syndrome. Orthopedics 14:1209–1217, 1991.

10. Agre JC, Rodriguez AA, Sperlina KB: Plasma lipid and lipid concentrations in symptomatic post-polio patients. Arch Phys Med Rehabil 71:393–394, 1990.

11. Gawne AC, Wells KD, Wilson K: Cardiac risk factors in polio survivors. Arch Phys Med Rehabil 84:694–696, 2003.

12. Windebank AJ, Daube JR, LichtyWJ, et al: Late effects of paralytic poliomyelitis in Olmsted County, MN. Neurology 41:27–38, 1991.

13. Nelson KR: Creatine kinase and fibrillation potentials in patients with late sequelae of polio. Muscle Nerve 13:722–725, 1990.

14. Vasiliadis HM, Collet JP, Shapiro S, et al: Predictive factors and correlates for pain in post-poliomyelitis syndrome patients. Arch Phys Med Rehabil 83:1109–1115, 2002.

15. Halstead LS,Gawne AC, Pham BT: The National Rehabilitation Hospital Limb Classification for Exercise: Research and clinical trials in post-polio patients. Ann N Y Acad Sci 753:343–353, 1995.

16. Gawne AC, Pham BT, Halstead LS: Electrodiagnostic findings in 108 consecutive patients evaluated in a post-polio clinic: The value of routine electrodiagnostic testing. Ann N Y Acad Sci 753:383–385, 1995.

17. Gawne AC: Pain in post-polio syndrome. Polio Netw News (winter):1–3, 1997.

18. Trojan DA, Cashman NR: Fibromyalgia is common in a postpoliomyelitis clinic. Arch Neurol 52:620–624, 1995.

19. Smith LK, Bonck J, Macrae A: Current issues in neurological rehabilitation. In Umphred DA (ed): Neurological Rehabilitation, 2nd ed. St. Louis, Mosby, 1990, pp 509–528.

20. Klein MG, Whyte J, Keenan MA, et al: Strength changes in polio survivors over time. Arch Phys Med Rehabil 81:1959–1064, 2000.

21. Nollet F, Beelan A: Strength assessment in post-polio syndrome: Validity of a hand held dynamometer. Arch Phys Med Rehabil 80:1316–1323, 1999.

22. Fisher SV, Gullicksen G: Energy cost of ambulation in health and disability: A review. Arch Phys Med Rehabil 59:124–132, 1978.

23. Roosevelt Warm Springs Institute for Rehabilitation: Energy Conservation: The 5 P's. Warm Springs, GA, Roosevelt Warm Springs Institute for Rehabilitation.

24. Young GR: Energy conservation, occupational therapy and the treatment of post-polio sequelae. Orthopedics 14:1233–1239, 1991.

25. Sobel E, Giogini RJ: Podiatric management of the neuromuscular patient. Podiatry To-day.com (Jan):1–10, 2001.
26. Meyer PR: Lower limb orthotics. Clin Orthop Rel Res 102:58–72, 1974.
27. Janisse DJ: Footwear for polio survivors. Polio Netw News 17:6–9, 2000.
28. Waring WP, et al: Influence of appropriate lower extremity orthotic management on am-bulation, pain and fatigue in a post-polio population. Arch Phys Med Rehabil 70: 371–375, 1989.
29. Gawne AC, Bernstein BH: Foot problems in polio survivors [abstract]. Arch Phys Med Rehabil 82:1317, 2001.
30. Maynard FM, Roller S: Recognizing typical coping styles of polio survivors can improve re-rehabilitation: A commentary. Am J Phys Med Rehabil 70:70–72, 1991.
31. Backman M: The post-polio patient: Psychological issues. J Rehabil 53:23–26, 1987.
32. Roller S: Post-polio memorandum. Polio Perspect 2:1–2, 1987.
33. Bruno RL, Frick NM: The psychology of polio as a prelude to post-polio sequalae: Be-havior modification and psychotherapy. Orthopedics 14:1185–1193, 1991.
34. Bruno RL: Predicting pain management program outcome: The Reinforcement Motiva-tion Survey. Arch Phys Med Rehabil 10:785, 1990.
35. Beck AT, Ward CH, Mendelson M, et al: An inventory for measuring depression. Arch Gen Psychiatry 4:561–571, 1961.
36. Freidenberg DL, Freeman D, Huber SJ, et al: Postpoliomyelitis syndrome: Behavioral features. Neuropsychiatry Neuropsychol Behav Neurol 2:272–281, 1989.
37. Myers JK, Weissman MM, Tischler OL, et al: Six month prevalence of psychiatric disor-ders in three communities. Arch Gen Psychiatry 41:959–967, 1984.
38. Roberts RE, Vernon SW: Depression in the community: Prevalence and treatment. Arch Gen Psychiatry 39:1407–1409, 1982.
39. Schleifer SJ, Macari M, Slater W, et al: Predictors of outcome after myocardial infarction: Role of depression. Circulation 74(suppl II):38, 1987.
40. Halstead LS, Rossi CD: New problems in old polio patients: Results of a survey of 539 polio survivors. Orthopedics 8:845–850, 1985.
41. Bach JR, Alba AS: Pulmonary dysfunction and sleep disordered breathing as post-polio sequelae: Evaluation and management. Orthopedics 14:1329–1337, 1991.
42. Saunders MH: Assessment of required nocturnal ventilatory assistance. Eur Respir Rev 2: 409–412, 1992.
43. Sanders MH, Kern N: Obstructive sleep apnea treated independently by adjusting inspi-ratory and expiratory pressures via nasal mask: Physiological and clinical implications. Chest 98:17–24, 1990.
44. Klefback B, Langerstrand L, Mattson E: Inspiratory muscle training in patients with prior polio who use part time assisted ventilation. Arch Phys Med Rehail 81:1065–1071, 2000.
45. Bernstein B, Gawne AC: Foot problems in polio survivors [abstract]. Submitted at the annual meeting of the American Academy of Physical Medicine and Rehabilitation, Orlando, FL, 2002.
46. Gawne AC, Wells KM, Wilson KS: Treatment of polio patients in the lipid care clinic [abstract]. Submitted at the annual meeting of the American Academy of Physical Medi-cine and Rehabilitation, Orlando, FL, 2002.
47. Baker AB, Matzhe HA, Brown JR: Poliomyelitis III: A study of medullary function. Arch Neurol 63:257, 1950.
48. Buckholtz DW, Jones B: Post-polio dysphagia: Alarm or caution. Orthopedics 14: 1303–1304, 1991.
49. Sonies BC, Dalakas MC: Dysphagia in patients with the post-polio syndrome. N Engl J Med 324:1162–1167, 1991.

50. Coelho CA, Ferranti R: Incidence and nature of dysphagia in polio survivors. Arch Phys Med Rehabil 72:1071–1075, 1991.
51. Buchholz DW, Jones B: Post-polio dysphagia: Alarm or caution. Orthopedics 14: 1303–1305, 1991.
52. Peach PE, Olejnik S: Effect of treatment and compliance on post-polio sequelae. Orthopedics 14:1199–1203, 1991.

Electrophysiology of Postpolio Syndrome

Neil R. Cashman, MD, and Daria A. Trojan, MD, MSc

Paralytic poliomyelitis is an acute viral disease of motor neurons in the spinal cord and brain stem. In North America, more than 600,000 people are survivors of acute paralytic poliomyelitis (APP).[1] Beginning with reports from Cornil and Raymond in 1875,[1a] it has been increasingly recognized that individuals recovering from APP develop a bewildering array of new symptoms, most commonly new weakness, fatigue (generalized fatigue as well as muscular fatigability), and pain.[2] The concurrence of these symptoms has been designated the postpolio syndrome (PPS).

The cause or causes of PPS have been widely debated for decades.[3] However, many authorities now agree that PPS is probably caused by distal axonal degeneration in the hugely enlarged axonal arborizations developing after APP. By this scheme, originally proposed by Weichers and Hubbell,[4] remaining healthy motor neurons are capable of sprouting extra axonal branches to reinnervate muscle fibers denervated during the APP. This motor unit enlargement is not indefinitely stable, however, and is accompanied by motor unit remodeling and eventual degeneration of terminal sprouts.

NEW WEAKNESS IN POSTPOLIO SYNDROME: A CONTROLLED STUDY

We examined a group of patients with well-defined PPS and compared them with a control group of individuals who had recovered from APP without new symptoms.[5] Patients were closely matched for severity of old polio, age, time since polio, and other factors. Study methodologies included conventional electromyography (EMG), single-fiber EMG (SFEMG), and muscle biopsy. SFEMG can be used to provide two convenient measures: fiber density, which can be interpreted as an indication of the severity of remote denervation of APP, and jitter, which has been thought to reflect terminal axonal instability in reinnervating axons.

We performed muscle biopsies, quantifying such features as fiber type grouping (a measure of remote denervation) and myofiber atrophy, which indicates permanent loss of motor innervation within the weeks before the biopsy. We also pioneered the use of immunohistochemisty for neural cell adhesion molecule (N-CAM) as an immunohistochemical indicator of denervation.[6]

We found ample evidence in electrophysiologic and biopsy studies of old denervation of APP in both PPS and control groups.[5] To our surprise, we also found no differences between PPS and polio control groups with regard to active ongoing denervation by electrophysiology and muscle biopsy, including increased jitter, acute myofiber atrophy, and widespread expression of N-CAM. We did find that evidence of remote denervation correlated well with evidence of ongoing denervation, which might suggest that the hugely overextended motor units from old polio were more vulnerable to undergo terminal axonal degeneration in later life.

FATIGUE AND FATIGABILITY: A NEUROLOGIC LESION?

One would anticipate that terminal axonal degeneration must be accompanied or preceded by terminal axonal dysfunction. We and others have assembled information suggesting that terminal axonal dysfunction is an important pathologic process in PPS. As noted, jitter is markedly increased in PPS compared with normal control subjects.[4,5] Although jitter in postpolio muscles has been used as an indirect indicator of the process of reinnervation,[7,8] it can also be regarded as measuring the adequacy of neuromuscular junction transmission, which can be defective in terminal axonal dysfunction.[8] N-CAM immunoreactivity on normal-sized myofibers might be regarded as an immunohistochemical indicator of terminal axonal dysfunction.[5,6] Certainly,

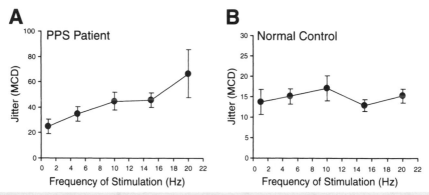

Figure 1. 1. Jitter response to stimulation frequency in a PPS patient and a normal control subject. Jitter (mean ± SEM) for each of five stimulation frequencies is illustrated. Jitter is measured (in μsec) as the mean consecutive difference (MCD) of latency from stimulation artifact to muscle fiber being studied. **A,** Jitter is increased with increased stimulation frequency in 10 quadriceps muscle fibers of a PPS patient. Mean jitter at high frequency stimulation (81.9 ± 27.0 μsec, mean ± SD) was significantly higher ($P < 0.001$) than mean jitter at low frequency stimulation (39.9 ± 22.5 μsec). **B,** Jitter does not change with increased stimulation frequency in five quadriceps muscle fibers of a normal control subject. Mean jitter at high-frequency stimulation (15.1 ± 4.43 μsec) was not significantly different from mean jitter at low-frequency stimulation (14.4 ± 5.38 μsec). (From Trojan DA, Gendron D, Cashman NR: Stimulation frequency-dependent neuromuscular junction transmission defects in patients with prior poliomyelitis. J Neurol Sci 118:150–157, 1993, with permission.)

"large" N-CAM+ myofibers are manifold more common in postpolio muscle biopsies than are atrophic myofibers, suggesting that permanent loss of innervation is rarer than partial or temporary loss of effective innervation.

In order to further assess the function of terminal axons, we have pioneered the use of stimulation SFEMG as a neuromuscular junction "stress test."[9] Jitter significantly increases at high rates of stimulation in about two thirds of PPS subjects; it is rare to see this finding in normal control subjects (Fig. 1). The likelihood of a positive "stress test" result increases with time after polio, suggesting that this defect represents an "acquired lesion" in PPS.[9]

One of the main functions of the motor nerve terminal is to release acetylcholine (ACh). We and others have obtained data to strongly suggest that ACh release is suboptimal in PPS. Beginning with reports in the 1940s,[10] it has been known that anticholinesterases can ameliorate decrement on repetitive stimulation of postpolio muscle. We have also observed that stimulation SFEMG jitter in PPS can be reduced by injection of edrophonium, a short-acting cholinesterase inhibitor (Fig. 2).[11] Moreover, subjects for whom the reduction of jitter was observed with edrophonium were

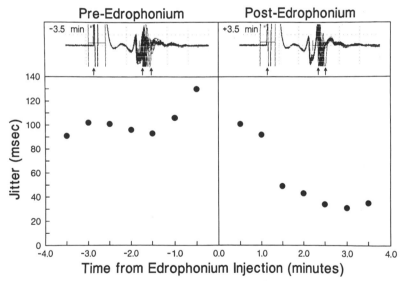

Figure 2. Pre- and post-edrophonium jitter on stimulation single-fiber electromyography in the vastus medialis muscle of a patient with PPS. *Upper panel* shows examples of raw data: the numerical jitter value is determined by the mean consecutive difference (MCD) between the stimulation artifact (*single arrow*) and the unstable potential (*double arrows*) in 50 superimposed stimulations. Jitter means (*lower panels*) were recorded every 30 seconds for 5 minutes before and 5 minutes after injection of edrophonium 10 mg (2-mg test dose followed by 8 mg 2 minutes later). Mean jitter for the 5 minutes before edrophonium injection (95.3 ± 5.09 μsec, mean ± SEM) significantly differed from mean jitter after edrophonium injection (47.6 ± 8.41 μsec, $P <$ 0.0001). Therefore, this patient was judged to have a significant reduction in jitter with edrophonium in the studied unstable potential. (From Trojan DA, Gendron D, Cashman NR: Anticholinesterase-responsive neuromuscular junction transmission defects in postpoliomyelitis fatigue. J Neurol Sci 114:170–177, 1993, with permission.)

also subjects with reduction of symptomatic fatigue when taking pyridostigmine, suggesting a link between this symptom and the electrophysiologic phenomena.[11]

CONCLUSION

It seems plausible that terminal axonal disease may be the source of two major clinical features of PPS. First, permanent degeneration of motor nerve terminals may underlie the slowly progressive new weakness observed in patients with PPS. Second, a "fluctuating lesion," caused by dysfunction of nerve terminals, appears associated with the symptoms of muscle fatigability and generalized fatigue. Many physiologic processes in the nerve terminal—including neurotransmitter synthesis and release—might be expected to provide novel "targets" for pharmacologic approaches to improve the symptoms of patients with PPS.[12]

References

1. Parsons PE: [letter]. N Engl J Med 325:1108, 1991.
1a. Cornil L: Sur un cas de paralysie générale spinal antérieure subaigne, suivi d'autopsie. Gaz Med (Paris) 4:127, 1875.
2. Trojan DA, Cashman NR: Current Trends in Postpoliomyelitis Syndrome. New York, Milestone Medical Communications (a division of Ruder-Finn), 1996.
3. Jubelt B, Cashman NR: Neurologic manifestations of the postpoliomyelitis syndrome. CRC Crit Rev Clin Neurobiol 3:199–220, 1987.
4. Wiechers DO, Hubbell SL: Late changes in the motor unit after acute poliomyelitis. Muscle Nerve 4:524–528, 1981.
5. Cashman NR, Maselli R, Wollmann RL, et al: Late denervation in patients with antecedent paralytic poliomyelitis. N Engl J Med 317:7–12, 1987.
6. Cashman NR, Covault J, Wollmann RL, Sanes J: Neural cell adhesion molecule (N-CAM) in normal, denervated and myopathic human muscle. Ann Neurol 21:481–489, 1987.
7. Dalakas MC, Elder G, Hallett M, et al: A long-term follow-up study of patients with post-poliomyelitis neuromuscular symptoms. N Engl J Med 314:959–963, 1986.
8. Stalberg E: Use of single fiber EMG and macro EMG in study of reinnervation. Muscle Nerve 13:804–813, 1990.
9. Trojan DA, Gendron D, Cashman NR: Stimulation frequency-dependent neuromuscular junction transmission defects in patients with prior poliomyelitis. J Neurol Sci 118:150–157, 1993.
10. Hodes R: Electromyographic study of defects of neuromuscular transmission in human poliomyelitis. Arch Neurol Psychiatry 60:457–473, 1948.
11. Trojan DA, Gendron D, Cashman NR: Anticholinesterase-responsive neuromuscular junction transmission defects in postpoliomyelitis fatigue. J Neurol Sci 114:170–177, 1993.
12. Cashman NR, Trojan DA: Correlation of electrophysiology with pathology, pathogenesis, and anticholinesterase therapy in post-polio syndrome. Ann N Y Acad Sci 753:138–150, 1995.

Joint and Muscle Pain

Frederick M. Maynard, MD, and Anne C. Gawne, MD

Postpolio syndrome (PPS) was initially defined as the clinical syndrome of new weakness, pain, and fatigue in patients who have recovered from acute polio.[12] More recently, new criteria for PPS have been developed, but fatigue and new weakness are essential elements.[13] Table 1 lists the most common symptoms recorded from a number of studies.[4,5,14,15,21] Muscle and joint pain are two of the most prevalent symptoms seen in PPS. Studies have found that the prevalence of muscle pain ranges from 38%[21] to 79%[15] and the prevalence joint pain ranges from 42%[21] to 80%.[15] In both these reports, either joint pain[21] or muscle pain[15] was the most prevalent complaint found in participants.

A correlation between muscle pain and weakness is believed to be either a measure of overuse or disuse that falls into a vicious cycle (Fig. 1). When musculoskeletal overuse occurs, pain develops. Rest and immobilization can relieve this pain, but this leads to decreased use of certain muscles, with development of disuse atrophy and further weakness. After this, relatively normal use of the muscle leads to pain and further disuse. Sometimes pain and subsequent weakness do not occur with activity. The fact that recent physical activity was not always associated with PPS may indicate that the intensity of the activity that is performed is more important. Frequent periods of activity with alternating periods of work and rest resulted in less evidence of local muscle fatigue, increased capacity to perform work, and increased ability to recover strength after activity in symptomatic postpolio patients,[1] Therefore, treatment of polio-related pain includes gentle paced exercises, preferably in water, bracing of unstable joints and limbs, and resting of muscles that are being overused.

Therefore, these authors suggest a causal relationship between symptoms of new weakness and musculoskeletal pain syndromes. This chapter covers research studies that offer various perspectives and varying support for this hypothesis. Possible causes for pain in polio survivors are examined in depth. The chapter also, reviews specific diagnoses for pain in polio survivors and examines outcome studies of useful treatments for specific pain syndromes.

SYMPTOM	CODD ET AL.[5] (N = 28)	HALSTEAD AND ROSSI[14] (N = 132)	CHETWYND AND HOGAN[4] (N = 694)	AGRE ET AL.[2] (N = 79)	RAMLOW[21] (N = 474)	HALSTEAD AND ROSSI[15] (N = 539)
Fatigue,%	59	89*	48	86	34	87*
Joint pain,%	74*	71	60*	77	42*	80
Muscle pain,%	48	71	52	86*	38	79
New weakness,%	71	N/A	47	69	38	N/A
In affected muscle,%	66	69	N/A	80	N/A	87
In unaffected muscle,%	15	50	N/A	53	N/A	77
Cold sensitivity,%	46	29	N/A	N/A	26	N/A

Table 1. COMPARISON OF MOST COMMON NEW SYMPTOMS IN SUBJECTS WITH A HISTORY OF PARALYTIC POLIO REPORTED IN SIX STUDIES

*Most frequent symptom.
Adapted from Gawne AC, Halstead LS: Post-polio syndrome: Pathophysiology and clinical management in CRC. Clin Rev Phys Med Rehabil 7:147–188, 1995.

CAUSE OF PAIN

The clinical finding of pain is correlated with the defining PPS symptom of new weakness. Trojan and colleagues used a case control study in order to determine which factors predispose polio survivors to develop PPS.[27] They evaluated weight gain; joint pain; muscle pain, either at rest or with exercise; degenerative joint disease (DJD); degenerative disc disease; age at presentation of acute polio; and degree of weakness initially, after recovery, and at presentation. Risk factors for the development of new weakness were determined by using an odds ratio. Factors predictive for PPS included variables consistent with chronic overuse such as length of time since polio (odds ratio [OR] = 1.6), recent weight gain, (OR = 6.4) muscle pain occurring with exercise (OR = 5.0), and joint pain (OR = 2.3). In addition, whereas the initial amount of weakness and present age were also correlated to PPS, gender and age of polio onset were not. The recent amount of physical activity and extent of recovery after acute polio were not correlated with the development of new weakness.

Maynard et al. reported a correlational analysis on secondary conditions associated with decreasing functional abilities among 120 postpolio subjects who participated in a clinical study, noting the prevalence of secondary conditions associated with PPS.[16] Significant correlations were found between new functional limitations and the following individual characteristics: (1) diagnosis of non–polio-related comorbidities, (2) reduced cardiovascular fitness, (3) obesity, (4) and elevated ratio of cholesterol to high-density lipoprotein level. Musculoskeletal problems of the upper and lower limbs were also notably prevalent (Table 2). Lower extremity weakness with gait de-

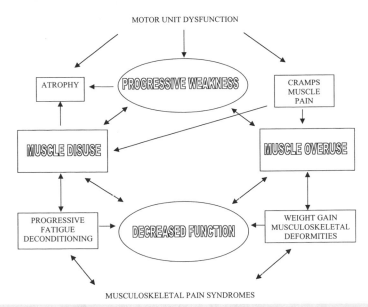

Figure 1. Vicious cycle of overuse or disuse leading to weakness and pain.

viations were significantly ($P < 0.05$) correlated with the presence of new functional limitations associated with declining functional capacity.

Gawne and colleagues studied the prevalence of postpolio muscle pain (PPMP) in 150 polio survivors using a pain questionnaire.[10] Participants answered questions regarding the intensity of the pain, temporal pattern, and relieving and exacerbating factors, and they completed the McGill Pain Questionnaire. Eighty percent of par-

Table 2. PREVALENCE OF SECONDARY MUSCULOSKELETAL PROBLEMS AMONG 120 POLIO SURVIVORS	
SECONDARY CONDITION	**PATIENTS, %**
Sensory loss in the hand	79
Median neuropathy at the wrist	58
Carpal tunnel syndrome (symptomatic)	24
Ulnar neuropathy at the wrist	31
Hand or wrist arthritis (radiograph)	48
Hand weakness	56
Impaired hand dexterity	52
Upper limb joint pain	56
Lower limb joint pain	49
Spinal pain	50
Gait abnormality	59

Adapted from Maynard FM: Managing the late effects of polio from a life-course perspective. Ann NY Acad Sci 753:354–360, 1995.

ticipants complained of pain. Of these, 64 patients (44%) met the criteria for PPMP. There were 23 men (36%) and 41 women (64%) with PPMP and 36 men (45%) and 44 women (55%) without PPMP. There were no significant differences between the groups with or without pain with respect to age or gender. These patients were significantly ($P < .0001$) more likely to have new weakness (90.2%) as opposed to the group with no pain (48.3%). Both polio groups with and without PPMP were statistically similar to each other with respect to exacerbating and relieving factors (Tables 3 and 4) and on the remaining responses on the McGill Pain Questionnaire.

The strongest evidence favoring musculoskeletal pain and a causative relationship to PPS is the prospective population based cohort study of polio survivors reported by Windebank et al.[35] Repeated detailed quantitative and electrophysiologic studies were done at 5-year intervals 30–55 years after patients experienced acute polio. These patients demonstrated no new weakness, but 60% of them were symptomatic. Among 20 of the 30 symptomatic patients, 16 had a musculoskeletal pain problem believed to explain their symptoms. Other medical conditions such as diabetes, obesity, alcoholism, and depression likely explained new weakness in 4 symptomatic patients. All symptomatic subjects had stable or improving neuromuscular function. Chronic overuse of muscles or muscles acting in a compensatory manner were suggested as predisposing factors for pain.

Smith et al. demonstrated further support for chronic musculoskeletal overuse in a study of 111 consecutive polio patients.[24] Gait deviations were seen in 100% of all patients. These included 53% who had an uneven pelvic base and 43% with major trunk oscillations. While standing, 69% of these patients had an absent lumbar curve and 38% of them were weight bearing on their stronger leg. Pain was the most prevalent complaint in this group of patients, occurring in 85% of those who walked unaided and 100% of those who used an assistive device or wheelchair.

Chronic overuse of weak muscles or weak muscles acting in a compensatory fashion was demonstrated by Perry et al., who evaluated the dynamic electromyography during gait analysis on 21 polio survivors with strength in the quadriceps greater than or equal to 4/5 and strength in the soleus of 0–3/5.[20] All patients had symptoms of PPS including fatigue, pain, and new weakness in the thigh or calf. They studied the gluteus maximus, long head of the biceps femoris, quadriceps, and soleus muscles. Overuse during walking (a total effort of greater than two standard deviations more than normal) was found in all four muscle groups. It was most common in the quadriceps followed by the gluteus maximus, and it was least common in the weaker soleus muscles. In addition to overuse, gait variations (e.g., genu recurvatum or flexion of the knee during the gait cycle) and equinus contractures were observed.

Additionally, joints of the upper limbs, especially the wrist and shoulder, are prone to DJD when assuming a weight-bearing role. This commonly occurs with the use of assistive devices, such as wheelchairs, crutches, and canes. Werner et al. studied 61 polio survivors ages 49 ± 6 years with a mean duration of disability of 35 ± 4 years.[33] They obtained radiographs of both hands and wrists in addition to a physical examination.[33] The prevalence of severe to moderate DJD of the hand or wrist was 13%, and mild DJD was present in 68% of patients. Risk factors associated with osteoarthritis

Table 3. FACTORS THAT RELIEVE PAIN

GROUP	MASSAGE	BRACE	SLEEP	WEIGHT LOSS	STRETCH	HEAT	ICE	REST	EXERCISE	INJECTION
PPMP,%	47	23	47	33	36	78	1	90	1	1
No PPMP,%	50	16	34	16	27	58	6	84	6	11*

* Significant $P < .001$

Table 4. FACTORS THAT EXACERBATE PAIN

GROUP	COLD	REST	EXERCISE	WEIGHT	STRESS	ACTIVITY
PPMP,%	68	3	61	39	53	78
No PPMP,%	56	10	51	32	46	78

Significant $P < .001$.

included advanced age, lower limb weakness, use of an assistive device, and severity of the disability.

Nerve compression syndromes, including carpal tunnel syndrome (CTS), ulnar mononeuropathy at the wrist or elbow, brachial plexopathy, and cervical or lumbo-sacral radiculopathy, are syndromes that can cause pain as well as neurologic deficits in postpolio individuals.[32] These neuropathies can be detected on electromyogram (EMG) and nerve conduction studies (NCS). These tests can also detect subclinical neuropathies (i.e., before the individual has the characteristic symptoms of CTS). To assess the prevalence of these conditions, Gawne et al. conducted a retrospective study of 100 consecutive patients seen in a postpolio clinic.[9] EMG and NCS, in-cluding routine studies of the median nerve, were performed on all patients. A total of 49% of the patients had an abnormal peripheral nerve study result. CTS, either alone or in conjunction with an ulnar nerve neuropathy, was the most prevalent finding in a total of 38% of all patients. Ulnar neuropathy at the wrist was seen in 22% of patients, and CTS and ulnar neuropathy together were found in 3% of pa-tients. A peripheral neuropathy was seen in 3% and either cervical or lumbosacral radiculopathy was present in 4% of all patients (Table 5).

In a similar study, Werner et al. looked at risk factors for the development of CTS in a retrospective study of 148 consecutive postpolio patients.[32] Electrodiag-nostic tests were done only on the patients who had classic signs and symptoms con-sistent with CTS such as nighttime numbness or abnormal sensory findings in the median nerve distribution, or a positive Tinel's or Phalen's sign. Of the 148 subjects, only 50% underwent sensory NCS. CTS was found in 33 patients (22%). There was no difference in age, gender, work status, or duration of disability in those with or without CTS. Risk factors for the development of CTS included use of an assistive device (cane, crutch, or wheelchair), with use of more than one device increasing the risk even further.

Muscle pain may be a sign of overuse, causing breakdown products such as creati-nine kinase (CK) to accumulate. Waring et al. found elevated CK levels in PPS pa-tients;[30] however, other studies failed to demonstrate this relationship. Nelson found that the incidence of an elevated CK level in a group of polio patients with delayed

Table 5. ELECTRODIAGNOSTIC FINDINGS IN 100 CONSECUTIVE POSTPOLIO PATIENTS		
FINDING	**PATIENTS, N**	**PATIENTS,%**
Carpal tunnel syndrome (CTS)	35	35
Ulnar neuropathy at the wrist	2	2
CTS and ulnar neuropathy	3	3
Peripheral neuropathy	3	3
Brachial plexopathy	1	1
Tibial neuropathy	1	1
Radiculopathy	4	4
Total	49	49

weakness (15 of 29) did not differ from polio patients without delayed weakness.[16] Trojan et al. also failed to demonstrate a relationship between muscle pain and elevated CK levels.[26] Further study is required in order to demonstrate a correlation between new weakness, pain, and measurable laboratory values of CK.

In another study by Willen and Grimby, 32 consecutive postpolio subjects were evaluated for pain.[36] Twenty-two patients fit the criteria for PPS, and 10 did not. Pain was assessed using a visual analog scale (VAS) on a scale of 0 (no pain) to 100 (worst possible pain). Of these individuals, 29 (91%) reported pain from muscles used for ambulation, 11 had joint pain at rest, and 12 reported muscle pain at rest. Pain symptoms were not related to whether the patient had PPS (new weakness) or to the presence of weakness in that limb; rather, they were correlated to the level of activity. The examiners found that the weaker patients experienced less pain. This study suggests that the more active an individual is, the more pain he or she experiences, as measured by the VAS. It also demonstrates that characteristics of the pain varied by site, with polio survivors describing a cramping, aching pain in the lower limbs and an aching pain in the trunk and non–polio-affected upper limbs.

In another study of 875 patients seen at a community postpolio clinic, Yarnell reported that pain was the most common complaint, occurring in 79% (693) of those studied.[39] Of the participants who complained of pain, 99% complained of pain associated with scoliosis. Yarnell proposed that scoliosis together with gait deviations could lead to DJD (44%), facet arthropathy (32%), mechanical low back pain (20%), spinal stenosis (10%), radiculopathy (5%), or sacroiliac joint dysfunction (4%) (participants could choose more than one option, so the numbers add up to 100%). In addition, causes of articular pain included DJD of the shoulder (19%) knee (16%), hip, ankle, and wrist. Nonarticular causes of pain included tendonitis, bursitis (28%), CTS (19%), myofascial pain (13%), tension headaches (11%), ulnar compression neuropathy (25%), and lateral femoral cutaneous neuropathy (25%). Wear and tear of the peripheral joints, especially the knees and shoulders, was a frequent cause of pain. Biomechanically, the shoulders are not suited to weight bearing, yet many polio survivors use their shoulders to walk with crutches, transfer, and push wheelchairs. Biomechanical abuse of unbraced knees, especially in those with genu recurvatum or valgus, commonly results in significant abnormalities, especially degenerative joint changes and pain.

Trojan et al. used a cross-sectional design with 126 polio survivors to identify predictive factors and correlates of muscle and joint pain.[28] They found that muscle pain was correlated with female gender, longer duration of general fatigue, and poorer physical and mental health. Predictive factors for joint pain were female gender, older age, higher body mass index (obesity), longer duration of stability after acute polio, greater weakness after acute polio, weaker lower limbs at the time of examination, and poorer general and mental health. Again, greater weakness, especially in the lower limbs, appears to be correlated with greater joint pain. The finding of a significant female prevalence has not been found in other studies, but both of these studies had a nonsignificant prevalence of women.[10,36]

In 1989, Waring et al. did a retrospective study of 104 ambulatory postpolio patients (43 men and 61 women) seen at the University of Michigan with clinical and EMG evidence of previous polio and the ability to ambulate.[31] Of these patients, 77% reported pain as a symptom. Associated medical conditions included 26 participants with genu recurvatum, 26 with DJD of the knee and 10 with DJD in other locations, 19 with CTS, and seven with a history of a knee injury. The average walking distance had decreased considerably at the time of the evaluation compared with the time of their initial recovery from polio.

Although all these studies demonstrate a significant relationship between musculoskeletal pain and PPS (i.e., the presence of new weakness and declining function), causation is not established because either problem could lead to the other through the vicious cycle described previously. However, these studies do show that pain and, in particular, PPMP and joint pain are common problems in the postpolio population

DIAGNOSIS

Because PPS is a diagnosis of exclusion, nonmusculoskeletal and neurologic pain syndromes must first be ruled out. Imaging studies and electrodiagnostic studies are usually necessary. For example, thyroid disease, heart disease, and rheumatologic syndromes must often be excluded. Frequently, studies demonstrate one or more comorbidity.[8]

In order to facilitate diagnoses and treatment of pain in polio survivors, a pain classification has been proposed by Gawne and colleagues.[11] **Type I** pain, or PPMP, occurs only in muscles affected by polio. It is described as a superficial aching pain that many patients say is similar to muscle pain they experienced during acute polio. It is characterized by muscle cramps, fasiculations, or a crawling sensation. It typically occurs at the end of the day or at night when the patient tries to relax. Physical activity, stress, and cold temperatures exacerbate the pain.

Type II, or overuse, pain includes injuries to soft tissue, muscles, tendons, bursa, and ligaments. Common examples are rotator cuff tendinitis; subacromial and greater trochanteric bursitis; and myofascial pain, especially in the upper and lower back. Myofascial pain in postpolio patients is similar to myofascial pain in other patients and is characterized by bands of taut muscles and discrete trigger points that elicit a jump response when palpated. These occur because of poor posture or improper body mechanics.[6]

Type III, or biomechanical, pain presents as DJD, low back pain, or pain from nerve compression syndromes. Weakness induced by polio-affected muscles and by poor body mechanics makes the joints, especially of the lower limbs, more susceptible to the development of DJD. In addition, years of ambulating on unstable joints and supporting tissue increase the stress and the energy expenditure to perform a given task. These costs accumulate slowly until they cross a critical threshold. In a study of 40 consecutive patients seen in a multidisciplinary postpolio clinic, 95% of all patients had pain complaints.[11] Of these patients, 17% had PPMP, 47% had overuse pain, and 77% had biomechanical pain. (Some patients had more than one type of pain; therefore, totals add up to > 100%.) In a larger study of 150 patients, 44% met the criteria for PPMP.[10]

Finally, another pain syndrome seen in polio survivors is fibromyalgia, which is pain similar to postpolio muscle pain and myofascial pain. It is classified according to the following criteria[38]: widespread pain in all four quadrants of the body for a minimum of 3 months and at least 11 of the 18 specified tender points (Fig. 2).

Although these criteria focus on tender point count, a consensus of 35 fibromyalgia experts have recently determined that a person does not need to have the required 11 tender points to be diagnosed and treated for fibromyalgia syndrome. This criterion was created for research purposes, and people may still meet criteria with < 11 of the required tender points as long as widespread pain and many of the common symptoms associated with fibromyalgia are present. Commonly associated symptoms include:

Fatigue

Temporal mandibular joint
    dysfunction

Skin sensitivities

Chronic headaches (tension type or
    migraines)

Morning stiffness

Dizziness or impaired coordination

Sleep disorder (or sleep that is unrefreshing)

Postexertion malaise and muscle pain

Numbness and tingling sensations

Irritable bowel syndrome

Cognitive or memory impairment

Menstrual cramping and/or
    premenstrual syndrome

Trojan and Cashman studied the prevalence of fibromyalgia in polio survivors by evaluating 95 patients seen at a university-affiliated postpolio clinic.[26] Using the diagnostic criteria for fibromyalgia listed previously, they found that 10.5% of all patients had fibromyalgia. In addition, another 10.5% met the criteria for borderline fibromyalgia. In summary, a fibromyalgia-like syndrome was present in 25% of all patients who met the criteria for PPS and in 21% of all polio patients who attended that clinic.

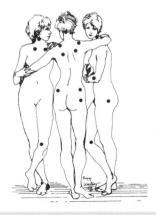

Figure 2. Tender points for diagnosis of fibromyalgia. (From Wolfe F, Smythe HA, Yanus MB: American College of Rheumatology clinical criteria for the diagnosis of fibromyalgia. Arthritis Rheum 33:160–172, 1990, with permission.)

In the Gawne et al. study of 150 polio survivors, pain descriptors were measured using the McGill Pain Questionnaire.[10] A total of 114 individuals with fibromyalgia and 94 persons with rheumatoid arthritis served as a comparison group. Both polio groups were statistically similar in their responses to this questionnaire to a group of patients with fibromyalgia, ($P < 0.01$), but they were different than patients with rheumatoid arthritis. This study suggests that the quality of pain in polio survivors is similar to fibromyalgia. This raises the possibility that fibromyalgia may be more prevalent in polio survivors than previously believed or that some of the other symptoms (e.g., fatigue, sleep disorders) that polio patients experience may be caused by fibromyalgia.

Windebank et al. did another study that demonstrated a significant incidence of fibromyalgia.[34] They examined 30 symptomatic patients and found causes for pain and fatigue in 20 patients. Among the 10 who did not have another condition to explain the symptoms of fatigue, pain, and new weakness, the symptom pattern was similar to chronic fatigue syndrome or fibromyalgia.

Although the causes of PPS and fibromyalgia are unclear, a reduction of growth hormone secretion with a resultant disruption of normal muscle repair can contribute to the coexistence of these conditions and to symptoms of pain, fatigue, and weakness in patients with PPS. It has been postulated that 80% of growth hormone is secreted during stage 4 sleep and that disruption of sleep results in a reduced level of the secretion of growth hormone and somatemedin C, or insulinlike growth factor (IGF-1).[26] This hormone stimulates the synthesis of protein and nucleic acids in muscle cells as well as neurons and may possibly stimulate regeneration of peripheral nerves after injury. This reinnervation includes sprouting, which occurs to strengthen muscles and assist recovery.[23] Somatemedin C has been found to be low in patients with fibromyalgia as well as those with PPS. In 1991, Shetty et al. reported that the serum IGF-1 level was low in 10 postpolio subjects.[22] Later, they also found reduced levels of IGF-1 in 124 polio survivors compared with a group of healthy age-matched controls.[23] However, they found that there was no difference in IGF concentrations among those with functional decline compared with those who were stable. Sunnerhagen and colleagues found no significant difference in IGF levels in 87 patients with a history of polio compared with a reference group.[25] There is clearly a need to further explore the relationship between fibromyalgia, IGF-1 levels, and the effects of growth hormone.

TREATMENT OF MUSCULOSKELETAL PAIN

Pain management of patients with PPS is based on a few basic principles, supplemented by class-specific recommendations. These basic principles include making efforts to improve abnormal body mechanics, mechanically correct and minimize postural and gait deviations, relieve or support weakened muscles or joints, promote lifestyle modifications, and decrease the abnormally high work load of muscles relative to their limited capacity.[6]

Treatment of patients with PPMP includes decreasing activity throughout the day. Pain can be relieved with rest, application of moist heat, and gentle stretching. Stretching has a role in maintaining the extensibility of muscle and connective tissue; however, it must be performed judiciously because there are situations in which a polio survivor may derive greater functional benefit and move about more safely with tighter tendons and reduced joint range of motion. A variety of medications are used to treat postpolio muscle pain, including nonsteroidal anti-inflammatory drugs (NSAIDs), acetaminophen, tramadol, benzodiazepines, and (rarely) narcotics. The use of tricyclic antidepressants (TCAs), especially amitriptyline, can help with pain and fatigue.

Treatment for overuse pain includes modification of extremity use, followed by modalities such as ice, heat, ultrasound, transcutaneous electrical nerve stimulation, and NSAIDs. Treatment for myofascial pain consists of myofascial release techniques, including spray and stretch and trigger-point injections. Rest is often not possible because many patients rely on their upper extremities for both locomotion and self-care. In rare cases, corticosteroid injections or surgery may be needed.[7]

Treatment for biomechanical pain includes posture and back care education as well as decreasing weight bearing through the use of assistive devices such as braces, crutches, wheelchairs, and scooters. Abnormal biomechanics can often be modified with fairly simple and practical interventions such as cervical pillows, lumbar rolls, gluteal pads, dorsal-lumbar corsets, and heel lifts.[6] Biomechanical pain is usually improved by conservative measures aimed at reducing mechanical stress such as supporting weakened muscles, stabilizing abnormal joint movements, and improving body biomechanics. In particular, efforts should be directed at improving posture and body mechanics during routine daily activities such as sitting, standing, walking, and sleeping, as well as any repetitious activities at work. Anti-inflammatory agents are used commonly to supplement conservative measures, and joint injections can also be helpful. Weight bearing with the wrist hyperextended and radially deviated should be avoided.[7]

For those with CTS who must use a cane or crutch, an ergonomically designed grip such as an Ortho-ease (Lumex) or a "gel grip" (Superlite) is prescribed to place the wrist in a more neutral position and distribute weight-bearing on the palm. Superlite also has a Tornado Tip, which absorbs shock and can be placed on canes or crutches. The use of aluminum or "chromy steel" reduces the weight further, decreasing pressure on joints. Providing adequate support for weakened muscles and unstable joints can often be a difficult challenge; however, the basic orthotic principles are similar to those used in the management of patients with other neuromuscular diseases. For individuals with low back pain, lumbosacral corsets, a shoe lift, or pelvic lift can help improve biomechanics. For genu recurvatum (back knee) or genu valgus (knock knee) caused by quadriceps weakness or ligament instability, a knee ankle foot orthosis (KAFO) with a free ankle and an extension stop at the knee is used. Townsend has recently developed a "polio brace" specifically for this purpose. Constructed as a custom-made laminated knee orthoses, it controls hyperextension at the knee while allowing

free movement at the ankle. Polio survivors with dorsiflexor weakness or ankle instability can benefit from an athletic ankle splint, high-top shoes, or an ankle foot orthosis (AFO). Many individuals need an orthosis that combines strength and light-
ness. The new plastics and lightweight metals can often be used alone or in
combination. Some polio survivors prefer to repair and use their old braces rather
than start over with new ones. Others may resist using any kind of brace for cosmetic
and psychological reasons. Orthotics are recommended to improve safety by reducing
the risk of falls, to reduce pain, and to decrease fatigue by improving gait speed and
symmetry.

In Perry et al.'s study of muscle overuse, they concluded that the most expedient
way to reduce symptoms such as pain that occurred through overuse was the prescription of an appropriate AFO or a KAFO.[20] An AFO should preferably be a solid
shell, allowing 15–20° of plantar flexion to allow the foot to reach foot flat during the
stance phase of gait, reducing the demand for the use of the quadriceps. In this study
11 of 21 subjects wore AFOs, with 9 of the 11 reporting subjective improvements
with symptoms.

In Waring et al.'s study of 104 patients, 19% were using braces at the time of their
initial evaluation.[31] An additional 37 patients were prescribed braces, including AFOs
(31.4%), KAFOs with free offset knee joints (25.7%), and KAFOs with drop lock
knees (42.9%). Patients who were prescribed orthoses to correct their ambulation and
those who used them daily reported improved ability to walk, improved walking
safety, and reduced knee and overall pain ($P < 0.05$) compared with those who did
not wear orthoses. Those who did not use orthoses on a daily basis showed fewer improvements than those who did. Reasons for not wearing braces included fit, not
enough training, and that they "don't help." Reasons for not using a prescribed cane
or crutch included "don't want to," not enough training, pain, and "doesn't help."
This uncontrolled clinical observation study provides case series evidence for the effectiveness of a biomechanically oriented musculoskeletal intervention on PPS symptom reduction.

Many times, an assistive device is necessary to help with either pain or deformity.
In a recent study of 27 polio survivors (15 women and 12 men ages 46–82 years),
Bernstein and Gawne found that 74% reported foot pain and 89% reported foot deformity, ranging from limb length discrepancies to hammertoes, cavus feet, and equinus deformity.[7] All of the patients reported using some type of appliance, assistive device, special shoe, or brace for ambulation.

Peach and Olejnik studied 77 polio survivors, dividing them into compliers (complied with all recommendations), partial compliers (accepted some recommendations), and noncompliers.[18] At the time of follow-up (mean, 2.1 years later), the
complier group reported resolution of muscle pain in 28%, resolution of joint pain
in 41%, and improvement in symptoms of muscle pain in 72% and joint pain in
53%, but none were unchanged or worse. The noncompliers showed worsening or
progression of muscle pain in 29% and joint pain in 18%; only 14% had some improvement in muscle pain, and none had resolution of muscle or joint pain or improvement in joint pain. The partial compliance group demonstrated a wider range

of responses, either no change or some improvement but little resolution (3–4%). Muscle strength increased in compliers, but decreased in the other groups. Reasons for noncompliance included lifestyle and resistance to orthotics and other assistive devices.

Alternative treatments have been suggested for polio pain; they were recently tested by Valbano et al. in a study of 50 polio survivors with myofascial pain.[29] Biomagnets were placed over palpable "trigger points," and examiners found a significant difference between the treatment group and the control group. Whereas only four patients (19%) in the placebo group reported relief, 22 patients (76%) in the magnet group reported relief. Whether the pain was of a myofascial nature or arthritic nature, the patients responded well to the static magnetic field. The effect was noticed within 45 minutes from the onset of the application.

In their study of 150 polio survivors, Gawne et al.[10] found that the majority reported that pain-relieving strategies included rest, heat, massage and stretching. Braces were helpful in 16–23% of all those studied. Local injection was found to be significantly more effective in patients who had overuse or biomechanical pain, relieving pain in 11% of those patients but only 1% of those with PPMP (see Table 3). Things that were of little use or actually exacerbated pain included ice, exercise or activity, stress, and weight gain (see Table 4).

In a study that evaluated the effects of dynamic water exercise in individuals with PPS, Willen et al. compared both the effects of training on cardiovascular function as well as general well-being.[37] Pain was measured on the VAS using a 1-to-100 scale and the Nottingham Health Profile (NHP) that measures pain, sleep energy level, and other measures. They found that the group who participated in an 8-month period of water exercises 40 minutes long three times a week had a no significant change in the amount of pain on the VAS; however, there were significant differences on the NHP (37 pretraining, 18 posttraining) compared with the control group (41 pretraining, 46 posttraining). In addition, they reported increased well-being and improved fitness on the NHP as a positive aspect of the water exercise.

Medications that are used to treat pain associated with PPS include NSAIDs (e.g., ibuprofen, naproxen) and cyclooxygenase-2 (COX-2) inhibitors (e.g., rofecoxib or celecoxib).[19] These all raise the risk of gastrointestinal effects such as ulcers and renal side effects, but these are seen less frequently with COX-2 inhibitors. Less frequent side effects include edema, diarrhea, and cardiovascular complaints such as hypertension. Injectable corticosteroids (Celestone and Kenalog) can also be used. Muscle relaxants such as cyclobenzaprine or baclofen may be useful, especially when there is muscle spasm. However, they carry the risk of sedation and further fatigue. Nerve stabilizers such as carbamazepine and gabapentin are occasionally helpful, but they also carry the risk of sedation and dizziness. Substance P blockers such as capsaicin can be used for localized pain, but they may cause burning and stinging. Narcotics such as codeine, hydrocodone, and even oxycodone can be used in cases of severe pain, but they can cause constipation, tolerance, and sedation. TCAs such as amitriptyline or trazodone and minor tranquilizers such as diazepam and alprazolam can assist with sleep as well as depression and anxiety, but they also cause drowsiness.

Other antidepressants such as fluoxetine have been tried, and tramadol is also sometimes successful.

Trojan and Cashman recommend the use of low-dose amitriptyline, cyclobenzaprine, fluoxetine, NSAIDs, relaxation, heat, massage, injections, and aerobic exercise for the treatment of patients with fibromyalgia.[26] They found that low-dose amitriptyline was helpful in controlling symptoms in approximately 50% of those with fibromyalgia or borderline fibromyalgia. If this was insufficient, most patients benefited from an alternative therapy.

The medication and modality used depend on the type of pain the patient is experiencing as well as the intensity and duration of the pain. It is recommended that when a true analgesic is required, it should be given in moderate amounts and on a schedule, not just when the pain is so severe that a higher dose is necessary.[19] If taken together, mild muscle relaxants or anxiolytics may make painkillers work better and at a lower dose, but they do have their own side effects. Nonpharmacologic measures such as hot packs, ice packs, ultrasound, hypnosis, massage, acupuncture, and relaxation can be used to avoid the side effects medications may cause.

CONCLUSION

Physical disability secondary to polio causes increased energy rates while patients perform tasks such as ambulation and ADLs, as well as reduced movement economy compared with nondisabled individuals. Reduced movement economy may contribute to increased fatigue. In addition, polio patients commonly develop musculoskeletal overuse syndromes, such as muscle strains. This leads to pain, which is treated by and relieved by rest, leading to disuse weakness and atrophy. Weakness can further exacerbate pain, perpetuating that cycle. A vicious cycle can occur in which fatigue, weakness, pain, and loss of physical function restrict physical activity, which in turn leads to further muscle and cardiorespiratory deconditioning and further reduction in function. When patients were prescribed orthoses (e.g., braces) to correct their ambulation, those who use them daily reported improved ability to walk, improved walking safety, and reduced knee and overall pain. Additional measures that have been found to helpful for treatment of both pain and disability are water exercises; heat; rest; and a number of medications, particularly those that assist with sleep in cases of fibromyalgia and PPMP.

Pain can be reduced by altering biomechanics and by changing to a lifestyle that reduces physical activity. These strategies may be difficult to accomplish, however, because they often require developing behaviors that are different than old familiar ones. Altering the pace and intensity of discretionary activities and learning new ways to gain more control over when and how activities are performed are essential. Education in the proper use of orthotic devices is important to improve compliance with the recommendations. Restoration of function as well pain relief can be accomplished by an interdisciplinary team that includes the polio survivor, physical therapist, occupational therapist, psychologist, orthotist, rehabilitation engineer, and physician.

The available research favors a causal relationship between symptoms of new weakness and musculoskeletal pain syndromes. Commonly accepted clinical thinking and practice regarding musculoskeletal pain syndromes and syndromes of fatigue and new weakness further support this relationship. Demonstrated effectiveness of treatments for patients with musculoskeletal pain syndromes offers further support for a likely causal relationship.

References

1. Agre JC, Rodriquez AA: Intermittent isometric activity: its effect on muscle fatigue in post-polio patients. Arch Phys Med Rehabil 72:971–975, 1991.
2. Agre JC, Rodriquez, AA, Sperling KB: Symptoms and clinical impressions of patients seen in a post-polio clinic. Arch Phys Med Rehabil 70:367–370, 1989.
3. Caroni P, Grandes P: Nerve sprouting in innervated adult skeletal muscle by exposure to elvated levels of insulin-like growth factor. J Cell Biol 110:1307–1317, 1990.
4. Chetwynd J, Hogan D: Post-polio syndrome in New Zealand: A survey of 700 polio survivors. N Z Med J 106:406–408, 1993.
5. Codd MP, Mulder DW, Kurland LT, et al: Poliomyelitis in Rochester, MN: 1935 to 1955. Epidemiology and long term sequelae: A preliminary report. In Halstead LS, Weicher DO (eds): Late Effects of Poliomyelitis. Miami, Symposium Foundation, 1985, pp 121–133.
6. Gawne AC: Pain in PPS. Polio Netw News (winter):1–3, 1986.
7. Gawne AC, Bernstein B: Foot problems in polio survivors. Arch Phys Med Rehabil 11: 1317, 2001.
8. Gawne AC, Halstead LS: Post-polio syndrome: Pathophysiology and clinical management in CRC. Clin Rev Phys Med Rehabil 7:147–188, 1995.
9. Gawne AC, Pham BT, Halstead LS: Electrodiagnostic findings in 108 consecutive patients evaluated in a post-polio clinic: The value of routine electrodiagnostic testing. Ann N Y Acad Sci 753:383–385, 1995.
10. Gawne AC, Richards RS, Petroski G: Post-polio muscle pain in polio survivors. Arch Phys Med Rehabil 81:1621, 2000.
11. Gawne AC, Yildez EO, Halstead LS: Pain syndromes in 40 consecutive post-polio patients: A guide to evaluation and treatment. Arch Phys Med Rehabil 74:1263–1264, 1993.
12. Halstead LS: Assessment and differential diagnosis for post-polio syndrome. Orthopedics 14:1209–1217, 1991.
13. Maynard FM: Managing the late effects of polio from a life-course perspective. Ann NY Acad Sci 753:354–360, 1995.
14. Halstead LS, Rossi CD: Post-polio syndrome: Clinical experience with 132 consecutive outpatients. In Halstead LS, Weichers DO (eds): Research and Clinical Aspects of the Late Effects of Poliomyelitis. White Plains, NY, March of Dimes Birth Defects Foundation, 1987, pp 13–26.
15. Halstead LS, Rossi CD: Post-polio syndrome: Results of a survey of 350 survivors. Orthopedics 8:845–859, 1995.
16. Maynard FM, Forcheimer M, Roller S, et al: Secondary conditions associated with declining functional abilities among polio survivors. Arch Phys Med Rehabil 72:795, 1991.
17. Nelson KR: Creatine kinase and fibrillation potentials in patients with late sequelae of polio. Muscle Nerve 13:722–725, 1990.
18. Peach PE, Olejnik S: Effect of treatment and compliance on post-polio sequelae. Orthopedics 14:1199–1203, 1991.
19. Perlman S: Use of medication in people with post-polio syndrome. Polio Netw News 15:1, 1999

20. Perry J, Fontaine JD, Mulroy S: Findings in post-poliomyelitis syndrome: Weakness of the muscles of the calf as a source of late pain and fatigue of muscles of the thigh after poliomyelitis. J Bone Joint Surg 77(A):1148–1153, 1995.
21. Ramlow J, Alexander M, Laporte R, et al: Epidemiology of the post-polio syndrome. Am J Epidemiol 136:769–784, 1992.
22. Shetty KR, Mattson DE, Rudman IE, et al: Hyposomatomedinemia in men with post-poliomyelitis syndrome. J Am Geriatr Soc 39:185–191, 1991.
23. Shetty KP, Rao UP, Gupta KL, Ridman D: Studies of growth hormone and insulin-like growth factor in polio survivors. Ann NY Acad Sci 753:276–284, 1995.
24. Umphred DA (ed): Neurological Rehabilitation, 2nd ed. St. Louis, Mosby, 1990, pp 509–528.
25. Sunnerhagen KS, Bengtsson BA, Lundberg PA, et al: Normal concentrations of serum insulinlike growth factor-1 in late polio. Arch Phys Med Rehabil 76:732–735, 1995.
26. Trojan DA, Cashman NR: Fibromyalgia is common in a post-poliomyelitis clinic. Arch Neurol 52:620–624, 1995.
27. Trojan DA, Cashman NR, Shapiro ST, et al: Predictive factors for post-poliomyelitis syndrome. Arch Phys Med Rehabil 75:770–775, 1994.
28. Trojan D, et al: Predictive factors and correlates for pain in post-poliomyelitis patients. Arch Phys Med Rehabil 83:1109–1115, 2002.
29. Valbano C, Hazelwood CF, Jurida G, et al: Response of pain to static magnetic fields in post-polio patients: A double blind pilot study. Arch Phys Med Rehabil 78:1200–1203, 1997.
30. Waring WP, Davidoff G, Werner RA: Serum creatine kinase in the post-polio population. Am J Phys Med Rehabil 68:86–90, 1989.
31. Waring WP, Maynard F, Grady W, et al: Influence of appropriate lower extremity managenemt on ambulation, pain and fatigue in a post-polio population. Arch Phys Med Rehabil 70:371–375, 1989.
32. Werner R, Waring W, Davidoff G: Risk factors for median mononeuropathy of the wrist in postpoliomyelitis patients. Arch Phys Med Rehabil 70:464–467, 1989.
33. Werner RA, Waring W, Maynard F: Osteoarthritis of the hand and wrist in the post-poliomyelitis population. Arch Phys Med Rehabil 73:1069–1072, 1992.
34. Windebank AJ, Daube JR, Lichty WJ, et al: Late effects of paralytic poliomyelitis in Olmsted County, MN. Neurology 41:27–38, 1991.
35. Windebank AJ, Lichty WJ, Daube JR, Iverson RA: Lack of progression of neurological deficit in survivors of paralytic polio. Neurology 46:80–84, 1996.
36. Willen C, Grimby G: Pain, physical activity and disability in individuals with late effects of polio. Arch Phys Med Rehabil 79:915–919, 1998.
37. Willen C, Sunnerhagen KS, Grimby G: Dynamic water exercise in individuals with late poliomyelitis. Arch Phys Med Rehabil 82:66–72, 2001.
38. Wolfe F, Smythe HA, Yanus MB: American College of Rheumatology clinical criteria for the diagnoses of fibromyalgia. Arthritis Rheum 33:160–172, 1990.
39. Yarnell S: The late effects of polio. In Sine R (ed): Basic Rehabilitation Techniques: A Self-Instructional Guide, 4th ed. New York, Aspen, 2000, p 60.

Postpolio Fatigue

Kristian Borg, MD, PhD

Many polio patients experience new or increased symptoms long after the acute polio infection, a condition known as late effects of polio or postpolio syndrome (PPS).[24, 44] Fatigue (i.e., an unusual tiredness) has been reported to be one of the most common new health problems found in 86% to 87% of PPS patients in different surveys, which is considerably higher than fatigue in healthy individuals.[2,17,50,70] PPS patients differentiate between a central, mental fatigue and physical, focal (i.e., limb) tiredness combined with decreased endurance.[17] This is supported by the neurophysiologic findings reported by Rodriquez and Agre, who found that the ability to recover from fatiguing exercise was related to local muscular factors and not to central ones.[60] Thus, the postpolio fatigue may be divided into central fatigue evolving from the central nervous system (CNS) and peripheral fatigue evolving from the peripheral nervous system (i.e., the motor unit). According to Schanke and Stanghelle, physical, peripheral fatigue was found to be a greater problem for the patients than mental, central fatigue.[63]

CENTRAL FATIGUE

CNS dysfunction with subjective reports of difficulty regarding cognition, concentration, memory, attention, word finding, maintaining wakefulness, and thinking clearly has been reported in PPS patients.[14,15,17,21] A possible common pathophysiology with the chronic fatigue syndrome has been suggested,[20,30] and Bruno et al. have suggested that the postpolio fatigue is caused by an affection of the CNS caused by brain damage induced by the poliovirus infection.[17] The parts of the brain affected by the poliovirus with implications for the development of fatigue are the parts responsible for cortical activation (i.e., the reticular activating system [RAS].[15–17,20] Other parts of the brain affected are the basal ganglia and substantia nigra.[14,17] Neuropsychologic testing has shown impairment of attention and information processing speed on tests which measure attention like the Double Letter Cancellation and Trail Making Tests.[15,17] Magnetic resonance imaging (MRI) studies have revealed abnormalities in different areas of the brain, including the RAS in about 50% of postpolio patients with fatigue: no abnormalities were found in patients reporting low fatigue.[16]

The possible disturbance of the CNS functions has been described by Bruno et al. and the results of the studies have not yet been repeated.[17] Thus, because it is of clinical importance for the PPS patients to recognize this kind of symptom, efforts should be done in order to further evaluate a possible CNS dysfunction.

Another possible factor causing the central fatigue may be an inflammation of the CNS. Immunologic factors, such as inflammation of the spinal cord[52,58] in muscle[26] as well as abnormal peripheral blood lymphocyte subsets[38] and high interleukin, interleukin 2 receptors,[64] oligoclonal bands,[27,64] and increased levels of different cytokines[39] in the cerebrospinal fluid of PPS patients have been reported. A poliovirus persistence in neural cells by means of several different mechanisms has been suggested[23] and has been discussed as being of importance for the pathophysiology of the ongoing denervation.[25,49,54,64] One may, thus, speculate that an inflammation and a persistent polio infection of the CNS may contribute to the development of central fatigue in PPS patients. However, other authors have failed to show a persistent polio infection in PPS patients.[27,46,48,62]

Thus, there are conflicting data, and the question of an inflammatory reaction and a possible persistent infection of polio virus in the CNS should be further investigated. The results may shed further light on postpolio fatigue.

Other factors that may cause or contribute to a general fatigue are restricted lung function caused by scoliosis or weak respiratory muscles and secondary effects of decreased lung function, pneumonia, and cor pulmonale.[6,45] A decrease of the peak oxygen uptake[67] and an increase in arterial carbon dioxide tension[51] have been shown in follow-up studies in PPS patients (i.e., during the same period of time as there has been an increase of fatigue).

Sleep pattern disturbances have been reported.[6,19,29,45] In the study by Bruno,[19] half of the PPS patients reported sleep disturbance caused by periodic movements and restless legs. Dean et al.[29] reported sleep apnea, most often seen in patients with bulbar involvement. Bach[6] noted both the occurrence of sleep disordered breathing and sleep apnea, and Hsu and Staats described obstructive sleep apnea and hypoventilation and a combination of both in a retrospective study.[45] Sleep-disordered breathing may influence daytime functioning and, thus, contribute to postpolio fatigue.[79]

Furthermore, a reduced physical work capacity related to weight gain and cardiorespiratory deconditioning was reported in PPS patients in a follow-up study by Stanghelle and Festvåg.[67] These are factors that also may contribute to postpolio fatigue.

One must also consider the last criterion of PPS: that other medical conditions should be ruled out as explanation for the increase of symptoms. Thus, other conditions such as depression and endocrinologic disorders (e.g., example hypothyroidism) should be considered before the fatigue is diagnosed as caused by PPS.

TREATMENT OF CENTRAL FATIGUE

Based on the hypothesis of a disturbance in the activating system of the brain, Bruno et al. administered bromocriptine, a postsynaptic dopamine 2 receptor agonist, to PPS patients with fatigue.[18] A decreased general fatigue was reported from three of five treated patients. Furthermore, two PPS patients receiving selegiline, a monoaminoxidase inhibitor, reported improvement of symptoms.[7]

Different treatments directed against a possible inflammation or a persistent poliovirus infection have been tried in PPS patients. Stein et al. found that the antiviral agent amantadine improved general fatigue in 54% of the PPS patients but also in 43% of control subjects.[68] Improvement was reported in a few patients treated with steroids, but patients given interferon or immunosuppressants (e.g., prednisone) showed no improvement.[13,28] In a double-blind, randomized study on treatment with high-dose prednisone, a modest trend of increased muscle strength was found at high doses, which, however, eroded as the prednisone was discontinued.[31]

PERIPHERAL FATIGUE

The loss of anterior horn cells and of motor units caused by the acute polio infection leads to muscle weakness. The denervation is compensated by reinnervation leading to a recovery of muscle function. There is sometimes full recovery of strength, but a paresis remains in some patients. Data from different studies indicate that the new or increased muscle weakness (i.e., PPS) is caused by denervation. Neurophysiologic studies have shown signs of ongoing denervation, such as fibrillations or positive sharp waves.[22,25,80] which is also supported by findings of atrophic muscle fibers in muscle biopsies.[9,11,25,26] However, the signs of denervation are seen in both stable muscles as well as in those with new weakness. Macro electromyographic (EMG) studies have shown that the motor units in PPS patients are five to 20 times larger than normal.[33,42,66,74] In follow-up studies, small motor units had increased, suggesting an ongoing denervation-reinnervation process, and the largest motor units had decreased over time, suggesting a failing reinnervation in these PPS patients.[42,66] Thus, the new or increasing muscle weakness in PPS patients may be caused by a denervation-reinnervation process that has reached its upper limit (i.e., the insufficiently compensated denervation leads to muscle weakness),[8,42] which has been shown earlier to appear in denervation experiments in animal studies.[47]

Nollet et al. showed a severely reduced submaximal work capacity in polio patients, leading to a premature fatigue during sustained activity.[55] It is possible that the peripheral muscular fatigue is secondary to the muscle weakness (i.e., the motor units have to be driven harder in order to produce the power needed for example locomotion). However, the muscular fatigue in PPS patients may increase over a period of time,[41,42] when muscle strength remains unchanged. Edwards et al. pointed out that muscle fatigue and muscle weakness may be separated in normal human muscle.[32] Thus, there might be different pathophysiologic reasons to the muscle weakness and muscle fatigue. Furthermore, Agre et al. found that PPS patients with declining muscle strength had a longer recovery time after exhausting muscular exercise compared with patients with stable symptoms.[5] This implies that patients with an active reconstruction of motor units experience fatigue, but those who are stable do not. Possibly, the reconstruction and the compensatory and adaptive phenomena of the motor unit may be responsible for the development of muscular fatigability. Although compensatory and adaptive mechanisms all aim at ameliorating the neuromuscular function, they may instead lead to a neuromuscular dysfunction such as muscular fatigue, but the muscle power may remain unchanged.

Reinnervation is the most powerful compensatory mechanism leading to an increase of the motor unit area, which, in turn, leads to impaired neuromuscular transmission with increased jitter and blocking.[59,61,76,80] This may cause decreased endurance (i.e., local muscle fatigue). Trojan et al. reported that anticholinesterases (e.g., edrophonium and pyridostigmine) ameliorate clinical muscle fatigue and increase muscle strength.[75,77] However, they recently published results from a larger double-blind, placebo-controlled, multicenter study of 126 PPS patients that showed no effect of pyridostigmine on muscle strength and fatigue.[78] The importance of an impaired transmission over the neuromuscular junction is currently uncertain and should be further elucidated.

Besides reinnervation, there are other compensatory and adaptive mechanisms in muscles of PPS patients that increase the contractile tissue or change the contractile properties of the motor unit. In patients with a critical degree of paresis, an overuse of remaining motor units has been described and suggested to be the cause of muscle dysfunction.[9,10,57] Borg et al.,[9,10] Einarsson et al.,[34] and Grimby et al.[40] reported groups of PPS patients in whom a muscle fiber hypertrophy and an increased frequency of type I (slow twitch) muscle fibers, due to a muscle fiber transformation, were found in the anterior tibial (TA) and vastus lateralis (VL) muscles. Borg and Henriksson found a decreased number of capillaries per area unit in the hypertrophic muscle fibers, leading to an increased diffusion distance.[12] Furthermore, in muscle fiber homogenates, a low oxidative enzyme capacity was found in both TA and VL muscles,[12,40] and a low level of glycolytic enzymes was found in TA.[12] This may, thus, lead to muscle dysfunction, including muscle fatigue and muscle pain.

Tollbäck et al.[73] found that muscle fibers from PPS patients with overuse of remaining motor units and muscular fatigue had abnormal contractile properties. Neither central factors nor peripheral blocking was found. The fatigue was ascribed to high energy utilization and low energy resynthesis, suggesting that there is a higher rate of consumption than resynthesis of adenosine triphosphate.[43] Furthermore, the overused motor units had lost their differentiation and were activated in an all-or-none fashion. The motor unit adaptation was toward a uniform type with intermediate properties favoring strength to endurance and driven into contractile fatigue more easily than normal units.[72] Sunnerhagen et al. showed that the fatigue was not caused by neuromuscular blocking and suggested that the slow recovery was caused by both peripheral and central fatigue.[69] One must, thus, consider central components as at least partly responsible for peripheral fatigue.

TREATMENT OF PERIPHERAL FATIGUE

On the basis of the hypothesis presented above, the way of "treating" the muscular fatigability is primarily by using physical therapy to obtain optimal muscle function. There have been encouraging results of muscle strengthening exercise, both of low and high intensity in PPS patients (see Chapter 9). Feldman[36] showed improvement of function using nonfatiguing exercise, and Owen and Jones[56] reported improvement with aerobic conditioning. In a long-term (every other day for 1 to 2 years) training study with nonfatiguing resistant exercise, Fillyaw et al. found improvement of muscle strength in 16 of 17 PPS patients; however, there was no effect on endurance.[37] In the study by Agre et al., PPS patients performed a low-intensity, alternate-day, 12-week exercise program. Improved muscle performance was found with no adverse effects regarding EMG and serum creatine kinase.[3] When performing a 12-week strengthening exercise home program in these patients, Agre et al. found an increase in muscle strength and endurance.[4] Ernstoff et al. reported improvement of muscle strength and increase of work performance after endurance training.[35] Einarsson performed a study on the effects of high-intensity training.[33] A maximal effort isokinetic and isometric exercise program was performed, and significant increases of both isometric and isokinetic strength were found. Spector et al. reported an increased muscle strength after a progressive resistance training program.[65] Rodriquez and Agre reported that intermittent activity (work–rest interval programs) resulted in less evident muscle fatigue and an increased capacity to perform work.[60]

Thus, some data indicate improvement of muscle function in PPS patients after both low- and high-intensity exercise training programs as well as pacing programs. There is reason to believe that muscle fatigue will be reduced because of training programs if individual programs are applied to different patients, taking into account, for example, the degree of paresis.[81]

Another way of treating PPS patients is to increase the contractile properties of the muscle fibers by means of enhancing the energy metabolism of the muscle fiber. Mizuno et al. found an effect on muscle energy metabolism using coenzyme Q.[53] However, only three PPS patients were included in the study and, thus, this treatment has to be further evaluated. In a pilot study, Tarnopolsky and Martin reported an increase of high-intensity strength in PPS patients using creatine monohydrate.[71]

Lastly, when recommending a treatment to a postpolio patient, one must consider the patient's own clinical situation. The patient may favor, for example, changes in his or her daily living, including energy conservation, pacing, appropriate orthosis, avoiding weight gain, and losing weight.[1]

References

1. Agre JC: The role of exercise in the patient with post-polio syndrome. In Dalakas MC, Bartfeld H, Kurland LT (eds): The Post-Polio Syndrome: Advances in the Pathogenesis and Treatment. New York, New York Academy of Sciences, 1995, pp 321–334.
2. Agre JC: Rationale for treatment of new fatigue. Disabil Rehabil 18:307–310, 1996.
3. Agre JC, Rodriquez AA, Franke TM, et al: Low-intensity, alternate-day exercise improves muscle performance without apparent adverse effects in post-polio patients. Am J Phys Med Rehabil 75:50–58, 1996.
4. Agre JC, Rodriquez AA, Franke TM: Strength, endurance, and work capacity after muscle strengthening exercise in postpolio subjects. Arc Phys Med Rehab 78:681–686, 1997.
5. Agre JC, Rodriquez AA, Franke TM: Subjective recovery time after exhausting muscular activity in postpolio and control subjects. Am J Phys Med Rehab 77:140–144, 1998.
6. Bach JR: Management of post-polio repiratory sequelae. In Dalakas MC, Bartfeld H, Kurland LT (eds): The Post-Polio Syndrome: Advances in the Pathogenesis and Treatment. New York, New York Academy of Sciences, 1995, pp 96–102.

7. Bamford CR, Montgomery EB Jr, Munoz JE, et al: Postpolio syndrome: Response to de-prenyl (selegiline). Intern J Neurosci 71:183–188, 1993.
8. Borg K: Workshop report. Post-polio muscle dysfunction. Neuromusc Disord 6:75–80, 1998.
9. Borg K, Borg J, Edström L, Grimby L: Effects of excessive use of remaining muscle fibers in prior polio and LV lesion. Muscle Nerve 11:1219–1230, 1988.
10. Borg K, Borg J, Dhoot GK, et al: Motoneurone firing and isomyosin type of muscle fi-bres in prior polio. J Neurol Neurosurg Psychiatry 52:1141–1148, 1989.
11. Borg K, Edström L: Prior poliomyelitis: An immunohistochemical study of cytoskeletal proteins and a marker for muscle fibre regeneration in relation to usage of remaining mo-tor units. Acta Neurol Scand 87:128–132, 1993.
12. Borg K, Henriksson J: Prior poliomyelitis-reduced capillary supply and metabolic enzyme content in hypertrophic slow-twitch (type I) muscle fibres. J Neurol Neurosurg Psychia-try 54:236–240, 1991.
13. Brown S, Patten BM: Post-polio syndrome and ALS: A relationship more apparent than real. In Halstead LS, Wiechers DO (eds): Research and Clinical Aspects of the Late Ef-fects of Poliomyelitis. White Plains, NY, March of Dimes Birth Defects Foundation, 1987, pp 83–98.
14. Bruno RL, Frick NM, Cohen J: Polioencephalitis, stress and the etiology of post-polio se-quelae. Orthopedics 14:1185–1193, 1991.
15. Bruno RL, Galski T, DeLuca J: Neuropsychology of post-polio fatigue. Arch Phys Med Rehabil 74:1061–1065, 1993.
16. Bruno RL, Cohen J, Galski T, Frick NM: The neuroanatomy of post-polio fatigue. Arch Phys Med Rehabil 75:498–504, 1994.
17. Bruno RL, Sapolsky R, Zimmerman JR, Frick NM: Pathophysiology of a central cause of post-polio fatigue. In Dalakas MC, Bartfeld H, Kurland LT (eds): The Post-Polio Syndrome: Advances in the Pathogenesis and Treatment. New York, New York Academy of Sciences, 1995, pp 257–275.
18. Bruno RL, Zimmerman JR, Creange SJ, et al: Bromocriptine in the treatment of post-polio fatigue: A pilot study with implications for the pathophysiology of fatigue. Am J Phys Med Rehabil 75:340–347, 1996.
19. Bruno RL: Abnormal movements in sleep as a post-polio sequelae. Am J Phys Med Re-habil 77:339–343, 1998.
20. Bruno RL, Creange SJ, Frick NM: Parallels between post-polio fatigue and chronic fa-tigue syndrome: a common pathophysiology? Am J Med 105:66–73, 1998.
21. Bruno RL, Zimmerman JR: Word finding difficulties as a post-polio sequela. Am J Phys Med Rehabil 79:343–348, 2000.
22. Cashman NR, Maselli R, Wollman RL, et al: Late denervation in patients with an-tecedent paralytic poliomyelitis. N Engl J Med 317:7–12, 1987.
23. Colbere-Garapin F, Duncan G, Pavlo N, et al: An approach to understanding the mech-anisms of poliovirus persistence in infected cells of neural or non-neural origin. Clin Di-agn Virol 9:107–113, 1998.
24. Dalakas MC: New neuromuscular symptoms after old polio ("the post-polio syndrome"): Clinical studies and pathogenetic mechanisms. In Halstead LS, Wiechers DO (eds): Re-search and Clinical Aspects of the Late Effects of Poliomyelitis. White Plains, NY, March of Dimes Birth Defects Foundation, 1987, pp 241–264.
25. Dalakas MC: Morphologic changes in the muscles of patients with postpoliomyelitis neu-romuscular symptoms. Neurology 38:99–104, 1988.
26. Dalakas MC: Pathogenetic mechanisms of post-polio syndrome: Morphological, electro-physiological, virological, and immunological correlations. In Dalakas MC, Bartfeld H,

Kurland LT (eds): The Post-Polio Syndrome: Advances in the Pathogenesis and Treatment. New York, New York Academy of Sciences, 1995, pp 167–185.

27. Dalakas MC, Sever JL, Madden DL, et al: Late postpoliomyelitis muscular atrophy: Clinical virologic and immunologic study. Rev Infect Dis 6(suppl 2):62–567, 1984.

28. Dalakas MC, Elder G, Hallett M, et al: A long-term follow-up study of patients with post-poliomyelitis neuromuscular symptoms. N Engl J Med 314:959–963, 1986.

29. Dean AC, Graham BA, Dalakas MC, Sato S: Sleep apnoea in patients with post-polio syndrome. Ann Neurol 43:661–664, 1998.

30. Dickinson CJ: Chronic fatigue syndrome: Aetiological aspects. Eur J Clin Invest 27: 257–267, 1997.

31. Dinsmore S, Dambrosia J, Dalakas MC: A double-blind, placebo-controlled trial of high-dose prednisone for the treatment of post-poliomyelitis syndrome. In Dalakas MC, Bartfeld H, Kurland LT (eds): The Post-Polio Syndrome: Advances in the Pathogenesis and Treatment. New York, New York Academy of Sciences, 1995, pp 303–313.

32. Edwards RH, Hill DK, Jones DA, Merton PA: Fatigue of long duration in human skeletal muscle after excercise. J Physiol 272:769–778, 1977.

33. Einarsson G: Muscle conditioning in late poliomyelitis. Arch Phys Med Rehabil 72:11–14, 1991.

34. Einarsson G, Grimby G, Stålberg E: Electromyographic and morphological compensation in late poliomyelitis. Muscle Nerve 13:165–171, 1990.

35. Ernstoff B, Wetterqvist H, Kvist H, Grimby G: Endurance training effect on individuals with postpoliomyelitis. Arch Phys Med Rehabil 77:843–848, 1996.

36. Feldman RM: The use of strengthening exercises in post-polio sequelae: Methods and results. Orthopedics 8:889–890, 1985.

37. Fillyaw MJ, Badger GJ, Goodwin GD et al: The effects of long-term non-fatiguing resistance exercise in subjects with post-polio syndrome. Orthopedics 14:1253–1256, 1991.

38. Ginsberg AH, Gale MJ, Rose LM, Clark EA: T-cell alteration in late post-poliomyelitis. Arch Neurol 46:497–501, 1989.

39. Gonzalez H, Khademi M, Andersson M, et al: Chronic cytokine production in the central nervous system in patients with prior poliomyelitis. J Neurol Sci 205:9–13, 2002.

40. Grimby G, Einarsson G, Hedberg M, Aniansson A: Muscle adaptive changes in post-polio subjects. Scand J Rehab Med 21:19–26, 1989.

41. Grimby G, Hedberg M, Henning G-B: Changes in muscle morphology, strength and enzymes in a 4–5-year follow-up of subjects with poliomyelitis sequelae. Scand J Rehab Med 26:121–130, 1994.

42. Grimby G, Stålberg E, Sandberg A, Stibrant-Sunnerhagen K: An 8-year longitudinal study of muscle strength, muscle fiber size, and dynamic electromyogram in individuals with late polio. Muscle Nerve 21:1428–1437, 1998.

43. Grimby L, Tollbäck A, Müller U, Larsson L: Fatigue of chronically overused motor units in prior polio patients. Muscle Nerve 19:728–737, 1996.

44. Halstead LS, Rossi CD: Post-polio syndrome: Clinical experience with 132 consecutive outpatients. In Research and Clinical Aspects of the Late Effects of Poliomyelitis. Halstead LS, Wiechers DO (eds.). Birth Defects: Original Article Series 23:13–26, 1987.

45. Hsu AA, Staats BA: "Postpolio" sequelae and sleep-related disordered breathing. Mayo Clin Proc 73:216–224, 1998.

46. Jubelt B, Salazar-Grueso EF, Roos RP, Cashman NR: Antibody titer to the poliovirus in blood and cerebrospinal fluid of patients with post-polio syndrome. In Dalakas MC, Bartfeld H, Kurland LT (eds): The Post-Polio Syndrome: Advances in the Pathogenesis and Treatment. New York, New York Academy of Sciences, 1995, pp 201–207.

47. Kugelberg E, Edström L, Abbruzzese M: Mapping of motor units in experimentally rein-nervated rat muscle. J Neurol Neurosurg Psychiatry 33:319–329, 1970.
48. Leon Monzon ME, Dalakas MC: Detection of poliovirus antibodies and poliovirus genome in patients with the postpolio syndrome. In Dalakas MC, Bartfeld H, Kurland LT (eds): The Post-Polio Syndrome: Advances in the Pathogenesis and Treatment. New York, New York Academy of Sciences, 1995, pp 208–218.
49. Leparc-Goffart I, Julien J, Fuchs F, et al: Evidence of poliovirus genomic sequences in cerbrospinal fluid from patients with postpolio syndrome. J Clin Microbiol 34:2023–2026, 1996.
50. Lonnberg F: Late onset polio sequelae in Denmark: Presentation and results of a nation-wide survey of 3607 polio survivors. Scand J Rehab Med Suppl 28:7–15, 1993.
51. Midgren B: Lung function and clinical outcome in postpolio patients: A prospective co-hort study during 11 years. Europ Resp J 10:146–149, 1997.
52. Miller DC: Post-polio syndrome spinal cord pathology. Case report with immunopathol-ogy. In Dalakas MC, Bartfeld H, Kurland LT (eds): The Post-Polio Syndrome: Advances in the Pathogenesis and Treatment. New York, New York Academy of Sciences, 1995, pp 186–193.
53. Mizuno M, Quistorff B, Theorell H, et al: Effects of oral supplementation of coenzyme Q 10 on 31P-NMR detected skeletal muscle energy metabolism in middle-aged post-polio subjects. Mol Asp Med 18(suppl):291–298, 1997.
54. Muir P, Nicholson F, Sharief MK, et al: Evidence for persistent enterovirus infection of the central nervous system in patients with previous paralytic poliomyelitis. In Dalakas MC, Bartfeld H, Kurland LT (eds): The Post-Polio Syndrome: Advances in the Patho-genesis and Treatment. New York, New York Academy of Sciences, 1995, pp 219–232.
55. Nollet F, Beelen A, Sargeant AJ, et al: Submaximal exercise capacity and maximal power output in polio subjects. Arch Phys Med Rehabil 82:1678–1685, 2001.
56. Owen RR, Jones D: Polio residuals clinic: Conditioning exercise program. Orthopedics 8:882–883, 1985.
57. Perry J, Barnes G, Gronley JK: The post-polio syndrome: An overuse phenomenon. Clin Orthop 233:145–162, 1988.
58. Pezeshkpour GH, Dalakas MC: Pathology of spinal cord in post-poliomyelitis muscular atrophy. In Halstead LS, Wiechers DO (eds): Research and Clinical Aspects of the Late Effects of Poliomyelitis. White Plains, NY, March of Dimes Birth Defects Foundation, 1997, pp 229–236.
59. Ravits J, Hallett M, Baker M, et al: Clinical and electromyographic studies of pospo-liomyelitis muscular atrophy. Muscle Nerve 13:667–674, 1990.
60. Rodriquez AA, Agre JC: Electrophysiologic study of the quadriceps muscles during fa-tiguing exercise and recovery: A comparison of symptomatic and non-symptomatic post-polio patients. Arch Phys Med Rehabil 72:993–997, 1991.
61. Rodriquez AA, Agre JC, Franke TM: Electromyographic and neuromuscular variables in unstable postpolio subjects, postpolio subjects and control subjects. Arch Phys Med Re-habil 78:986–991, 1997.
62. Roivanen M, Kinnunen E, Hovi T: Twenty-one patients with strictly defined postpo-liomyelitis syndrome: No poliovirus-specific IgM antibodies in the cerebrospinal fluid. Ann Neurol 36:115–116, 1994.
63. Schanke AK, Stanghelle JK: Fatigue in polio survivors. Spinal Cord 39:243–251, 2001.
64. Sharief MK, Hentges R, Ciardi M: Intrathecal immune response in patients with the post-polio syndrome. N Engl J Med 325:748–755, 1991.

65. Spector SA, Gordon PL, Feuerstein IM, et al: Strength gains without muscle injury after strength training in patients with postpolio muscular atrophy. Muscle Nerve 19:1287–1290, 1996.
66. Stålberg E, Grimby G: Dynamic electromyography and muscle biopsy changes in a 4-year follow-up study of patients with a history of polio. Muscle Nerve 18:699–707, 1995.
67. Stanghelle JK, Festvåg LV: Postpolio syndrome: a 5 year follow-up. Spinal Cord 35:503–508, 1997.
68. Stein DP, Dambrosia JM, Dalakas MC: A double-blind, placebo-controlled trial of amantadine for the treatment of fatigue in patients with the post-polio syndrome. In Dalakas MC, Bartfeld H, Kurland LT (eds): The Post-Polio Syndrome: Advances in the Pathogenesis and Treatment. New York, New York Academy of Sciences, 1995, pp 296–302.
69. Sunnerhagen KS, Carlsson U, Sandberg A, et al: Electrophysiologic evaluation of muscle fatigue development and recovery in late polio. Arch Phys Med Rehabil 81:770–776, 2000.
70. Sunnerhagen KS, Grimby G: Muscular effects in late polio. Acta Physiol Scand 171:335–340, 2001.
71. Tarnopolsky M, Martin J: Creatine monohydrate increases strength in patients with neuromuscular disorders. Neurology 52:854–857, 1999.
72. Tollbäck A: Neuromuscular compensation and adaptation to loss of lower motoneurons in man: Studies in prior-polio subjects [thesis]. Stockholm, Karolinska Institute, 1995.
73. Tollbäck A, Knutsson E, et al: Torque-velocity and muscle fibre characteristics of foot dorsiflexors after long-term overuse of residual muscle fibres due to prior poliomyelitis and LV lesion. Scand J Rehab Med 24:151–156, 1992.
74. Tollbäck A, Borg J, Borg K, Knutsson E: Isokinetic strength, macro EMG and muscle biopsy of paretic foot dorsiflexors in chronic neurogenic paresis. Scand J Rehab Med 25:183–187, 1993.
75. Trojan DA, Gendron D, Cashman NR: Anticholinesterase-responsive neuromuscular junction transmission defects in post-poliomyelitis fatigue. J Neurol Sci 114:170–177, 1993.
76. Trojan DA, Gendron D, Cashman NR: Stimulation frequency-dependent neuromuscular junction transmission defects in patients with prior poliomyelitis. J Neurol Sci 118:150–157, 1993.
77. Trojan DT, Cashman NR: Anticholinesterases in post-poliomyelitis syndrome. In Dalakas MC, Bartfeld H, Kurland LT (eds): The Post-Polio Syndrome: Advances in the Pathogenesis and Treatment. New York, New York Academy of Sciences, 1995, pp 285–295.
78. Trojan DA, Collet JP, Shapiro S, et al: A multicenter randomized double-blinded trial of pyridostigmine in postpolio syndrome. Neurology 53:1225–1233, 1999.
79. Van Kralingen KW, Ivanyi B, van Keipema AR, et al: Sleep complaints in postpolio syndrome. Arch Phys Med Rehabil 77:609–611, 1996.
80. Wiechers DO, Hubbel SL: Late changes in the motor unit after acutepoliomyelitis. Muscle Nerve 4:524–528, 1981.
81. Willen C, Cider A, Sunnerhagen KS: Physical performance in inviduals with late effects of polio. Scand J Rehab Med 31:244–249, 1999.

Postpolio Pulmonary Dysfunction

John R. Bach, MD, and Jose Vega, MD, PhD

R espiratory morbidity and mortality are common, yet avoidable, for postpolio survivors. Besides respiratory muscle weakness, poliomyelitis survivors have a high incidence of scoliosis, obesity, sleep-disordered breathing, and bulbar muscle dysfunction. These factors often result in or exacerbate chronic alveolar hypoventilation (CAH). The risk of pulmonary complications is inversely related to the ability to cough (peak cough flows [PCFs]) and take deep breaths. Hypercapnia and inadequate cough flows are usually not recognized until acute respiratory failure is caused by airway secretion encumberment during otherwise benign upper respiratory tract infections. With the use of noninvasive inspiratory and expiratory muscle aids, acute respiratory failure, hospitalizations for respiratory complications, and the need to resort to tracheal intubation can be avoided. Timely introduction of noninvasive aids, including noninvasive ventilation, manually assisted coughing, and mechanical insufflation-exsufflation (MI-E) can be critical for avoiding complications and maintaining optimal quality of life.

PATHOPHYSIOLOGY OF RESPIRATORY SEQUELAE

Between 1928 and 1962, more than 500,000 people were afflicted with poliomyelitis in the United States.[45] About 12.5% of those who required ventilator use could not be weaned, and many are still alive and have been continuously ventilator supported by noninvasive means, for more than 40 years.[52] Others who weaned from ventilator use initially, have once again developed respiratory symptoms and new breathing problems.[36,41] The total number of patients who now require ventilator use is increasing. Chronic ventilatory insufficiency and the need for long-term ventilatory assistance has begun 18 years after the diagnosis of acute poliomyelitis.[13,38,47] Thus, a large number of patients are now supported by mechanical ventilation because of weakness of their inspiratory and expiratory muscles.

Both inspiratory and expiratory musculature weaken as late effects of polio. This results in the loss of vital capacity (VC) at rates that are 60–90% greater than normal.[21,38] Decreases in VC, tidal volumes, maximum inspiratory and expiratory pressures, and inability to take occasional deep breaths lead to chronic microatelectasis, decreased pulmonary compliance, and increased stiffness of the chest wall and work of breathing.[33,37] Fortunately, bulbar muscle function is rarely lost to the extent that loss of airway control necessitates tracheotomy.

Hypercapnia becomes likely when the VC falls below 55% of predicted normal.[28] It is insidiously progressive. Hypoxia, hypercapnia, and rate of loss of VC are exacerbated when intrinsic lung disease, kyphoscoliosis, or obesity complicate inspiratory muscle weakness.[20,55] In addition, respiratory muscles can be expected to weaken with age, fatigue, and ultimately with the death or dysfunction of overworked anterior horn cells that survived the original insult by the poliovirus. When the muscles are not relieved by use of inspiratory muscle aids, respiratory control centers accommodate hypercapnia,[11] and a compensatory metabolic alkalosis develops. The resulting elevated central nervous system bicarbonate levels contribute to depress the ventilatory response to hypoxia and hypercapnia. This permits worsening of CAH and may decrease the effectiveness of the nocturnal use of inspiratory muscle aids after they are instituted.[20]

Although almost always ignored, *expiratory muscle weakness is usually the key factor that causes acute respiratory failure.* Expiratory and bulbar muscle weakness can result in severely decreased PCFs that prevent effective elimination of airway secretions, particularly during intercurrent respiratory tract infections. Whether attained by autonomous coughing or by the use of manually or mechanically assisted coughing, PCFs of at least 3 L/s are necessary for effective airway secretion and mucus clearance.[4] Adequate PCFs are most important during respiratory tract infections. Likewise, bulbar muscle dysfunction and the inability to close or fully open the vocal cords can result in greatly diminished cough flows by preventing the retention of optimal lung volumes and causing upper airway obstruction. It can also lead to aspiration of food and saliva. Laryngeal dysfunction can not only result from the primary neuromuscular process but also from complications of translaryngeal intubation and tracheostomy. Likewise, fixed lower airway obstruction from concomitant chronic obstructive pulmonary disease (COPD), the presence of tracheal stenosis, or any other irreversible impediment to the generation of optimal PCF greatly increases the risk of pulmonary morbidity. Because average cough volumes are 2.3 liters, PCFs are also decreased by any inspiratory muscle weakness that decreases the inspiratory capacity below this level.[54]

Smoking, the presence of an endotracheal cannula, or bronchorrhea for any other reason increases the tendency to develop chronic mucus plugging in people with diminished PCFs. This, in turn, leads to ventilation/perfusion imbalance, atelectasis, pneumonias, pulmonary scarring, and further loss of lung compliance and functioning respiratory exchange membrane. A large mucus plug can cause sudden death. Polio survivors with chronic mucus plugging can require repeated intubation and bronchoscopy and are usually thought to need tracheotomy.

Polio survivors may also be particularly susceptible to the development of sleep-disordered breathing,[40,48,69] a condition reported to have a high incidence in this population[13,38] because of bulbar muscle dysfunction, which can increase susceptibility to hypopharyngeal collapse and obstructive apneas during sleep and immobility-associated obesity. Damage to respiratory control centers might also have occurred from the encephalitic process of the primary viral infection.[44,46,62,63]

Sleep-disordered breathing is the occurrence of multiple central or obstructive apneas and hypopneas during sleep. Its incidence normally increases with age.[30] The obstructive sleep apnea syndrome (OSAS) is diagnosed when such individuals are symptomatic and have a mean of 10 or more apneas plus hypopneas per hour.[39,43] Sleep-disordered breathing alone can result in CAH, hypoxia, right ventricular strain, and (when severe), acute cardiopulmonary failure.

PATIENT EVALUATION

The evaluator requires a simple spirometer, peak flow meter, end-tidal CO_2 monitor, and oximeter. First, symptoms are assessed. The symptoms of CAH are essentially the same as those of sleep-disordered breathing and include fatigue, headaches, sleep disturbances, difficult arousals, hypersomnolence, impaired concentration, nightmares, irritability, anxiety, nocturnal urinary frequency, impaired intellectual function, depression, and memory impairment.[11] Generally, only patients able to walk complain of shortness of breath. CO_2 is retained and ventilatory centers reset by bicarbonate retention to avoid this symptom. During acute respiratory tract infections, wheelchair users with impending respiratory failure complain more often of anxiety and insomnia than of shortness of breath. The respiratory evaluation also takes into account any history of allergies, asthma, smoking, respiratory hospitalizations, intubations, and bronchoscopies.

The spirometer is used to assess the VC with the patient sitting, supine, sidelying, and when wearing thoracolumbar orthoses when applicable. A properly fitting orthosis can increase VC, but a poorly fitting one that restricts respiratory muscle movement will decrease it. The VC is often most reduced when the patient is supine because of inordinate diaphragm weakness. The presence of hypercapnia may not be suspected unless the VC is obtained in this position. Evaluation of forced expiratory flow in 1 second (FEV_1) should be done whenever COPD is suspected.

When the VC is less than predicted normal, this is analogous to a joint that does not go through full range of motion (ROM).[16] ROM is promoted for the lungs and chest wall by training in "air stacking." Air stacking facility is monitored by assessment of the maximum insufflation capacity (MIC). The MIC is the spirometric measure of the maximum volume of air that can be held with a closed glottis. To attain the MIC, the patient takes a deep breath and holds it with a closed glottis. He or she then receives delivered volumes of air from a manual resuscitator or portable volume ventilator, "air stacking" the volumes into the lungs to the point that no more can be held. The patient may also use maximum depth glossopharyngeal breathing (GPB) (see below) or perform some combination of these methods.[21] The MIC is a function of pulmonary compliance and bulbar muscle control. It is also useful for predicting the glossopharyngeal maximum single breath capacity (GPmaxSBC).[21] The greater the MIC, the better pulmonary compliance, GPB potential, voice volume during mouthpiece intermittent positive pressure ventilation (IPPV), the potential for using noninvasive alternatives to tracheostomy IPPV, and assisted PCF.

The peak flow meter is used to measure unassisted PCF, PCF generated from maximum lung volumes that are air stacked, and fully assisted PCF. The latter is most important because patients with encumbered airways often require fully assisted PCF. These are measured by having the patient air stack to approach the MIC and then timing an abdominal thrust to glottic opening as the patient coughs into the peak flow meter.

Any patient with a low supine VC and respiratory symptoms at rest deserves a trial of nocturnal nasal ventilation. Justification for this can derive from SpO_2 and possibly capnography or transcutaneous pCO_2 monitoring during sleep. Sleep monitoring by capnography and oximetry is warranted for patients with respiratory symptoms, daytime hypercapnia, a supine VC less than 40% of predicted normal or at least 30% less than that in the sitting position.[11] This noninvasive blood gas monitoring is most conveniently performed in the home. The oximeter should be capable of averaging data hourly.[11] Hourly SpO_2 means < 95% in a symptomatic patient without intrinsic lung disease is more than sufficient to make a presumptive diagnosis of CAH and initiate treatment with noninvasive ventilation. Maximum nocturnal pCO_2 > 50 mmHg is also a strong indication for treatment, especially when the disease course is clearly progressive or the patient has had recent pulmonary complications.

Although patients with CAH can have many transient and often severe oxyhemoglobin desaturations, a "sawtooth" pattern with more than ten transient 4% or greater desaturations per hour in a symptomatic patient with normal supine VC and mean SpO_2 may signal uncomplicated sleep-disordered breathing. For symptomatic patients, oximetry studies alone are highly sensitive in screening for this condition.[50,74] Polysomnography can assist in the evaluation of patients who may be symptomatic despite having inconclusive nocturnal oximetry and carbon dioxide studies and relatively normal VCs.[65] Patients should be reevaluated yearly or whenever there is a change in symptoms by spirometry, PCFs, and possibly nocturnal $EtCO_2$ and SpO_2.

Because of the availability of oximetry and capnography, arterial blood gas sampling is rarely warranted in the outpatient setting. Full batteries of pulmonary function studies and arterial blood gas sampling are unnecessary unless the patient is in acute respiratory failure with concomitant intrinsic lung disease.

GLOSSOPHARYNGEAL BREATHING

Both inspiratory and, indirectly, expiratory muscle function can be assisted by GPB.[8,9,22] Bach et al. studied polio, high-level tetraplegic, muscular dystrophy, and other patients and found that GPB can provide a patient with weak inspiratory muscles and no VC or breathing tolerance with normal alveolar ventilation and perfect safety when not using a ventilator (or in the event of sudden ventilator failure) day or night.[22] The technique involves the use of the glottis to add to an inspiratory effort by projecting (gulping) boluses of air into the lungs. The glottis closes with each "gulp." One breath usually consists of 6 to 9 gulps of 40 to 200 mL each (Fig. 1). During the training period, the efficiency of GPB can be monitored by spirometrically measuring the milliliters of air per gulp, gulps per breath, and breaths per minute. A training manual[32] and numerous videos are available,[31] the most comprehensive of which was produced in 1999 by Webber.[71]

Although severe oropharyngeal muscle weakness can limit the usefulness of GPB, this is rare in polio survivors. Approximately 60% of ventilator users with no autonomous ability to breathe and good bulbar muscle function can use GPB for breathing tolerance from minutes up to all day.[5,22] Although potentially extremely useful, GPB is rarely taught because there are few health care professionals familiar with the technique. GPB is also rarely useful in the presence of an indwelling tracheostomy tube. It can not be used when the tube is uncapped as it is during tracheostomy IPPV, and even when capped, the gulped air tends to leak around the outer walls of the tube and out the stoma as airway volumes and pressures increase during the GPB air-stacking process. The safety and versatility afforded by GPB are key reasons to eliminate tracheostomy in favor of noninvasive aids.

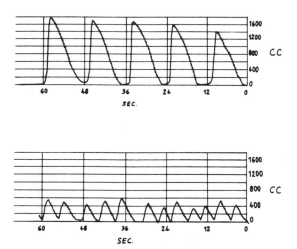

Figure 1. *Top,* Maximal GPB minute ventilation 8.39 L/min, GPB inspirations average 1.67 L, 20 gulps, 84 mL/gulp for each breath in a patient with a vital capacity of 0 mL. *Bottom,* Same patient with regular GPB minute ventilation 4.76 L/min, 12.5 breaths, average 8 gulps per breath, 47.5 mL/gulp performed over a 1-minute period.[1] (Courtesy of the March of Dimes.)

CONVENTIONAL MANAGEMENT

Polio survivor symptoms that may be largely caused by respiratory muscle weakness are often thought to result from sleep-disordered breathing. Patients are then sent for polysomnographies and, although the problem is often inspiratory muscle weakness rather than obstructive apneas, they are often inappropriately treated with continuous positive airway pressure (CPAP) or low-span (inspiratory minus expiratory positive airway pressure < 10 cm H_2O) bilevel (BiPAP). Although these modalities can relieve symptoms of uncomplicated central and obstructive apneas, they often inadequately assist weak respiratory muscles and do not prevent respiratory failure from occurring during periods of airway encumberment.

Respiratory muscle dysfunction is often undiagnosed and untreated until an otherwise benign intercurrent respiratory tract infection leads to acute respiratory failure. Obesity, abdominal distention, dehydration, undernutrition, and the respiratory infections themselves and possibly resulting hypercapnia decrease both inspiratory and expiratory muscle function.[59] Mucus plugs airways, and, when the patient cannot generate sufficient PCF to eliminate it, oxyhemoglobin desaturation occurs and supplemental oxygen is administered rather than effective airway secretion management. This results in atelectasis, ventilation perfusion mismatching, worsening hypercapnia, pneumonia, and acute respiratory failure.

The patients are then hospitalized and continue to receive supplemental oxygen rather than manually and mechanically assisted coughing (MAC) to eliminate airway secretions. This may maintain oxyhemoglobin saturation at the cost of life-threatening hypercapnia. Oxygen therapy can also prevent the signaling of bronchial mucus plugging–associated oxyhemoglobin desaturations by oximetry. This can eliminate oximetry as feedback to institute MAC to clear them. Patients may receive intermittent positive pressure breathing (IPPB) treatments but at inadequate pressures to provide the deep lung volumes needed for effective assisted coughing. Bronchodilators and methylxanthines are also often used but rarely useful in the absence of reversible bronchospasm. It is not surprising that patients treated in this manner often require translaryngeal intubation.

After intubation, the patient may not have sufficient respiratory muscle function for early ventilator weaning, particularly when mucus plugs are inadequately expulsed, respiratory control centers are dulled by supplemental oxygen administration, and muscle deconditioning and inadequate nutrition complicate the picture. Then, after perhaps refusing for years, the patient may succumb to tracheotomy. Weaning attempts from tracheostomy IPPV usually continue by some combination of assist control or synchronized intermittent mandatory ventilation (SIMV) used in combination with pressure support ventilation, positive end-expiratory pressure (PEEP), and supplemental oxygen. Occasionally, progressive ventilator-free breathing with T-piece supplemental oxygen and intermittent CPAP delivery is tried. The patient's carbon dioxide levels may increase during the weaning attempts. Thus, the failure to provide noninvasive respiratory muscle aids in a timely manner often leads to otherwise unnecessary hospitalization, intubation, tracheotomy, and bronchoscopies.

NONINVASIVE MANAGEMENT OF POSTPOLIO RESPIRATORY SEQUELAE

The key therapeutic goals are to maintain pulmonary compliance by providing ROM to the lungs and chest wall, maintain normal alveolar ventilation around the clock, and effectively clear airway secretions by augmenting PCF. Therapeutic options for accomplishing these goals should be presented and the patient ultimately trained and equipped. In addition, patients are cautioned to avoid dehydration, heavy meals, extremes of temperature, humidity, excessive fatigue, exposure to respiratory tract pathogens, obesity, sedatives, and narcotic use. Therapeutic exercise programs, extremity bracing, energy conservation, assistive equipment needs, and day-to-day functioning should also be addressed.[6,7] Appropriate flu and bacterial vaccinations are administered. Most importantly, patients are taught an oximetry, respiratory muscle aid protocol to prevent pneumonia and respiratory failure during intercurrent upper respiratory tract infections or other episodes of airway encumberment. Patients are also warned to avoid supplemental oxygen therapy unless receiving invasive respiratory support in the hospital setting. Likewise, local hospitals and family physicians need to be advised on the patient's needs in advance of any elective or unanticipated surgical procedures. To be able to accomplish the three key therapeutic goals, one must understand the use of inspiratory and expiratory muscle aids.

INSPIRATORY AIDS

Inspiratory muscle aids or ventilatory assistance can be provided by negative pressure body ventilators. These devices apply subatmospheric pressure changes around the chest and abdomen. These methods are cumbersome, less effective, and less practical, particularly for daytime aid, than noninvasive IPPV. They have been described elsewhere.[8] We have found them useful only for providing ventilatory support during tracheostomy site closure when switching patients with little or no ability to breathe from tracheostomy to noninvasive IPPV.[2,10]

Body ventilators that act directly on the body include the rocking bed and the intermittent abdominal pressure ventilator (IAPV).[14] The rocking bed is one of the least effective devices, but the IAPV continues to be useful. It consists of an inflatable bladder in an abdominal girdle (Fig. 2). The bladder is cyclically inflated by a portable positive pressure ventilator. The alternating pressure on the abdominal contents moves the diaphragm and ventilates the lungs. The IAPV generally augments the patient's autonomous tidal volumes by about 600 mL.[60] It is most effective in the sitting position at 75–85°. It is the method of choice for daytime ventilatory support for patients with less than 1 hour of ventilator-free breathing ability because it provides better appearance than any other method of ventilatory assistance and is ideal for concurrent GPB and wheelchair use.[14]

The inspiratory muscle aids that apply IPPV noninvasively to the airways are the most effective, most practical, and best tolerated alternatives to tracheostomy IPPV for patients with inspiratory muscle dysfunction who require assistance up to 24 hours a day.[15] They are also greatly preferred by patients and caregivers over the use of tracheostomy IPPV.[3]

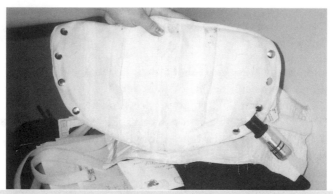

Figure 2. This air bladder is inside the abdominal girdle of a functioning intermittent abdominal pressure ventilator. The bladder is cyclically filled and emptied of air as abdominal displacement and the resulting diaphragm movement ventilate the lungs.

Noninvasive IPPV can be provided via oral,[15] nasal,[11] or oral–nasal[17] interfaces. For daytime ventilatory support, IPPV is most conveniently provided via simple mouthpieces that are held near the patient's mouth for easy accessibility. The mouthpiece might be fixed adjacent to the sip-and-puff or chin controls of a motorized wheelchair or simply kept in the mouth (Fig. 3). Oximetry feedback can be used and the patient told to take assisted breaths whenever necessary to maintain normal SpO_2. Thus, oximetry can guide the patient with CAH in using an appropriate schedule of IPPV to normalize ventilation during daytime hours.[6,15] The patient is usually instructed to keep the SpO_2 greater than 94% throughout daytime hours.[21,22] Patients use mouthpiece IPPV for increasing periods of time up to 24 hours a day as respira-

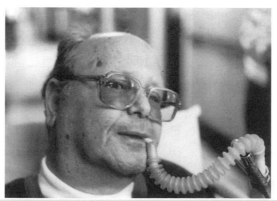

Figure 3. This polio survivor used mouthpiece IPPV continuously from 1955 until 1995, when he succumbed to leukemia.

tory muscles weaken with age or acute illness. It is the most effective and generally the preferred method of daytime support.[15]

For nocturnal use, many patients choose to use mouthpiece IPPV with lipseal retention (Fig. 4) (Puritan-Bennett, Boulder, CO); however, most patients prefer nasal IPPV.[11,29,53] Each patient tries at least three or four commercially available CPAP masks as interfaces for IPPV to determine the ones that best optimize fit, seal, and comfort. If none are adequate, custom interfaces are constructed. Transparent, durable, custom-molded, low-profile nasal interfaces can be prepared from a plaster moulage (Fig. 5).[58] They are lighter, durable, comfortable, and cosmetic in appearance but require several patient visits. Although pressure-cycled ventilators such as the BiPAP-ST can be used for nocturnal nasal or mouthpiece ventilation, they cannot be used for air stacking. This is the main reason that volume-cycled ventilators are preferred for patients with sufficient bulbar muscle function for air stacking.

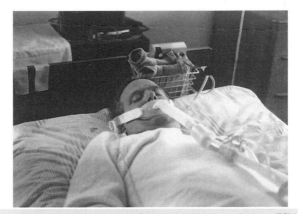

Figure 4. Use of lipseal retention for nocturnal mouthpiece IPPV.

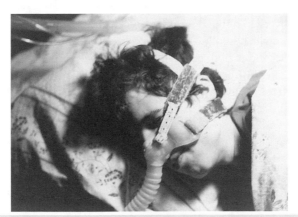

Figure 5. Nasal intermittent PPV provided via a custom-molded, low-profile acrylic nasal interface.

If nocturnal oximetry and possibly capnography do not demonstrate adequate improvement of ventilation using nasal IPPV, the problem is usually that the patient's lungs are underventilated during daytime hours. If this is the case, the patient is asked to use sufficient daytime aid to normalize daytime SpO_2. The patient can also be switched to nocturnal use of mouthpiece IPPV with lipseal retention. A custom-molded acrylic bite plate and outer shell (acrylic lipseal) can also be fabricated to decrease the risk of orthodontic deformity.[6,58] When using mouthpiece IPPV, a complete seal can be obtained by plugging the nose with cotton pledgets and tape, thus creating a closed system.

For ventilator users who live alone and who are unable to manage a strap retention system, a strapless interface can be constructed.[17,58] Oral and oronasal interfaces are often used with a bite plate rather than with strap retention. Thus, air can be delivered via comfortable custom-molded interfaces for nasal, oral, or oronasal IPPV.

EXPIRATORY AIDS

The expiratory muscles can be assisted by providing maximal insufflations by air stacking and then manually applying thrusts to the abdomen timed to glottic opening. Mechanical insufflation-exsufflation (MI- E) (Cough-Assist, J. H. Emerson Co., Cambridge, MA) can also be used.[4] MAC is the use of MI-E with an abdominal thrust timed to mechanical exsufflation. Manually assisted coughing with abdominal thrusts should not be used after meals because of the risk of regurgitation and aspiration of food. Because normal cough volumes are about 2.3 L and PCF diminish greatly when expiratory volumes are less than 1500 mL, a good rule of thumb is to provide a maximal insufflation for any patient whose VC is less than 1500 mL before applying the abdominal thrust to assist the cough.[4]

Mechanically assisted coughing is used when manual techniques are inadequate to eliminate airway secretions to maintain normal SpO_2. This can occur when the care provider cannot generate sufficient force for or effectively coordinate abdominal thrusts or when there is scoliosis or at least moderate bulbar muscle dysfunction. In addition, MI-E should be used with abdominal thrusts (MAC) when the stomach is empty. MI-E delivers an optimal insufflation via an oral–nasal mask, mouthpiece, or endotracheal tube, which is followed by a decrease in pressure, usually of about 80 cm H_2O over a 0.2-second period, to create a forced exsufflation of 10 L/s.[24,25] The abdominal thrust timed to the machine's exsufflation cycle is important to further increase PCF and maintain airway patency. These forced exsufflation flows carry airway secretions up into the mouth, mask, or tubing. This can increase VC, maximum pulmonary airflows, and SpO_2.[4] MAC can be necessary essentially around the clock during respiratory tract infections and after surgical anesthesia.[4,68]

Chest physical therapy techniques along with postural drainage may be useful for patients with airway encumberment. Other mechanical approaches for eliminating secretions include rapidly oscillating pressure changes or vibrations applied to the chest wall or airway. These methods may be particularly useful in combination with postural drainage techniques. Their use may also be helpful before using manually assisted coughing for some patients.[9,42] The Percussionaire, or Intrapulmonary Percussive Ventilator, pulses positive pressure into the airway at 2–5 Hz as the patient breathes spontaneously. The pulsed air tends to expulse secretions from peripheral airways.

Chest wall vibrators such as the Hayek Oscillator (Breasy Medical Equipment Inc., Stamford, CT) and ThAIRapy Vest (American Biosystems, Inc., St. Paul, MN) may also be useful for patients with acute airway encumberment. The ThAIRapy Vest provides oscillation at 5–25 Hz. Hayek Oscillator vibration is performed at frequencies up to 40 Hz. Vibration is applied during the entire breathing cycle or during expiration only. The adjustable I/E ratio of the Oscillator permits inspiratory and expiratory pressure changes (e.g., $+3$ to -6 cm H_2O) favoring higher exsufflation flow velocities to mobilize secretions. Baseline pressures can be set at negative, atmospheric, or positive values, thus commencing oscillation above, at, or below the functional residual capacity.

MAINTENANCE OF PULMONARY COMPLIANCE

After the VC has decreased below predicted normal in any position, patients are instructed to air stack and take maximum insufflations via a mouthpiece several times a day. A manual resuscitator is usually used to provide the deep insufflations. The goal is to approach the predicted maximum inspiratory capacity and thus provide ROM to the lungs and chest wall, maximize the MIC, reduce microatelectasis, accustom the user to receiving positive airway pressure via oral and nasal interfaces (noninvasive ventilation), and at least temporarily increase dynamic pulmonary compliance and decrease the work of breathing. It is very important that the clinician ascertain that the patient has learned this technique so that he or she can use mouthpiece IPPV to effectively ventilate the lungs during intercurrent respiratory tract infections. When patients use MI-E for maximum insufflations, they can also use it after PCF decreases below 4–4.5 L/s to treat bronchorrhea when airway mucus becomes a problem.[4]

THE OXIMETRY RESPIRATORY AID PROTOCOL

The oximetry respiratory aid protocol is the use of inspiratory and expiratory muscle aids to maintain normal alveolar ventilation and augment PCF to clear airway secretions sufficiently to maintain SpO_2 greater than 94% at all times.

During intercurrent respiratory infections, the VC decreases precipitously, and hypercapnia and hypoxemia can develop or worsen. The patient then needs a portable ventilator to use up to 24 hours a day, noninvasive IPPV, manually assisted coughing, a Cough-Assist (J. H. Emerson Company, Cambridge, MA) for MAC (if indicated), and an oximeter to signal hypoventilation and mucus plugging that require immediate attention. Provided that the patient maintains normal alveolar ventilation with or without the use of IPPV, acute oxyhemoglobin desaturation can only be explained by mucus plugging, atelectasis, or intrinsic lung disease. Sudden decreases in SpO_2 are usually caused by mucus plugging, and are reversed by using MAC to expulse secretions and return the SpO_2 to baseline. With effective elimination of airway secretions, baseline SpO_2—depressed to 92% to 94% by the presence of microatelectasis—normalizes over a period of days with these treatments and supportive medical therapy. If the baseline SpO_2 continues to decrease, pneumonia becomes likely and the patient usually requires hospitalization for more intensive and invasive therapy. This is uncommon, however, for patients using respiratory muscle aids and oximetry as described.

INSPIRATORY MUSCLE TRAINING

Muscle training for patients with any neuromuscular disorder is controversial as it has been suggested that overuse of already weakened muscles can have deleterious effects.[49] This is in agreement with a recent study that showed that exercise performance in postpolio patients induced an abnormal blood gas profile, indicating that the patients avoid diaphragm fatigue at the expense of hypoventilation.[1,72] In the few specific studies dedicated to the assessment of the potential benefits of respiratory muscle training on neuromuscular disease patients, short daily sessions of inspiratory resistive exercise alone were reported to have no effect on spirometry or maximum inspiratory or expiratory pressures.[35,57,66] However, in these studies, inspiratory resistive exercises improved respiratory endurance, provided that the VC at onset of exercise was 30% or more. A recent study by Klefbeck and colleagues confirmed similar findings in postpolio patients.[51] However, the overall clinical benefits of respiratory muscle training in patients with chronic muscle weakness are not clear. For example, in patients with COPD, despite similar results with inspiratory muscle training, there are no reports of fewer exacerbations or decreased risk of pulmonary complications.

TRACHEAL DECANNULATION AND WEANING

Many polio survivors with underlying respiratory muscle weakness undergo tracheotomy during an episode of respiratory failure triggered by an inability to clear airway secretions during an intercurrent respiratory tract infection. However, the patient, can be decannulated and switched to the use of strictly noninvasive respiratory muscle aids provided that he or she has assisted PCF > 160 L/m.[19] Decannulation and switching to noninvasive IPPV results in ventilator weaning to nocturnal-only use. For those with no breathing tolerance, decannulation permits the mastery of GPB for ventilator-free breathing. Patients using noninvasive methods of ventilatory support rather than tracheostomy also have significantly fewer hospitalizations for respiratory complications.[18]

The patient can first be switched to using a fenestrated cuffed tube. The cuff should be deflated and the ventilator-delivered volumes increased to compensate for insufflation leakage. Virtually all tracheostomy IPPV users with any residual bulbar muscle function can be adequately ventilated with the cuff fully deflated, day or night, provided that a tracheostomy tube with the proper diameter is used[12] and leakage is sufficiently compensated to maintain the same lung insufflation pressures with the cuff deflated as there were with the cuff inflated. The patient uses an inflated cuff only during MAC. Whether used via a facial interface or an endotracheal or tracheostomy tube, MI-E that eliminates airway secretions results in immediate increases in VC and SpO_2. Thus, these patients are aggressively exsufflated through the indwelling tubes and maintained free from supplemental oxygen.

The patient is then introduced to mouthpiece and nasal IPPV with the tracheostomy tube capped. After it has been learned[2,15] the tube can be removed, a tracheostomy button placed, and the PCF measured with the airway now clear. Mouthpiece IPPV is used during daytime hours, initially with oximetry feedback, and either nasal or lipseal IPPV is used overnight. Whether or not the patient has any breathing tolerance it is necessary to attain unassisted or assisted PCF of 160 L/m or more to use noninvasive ventilation indefinitely. After the patient is comfortable using noninvasive IPPV and adequate PCF has been documented, the button is removed and the tracheostomy site closed. If the site does not close completely on its own, it is sutured. Airway secretions will "dry up" within 1 week of tracheostomy closure unless the patient has postnasal drip, allergic bronchorrhea, or chronic bronchitis.

The patient and family are instructed to use the oximetry feedback respiratory aid protocol to maintain $SpO_2 > 94\%$ during future episodes of respiratory infection, distress, or fatigue. The patient is instructed to notify the physician at the first signs of infection or airway congestion for antibiotics and other supportive therapy but to avoid oxygen therapy and extensive medical evaluations unless the baseline SpO_2 decreases below 95%. Using MAC as necessary and oximetry as feedback, patients wean from continuous IPPV by taking fewer and fewer mouthpiece-assisted breaths while maintaining normal alveolar ventilation on room air until weaning is completed or until the extent of ongoing need for noninvasive IPPV is determined.

Patients may wean to nocturnal-only use of noninvasive IPPV or require daytime IPPV as well. Patients, however, wean themselves on their own schedules. This incurs less anxiety than weaning from tracheostomy IPPV using synchronized mandatory ventilation (SIMV) or periods of CPAP and free breathing because they know that they always have immediate access to deep breaths. Thus, the patient is first weaned from supplemental oxygen administration by using MAC to eliminate mucus plugging; then the tube is removed and the site allowed to close; and finally, if possible, the patient weans him- or herself from noninvasive IPPV.

If a patient who is experienced in taking deep insufflations via a mouthpiece or nasal interface is translaryngeally intubated, he or she can usually be safely extubated and switched to 24-hour mouthpiece or nasal IPPV and MAC. For patients who are untrained in noninvasive IPPV techniques, this should only be attempted if the patient has at least a few minutes of ventilator-free breathing tolerance or by using a negative-pressure body ventilator for effective ventilatory support during extubation and training in noninvasive IPPV techniques. For untrained individuals with little ability to breathe, extubation and attempts at supporting ventilation by noninvasive IPPV without backup body ventilator support can result in panic and reintubation.

SLEEP-DISORDERED BREATHING

There are patients for whom neither sleep disordered breathing, nor concurrent lung disease, nor respiratory muscle dysfunction are severe enough to warrant treatment but who, because of multiple conditions, require the use of respiratory muscle aids to remain healthy and symptom free. Any reversible conditions associated with obstructive sleep apnea syndrome (OSAS) should be identified and treated.[67] However, for the majority of patients with simple OSAS, nocturnal nasal CPAP is effective.[56] CPAP works as a pneumatic splint to maintain airway patency. CPAP of 5–15 cm H_2O is usually adequate. Independently varying the inspiratory (IPAP) and expiratory (EPAP) pressures with the use of a BiPAP-ST device (Respironics Inc., Murrysville, PA) can improve effectiveness and comfort.[70] The IPAP and EPAP difference is the BiPAP span. The greater the span, the greater the inspiratory muscle aid. Spans of 17–20 cm H_2O are usually required for full ventilatory support.

To optimize treatment efficacy, nocturnal recordings of SpO_2 can be done at various CPAP or BiPAP settings. For patients with a combination of neuromuscular ventilatory insufficiency and sleep-disordered breathing, both CPAP and low spans can be ineffective. Either high-span BiPAP or the use of volume-triggered ventilators are then used for noninvasive IPPV. Noninvasive IPPV supports the patient's ventilation, maintains upper airway patency, and most importantly, facilitates air stacking.[11,20,29,40,69]

PREPARATION FOR SURGICAL ANESTHESIA

Polio survivors require surgical intervention more frequently than the general population.[61] Mastery of the use of respiratory muscle aids before surgery can greatly decrease the risk of pulmonary morbidity. A hospital of the patient's choice is made aware of the patient's equipment and special needs. For the majority of hospitals that do not own portable ventilators or Cough-Assists, this will require advanced notice. Nursing and respiratory therapy in-services are required.

The VC, PCF, pCO_2 and SpO_2 are sensitive indicators of risk of postsurgical pulmonary complications. The lower the VC below 60% and the PCF below 5 L/s, the greater the likelihood of complications. Patients are trained in receiving maximum insufflations and noninvasive IPPV and in MAC in anticipation of postoperative difficulties. Access to MI-E is particularly important for patients who undergo abdominal surgery.[23,73] The use of MI-E requires no abdominal muscle effort, and abdominal pressures are increased 70% lower than during spontaneous coughing.[26]

General anesthesia should ideally be avoided in favor of local or regional anesthesia whenever possible, and nonessential elective procedures should be avoided. Simple inhalation anesthetic techniques should be used whenever possible. The use of opioids and muscle relaxants can diminish ventilatory drive, exacerbate hypercapnia, render nocturnal noninvasive IPPV ineffective; therefore, they should be used sparingly or avoided.[61]

Provided that the presurgical PCF exceeded 160 L/m and high-dose narcotics, sedatives, and supplemental oxygen are avoided, once the ventilator user is fully alert after anesthesia, he or she can be safely extubated whether or not capable of autonomous ventilation. Immediately upon extubation, the patient receives IPPV via a mouthpiece or nasal interface and uses nasal or lipseal IPPV during sleep with oximetry monitoring. Except during the surgical procedure itself, patients should be permitted to use their own portable equipment because, besides the differences in flow characteristics, the expiratory volume alarms of the usual hospital ventilators can make it impractical to use noninvasive IPPV. The secretions stimulated by the intubation and anesthesia can usually be efficiently eliminated by MAC, and pulmonary and laryngeal complications are averted by avoiding prolonged intubation and tracheostomy.

CONCLUSION

The failure to make timely appropriate management decisions often leads to episodes of acute respiratory failure and unnecessary hospitalizations, endotracheal intubations, bronchoscopies, and tracheostomies. The use of invasive IPPV instead of noninvasive IPPV and MAC adversely affects quality of life and can increase the risk of pulmonary complications and mortality for postpolio patients.[18,34] Episodes of acute respiratory failure, which most often result from otherwise benign upper respiratory tract infections, can be prevented or reversed by the timely use of noninvasive respiratory muscle aids.

References
1. Annane D, Chevrolet JC, Chevret S, Raphael JC: Nocturnal mechanical ventilation for chronic hypoventilation in patients with neuromuscular and chest wall disorders. Cochrane Database Syst Rev 2:CD001941, 2000.
2. Bach JR: Alternative methods of ventilatory support for the patient with ventilatory failure due to spinal cord injury. J Am Paraplegia Soc 14:158–174, 1991.
3. Bach JR: A comparison of long-term ventilatory support alternatives from the perspective of the patient and care giver. Chest 104:1702–1706, 1993.
4. Bach JR: Mechanical insufflation-exsufflation: Comparison of peak expiratory flows with manually assisted and unassisted coughing techniques. Chest 104:1553–1562, 1993.
5. Bach JR: New approaches in the rehabilitation of the traumatic high level quadriplegic. Am J Phys Med Rehabil 70:13–20, 1991.
6. Bach JR: Pulmonary rehabilitation. In DeLisa JD (ed): Rehabilitation Medicine: Principles and Practice. Philadelphia, JB Lippincott, 1993, pp 952–972.
7. Bach JR: Comprehensive rehabilitation of the severely disabled ventilator-assisted individual. Monaldi Arch Chest Dis 48:331–345, 1993.
8. Bach JR: Update and perspectives on noninvasive respiratory muscle aids: Part 1—the inspiratory muscle aids. Chest 105:1230–1240, 1994.
9. Bach JR: Update and perspectives on noninvasive respiratory muscle aids: Part 2—the expiratory muscle aids. Chest 105:1538–1544, 1994.
10. Bach JR, Alba AS: Noninvasive options for ventilatory support of the traumatic high level quadriplegic. Chest 98:613–619, 1990.
11. Bach JR, Alba AS: Management of chronic alveolar hypoventilation by nasal ventilation. Chest 97:52–57, 1990.
12. Bach JR, Alba AS: Tracheostomy ventilation: A study of efficacy with deflated cuffs and cuffless tubes. Chest 97:679–683, 1990.

13. Bach JR, Alba AS: Pulmonary dysfunction and sleep disordered breathing as post-polio sequelae: Evaluation and management. Orthopedics 14:1329–1337, 1991.
14. Bach JR, Alba AS: Total ventilatory support by the intermittent abdominal pressure ventilator. Chest 99:630–636, 1991.
15. Bach JR, Alba AS, Saporito LR: Intermittent positive pressure ventilation via the mouth as an alternative to tracheostomy for 257 ventilator users. Chest 103:174–182, 1993.
16. Bach JR, Kang SW: Disorders of ventilation: Weakness, stiffness, and mobilization. Chest 117:301–303, 2000.
17. Bach JR, McDermott I: Strapless oral-nasal interfaces for positive pressure ventilation. Arch Phys Med Rehabil 71:908–911, 1990.
18. Bach JR, Rajaraman R, Ballanger F, et al: Neuromuscular ventilatory insufficiency: The effect of home mechanical ventilator use vs. oxygen therapy on pneumonia and hospitalization rates. Am J Phys Med Rehabil 77:8–19, 1998.
19. Bach JR, Saporito LR: Criteria for extubation and tracheostomy tube removal for patients with ventilatory failure: A different approach to weaning. Chest 110:1566–1571, 1996.
20. Bach JR, Robert D, Leger P, Langevin B: Sleep fragmentation in kyphoscoliotic individuals with alveolar hypoventilation treated by nasal IPPV. Chest 107:1552–1558, 1995.
21. Bach JR, Alba AS, Bohatiuk G, et al: Mouth intermittent positive pressure ventilation in the management of postpolio respiratory insufficiency. Chest 91:859–864, 1987.
22. Bach JR, Alba AS, Bodofsky E, et al: Glossopharyngeal breathing and non- invasive aids in the management of post-polio respiratory insufficiency. Birth Defects 23:99–113, 1987.
23. Barach AL, Beck GJ: Exsufflation with negative pressure: Physiologic and clinical studies in poliomyelitis, bronchial asthma, pulmonary emphysema and bronchiectasis. Arch Intern Med 93:825–841, 1954.
24. Barach AL, Beck GJ, Bickerman HA, et al: Physical methods simulating mechanisms of the human cough. J Appl Physiol 5:825–841, 1952.
25. Barach AL, Beck GJ, Smith RH: Mechanical production of expiratory flow rates surpassing the capacity of human coughing. Am J Med Sci 226:241–248, 1953.
26. Beck GJ, Scarrone LA: Physiological effects of exsufflation with negative pressure. Dis Chest 29:1–16, 1956.
27. Birk T: Poliomyelitis and the post-polio syndrome. Med Sci Sports Exerc 25:466–472, 1993.
28. Braun NMT, Arora MS, Rochester DF: Respiratory muscle and pulmonary function in polymyositis and other proximal myopathies. Thorax 38:616–623, 1983.
29. Carroll N, Branthwaite MA: Control of nocturnal hypoventilation by nasal intermittent positive pressure ventilation. Thorax 43:349–353, 1988.
30. Carskadon M, Dement W: Respiration during sleep in the aged human. J Gerontol 36:420–425, 1981.
31. Dail CW, Affeldt JE: Glossopharyngeal Breathing [video]. Los Angeles, Department of Visual Education, College of Medical Evangelists, 1954.
32. Dail C, Rodgers M, Guess V, Adkins HV: Glossopharyngeal Breathing. Downey, CA, Rancho Los Amigos Department of Physical Therapy, 1979.
33. De Troyer A, Deisser P: The effects of intermittent positive pressure breathing on patients with respiratory muscle weakness. Am Rev Respir Dis 124:132–137, 1981.
34. De Boeck C, Zinman R: Cough versus chest physiotherapy: A comparison of the acute effects on pulmonary function in patients with cystic fibrosis. Am Rev Respir Dis 129:182–184, 1984.
35. DiMarco AF, Kelling JS, DiMarco MS, et al: The effects of inspiratory resistive training

on respiratory muscle function in patients with muscular dystrophy. Muscle Nerve 1985:8:284–290.

36. Elam JO, Hemingway A, Gullickson G, Visscher MB: Impairment of pulmonary function in poliomyelitis: Oximetric studies in patients with the spinal and bulbar types. Arch Intern Med 81:649–665, 1948.

37. Estenne M, De Troyer A: The effects of tetraplegia on chest wall statics. Am Rev Respir Dis 134:121–124, 1986.

38. Fischer DA: Poliomyelitis: Late respiratory complications and management. Orthopedics 8:891–894, 1985.

39. George CF, Millar TW, Kryger MH: Identification and quantification of apneas by computer-based analysis of oxygen saturation. Am Rev Respir Dis 137:1238–1240, 1988.

40. Guilleminault C, Motta J: Sleep apnea syndrome as a long-term sequelae of poliomyelitis. In Guilleminault C (ed): Sleep Apnea Syndromes. New York, KROC Foundation, 1978, pp 309–315.

41. Halstead LS, Wiechers DO, Rossi CD: Late effects of polio-myelitis: A national survey. In Halstead LS, Wiechers DO (eds): Late Effects of Poliomyelitis. Miami, Symposia Foundation, 1985, p 11.

42. Hardy KA: A review of airway clearance: New techniques, indications and recommendations. Respir Care 39:440–455, 1994.

43. He J, Kryger MH, Zorick FJ, et al: Mortality and apnea index in obstructive sleep apnea. Chest 94:9–14, 1988.

44. Hill R, Robbins AW, Messing R, Arora NS: Sleep apnea syndrome after poliomyelitis. Am Rev Respir Dis 127:129–131, 1983.

45. Historical Statistics of the United States: Colonial Times to 1970, Bicentennial Edition, Part 1. Washington, DC, U. S. Department of Commerce, Bureau of the Census, 1975, p 8, 77.

46. Hodes HL: Treatment of respiratory difficulty in poliomyelitis. In Poliomyelitis: Papers and Discussions Presented at the Third International Poliomyelitis Conference. Philadelphia, JB Lippincott, 1955, pp 91–113.

47. Howard RS, Wiles CM, Spencer GT: The late sequelae of poliomyelitis. Q J Med 66:219–232, 1988.

48. Hsu AA, Staats BA: "Postpolio" sequelae and sleep-related disordered breathing, Mayo Clin Proc 73:216–224, 1998.

49. Johnson EW, Braddom R: Over-work weakness in facioscapulohumeral muscular dystrophy. Arch Phys Med Rehabil 52:333–336, 1971.

50. Kaplan J, Fredrickson PA: Home pulse oximetry as a screening test for sleep-disordered breathing [abstract]. Chest 103(suppl):322, 1993.

51. Klefbeck B, Lagerstrand L, Mattsson E: Inspiratory muscle training in patients with prior polio who use part-time assisted ventilation. Arch Phys Med Rehabil 81:1065–1071, 2000.

52. Lassen HCA: The epidemic of poliomyelitis in Copenhagen, 1952. Proc R Soc Med 47:67–71, 1953.

53. Leger P, Jennequin J, Gerard M, Robert D: Home positive pressure ventilation via nasal mask for patients with neuromuscular weakness or restrictive lung or chest-wall disease. Respir Care 34:73–79, 1989.

54. Leith DE: Lung biology in health and desease: Respiratory defense mechainisms, part 2. In Brain JD, Proctor D, Reid L (eds): Cough. New York, Marcel Dekker, 1977, pp 545–592.

55. Lin MC, Liaw MY, Chen WJ, et al: Pulmonary function and spinal characteristics: The relationship in persons with idiopathic and postpoliomyelitic scoliosis. Arch Phys Med Rehabil 82:335–341, 2001.
56. Lombard R Jr, Zwillich CW: Medical therapy of obstructive sleep apnea. Med Clin North Am 69:1317–1335, 1985.
57. Martin AJ, Stern L, Yeates J, et al: Respiratory muscle training in Duchenne muscular dystrophy. Dev Med Child Neurol 28:314–318, 1986.
58. McDermott I, Bach JR, Parker C, Sortor S: Custom-fabricated interfaces for non-invasive intermittent positive pressure ventilation. Int J Prosthodontics 2:224–233, 1989.
59. Mier-Jedrzejowicz A, Brophy C, Green M: Respiratory muscle weakness during upper respiratory tract infections. Am Rev Respir Dis 138:5–7, 1988.
60. Miller HJ, Thomas E, Wilmot CB: Pneumobelt use among high quadriplegic population. Arch Phys Med Rehabil 69:369–372, 1988.
61. Patrick JA, Meyer-Witting M, Reynolds R, Spencer GT: Peri-operative care in restrictive respiratory disease. Anaesthesia 45:390–395, 1990.
62. Petrn K, Ehrenberg L: Etudes cliniques sur la poliomylite aigue. Nouv Inconog Salperiee 22:373, 546, 661, 1909.
63. Plum F, Swanson AG: Abnormalities in central regulation of respiration in acute and convalescent poliomyelitis. Arch Neurol Psych 80:267–285, 1958.
64. Ramlow J, Alexander M, LaPorte R, et al: Epidemiology of the post-polio syndrome. Am J Epidemiol 136:769–786, 1992.
65. Redline S, Tosteson T, Boucher MA, Millman RP: Measurement of sleep-related breathing disturbances in epidemiologic studies: Assessment of the validity and reproducibility of a portable monitoring device. Chest 100:1281–1286, 1991.
66. Rodillo E, Noble-Jamieson CM, Aber V, et al: Respiratory muscle training in Duchenne muscular dystrophy. Arch Dis Childhood 64:736–738, 1989.
67. Smolley LA: Obstructive sleep apnea: Avoiding diagnostic pitfalls. J Respir Dis 11:547–552, 1990.
68. Sortor S, McKenzie M: Toward Independence: Assisted Cough [video]. Dallas, Bio-Science Communications of Dallas, Inc., 1986.
69. Steljes DG, Kryger MH, Kirk BW, Millar TW: Sleep in postpolio syndrome. Chest 98:133–140, 1990.
70. Waldhorn RE, Herrick TW, Nguyen MC, et al: Long-term compliance with nasal continuous positive airway pressure therapy of obstructive sleep apnea. Chest 97:33–38, 1990.
71. Webber B, Higgens J: Glossopharyngeal breathing—what, when and how? [video]. Holbrook, Horsham, West Sussex, England, Aslan Studios Ltd., 1999.
72. Weinberg J, Borg J, Bevegard S, Sinderby C: Respiratory response to exercise in postpolio patients with severe inspiratory muscle dysfunction: Arch Phys Med Rehabil 80:1095–1100, 1999.
73. Williams EK, Holaday DA: The use of exsufflation with negative pressure in postoperative patients. Am J Surg 90:637–640, 1955.
74. Williams AJ, Yu G, Santiago S, Stein M: Screening for sleep apnea using pulse oximetry and a clinical score. Chest 100:631–635, 1991.

Speech and Swallowing in Postpolio Syndrome

Barbara C. Sonies, PhD

Evidence suggests that many polio survivors have changes in the oropharyngeal musculature that are similar to the changes in the proximal and distal muscle.[9] Because oropharyngeal deficits imply dysfunction of the bulbar muscles, it is important that individuals become aware of dysphagia and dysarthria and their evolution in polio survivors. The complications associated with swallowing difficulty, such as aspiration pneumonia, are not only serious but can also be life threatening; therefore, information on prevention and treatment needs to be disseminated.

Some controversy exists as to whether persons who did not have early bulbar symptoms would have new signs of speech and swallowing dysfunction.[3-6] A study by Sonies and Dalakas suggested that new swallowing symptoms may not always correspond to original symptoms and that persons with mild symptoms may not report them until they become moderate and compensations no longer work.[32] It is known that as many as 20–60% of persons who have had acute bulbar polio with or without symptoms of dysphagia or dysarthria can develop speech and swallowing problems decades after their initial symptoms.[15,25,27–30,33,36] It is probable that the late development of dysphagia and changes in speech and voice may relate to residual weakness of the oral, pharyngeal, or laryngeal muscles from the original insult or as the result of further neuronal degeneration associated with postpolio syndrome (PPS) that appears with increasing age or continual use of the surviving motor neuron axons. Normal aging in itself is not associated with oropharyngeal swallowing dysfunction; thus, any new signs of dysfunction are related to diseases or other conditions more commonly found as one ages.[32,32a]

This chapter reviews the findings of studies on PPS that relate to speech and swallowing and provides information relative to the role of speech-language pathologists in the evaluation and treatment of patients with these syndromes.

SPEECH AND VOICE

The majority of reports and articles reviewed for this chapter indicate that patients with acute bulbar polio have some late-appearing speech findings that reduce the intelligibility of their speech.[17,26,36] A review of the literature revealed that most of these studies are small case reports or observational studies in which the data were acquired from chart review. The commonly observed problems as a result of PPS were slurred speech, hypernasality, soft speaking voice, intermittent aphonia, and hoarseness.[1,12] These symptoms appeared to be present in some degree in the original acute episode and they often subsided, only to worsen decades later.

A study of three cases reported to have new laryngeal muscle weakness, progressive speech, and swallowing complaints all underwent surgical intervention to maintain the airway and optimize vocal quality.[26]

SWALLOWING

Swallowing consists of three interrelated phases (oral, pharyngeal, and esophageal) and an oral preparatory phase that act in concert to move food from the mouth to the stomach for further digestion. Varying degrees of change in strength, symmetry, coordination, and innervation of the muscles, nerves, and anatomic structures of the oropharynx, larynx, or esophagus can cause abnormal swallowing (dysphagia) in those with PPS.[7,11,18,19,21,24,32] Dysphagia is listed among the most common new manifestations of PPS in patients referred to postpolio clinics and is most likely caused by slowly progressive weakness in muscles that were previously affected but recovered, as well as in unaffected muscles.[17,24] Twenty patients were studied at the University of Michigan's postpolio clinic and followed for 2 years. Although only 10 had swallowing difficulties during their original attack of polio, new symptoms emerged in many other patients as they were followed.

THE OROPHARYNX

In our experience at the National Institutes of Health in evaluating postpolio patients, we find that fewer patients report oropharyngeal symptoms than problems with ambulation. It appears that swallowing is underreported because most persons have compensated for mild problems in transporting food and mild indigestion and have accepted these as common sequela of eating and mealtime experiences. Dysphagia is identified only when discomfort emerges and social eating is affected. The common signs that emerged in relation to the oropharyngeal swallowing in the 1995 follow-up study were that there was an increase in subjective complaints of difficulty swallowing (36% to 55%).[33] Increases in objective findings from the videofluoroscopic swallow study (VFS) and ultrasound showed that lingual pumping increased from 36% to 90%, delays in the total swallow increased from 36% to 100%, and abnormal hyoid elevation increased from 0% to 36% at 4 year follow-up. When the pharyngeal swallow was examined in these same patients, it was also evident that symptoms had progressed but no aspiration was noted. Pooling in the pyriform sinuses increased from

0% to 73%. Taken together, PPS had observable long-term effects on the oral swallow in agreement with most other long-term studies.

THE ESOPHAGUS

Several case studies of esophageal involvement have been reported in patients with PPS and may be more common in PPS combined with the effects of age. The esophagus is composed of striated muscles in the upper third and smooth muscles in the lower two thirds of this tubelike structure. It appears that a common finding of esophageal dysphagia in PPS is achalasia. This is "a motor disorder of the esophagus characterized by loss of esophageal peristalsis and failure of the lower esophageal sphincter (LES) to completely relax on deglutition."[37] In three reported studies of cases with PPS and achalasia, there was no original bulbar involvement.[2,10,23] In all of these cases of dilatation of the LES or myotomy, surgical interventions were performed with moderate success in alleviating the esophageal findings. No studies have established a direct causal relationship with PPS and the esophageal dysphagia.[5] Videofluorography (VF) is one of the primary radiologic methods used to evaluate the flow of barium through the esophagus and to diagnose esophageal function. The major esophageal findings in PPS revealed on VF are gastroesophageal reflux, pharyngeal reflux, Zenker's diverticulum, hiatal hernia, achalasia, and delayed relaxation of the upper esophageal sphincter.[20,23] In their 1995 4-year follow-up study, Sonies and Dalakas also found that esophageal reflux increased from 1% to 45% and delayed lower esophageal motility increased from 27% to 82%.[33]

It is difficult to determine if these findings are disease specific, but they are prevalent in PPS. However, it has been theorized that polio may cause a lesion in the dorsal motor nucleus of the vagus nerve that results in achalasia, this may add another component to the explanation for esophageal changes.

SYMPTOM PROGRESSION IN POSTPOLIO SYNDROME

The question of whether oropharyngeal function is affected by PPS has been addressed in several studies. In 1991, Sonies and Dalakas studied 32 patients with PPS using objective and repeated measures of swallowing and oral motor function in order to examine changes in a more reliable manner.[32] New symptoms that were not present in the original episode were revealed in 31 of 32 patients regardless of whether they were aware of these symptoms or whether there was bulbar involvement present when they were originally diagnosed with polio. Of these 32 patients, two had signs indicative of possible risk for aspiration. All 32 were reexamined 2 years later, and four had objective signs of worsening or new symptoms of oropharyngeal dysfunction. At their 4-year follow-up, minimal changes were found in oral motor function, but the average swallow severity rating on the modified barium swallow (MBS) changed from mild to moderate. The observed changes did not limit oral intake or increase the risk of aspiration because they were all using recommended compensatory swallowing strategies. In 1994, Ivanyi and colleagues followed eight patients with PPS using videofluoroscopy for 12 to 36 months who had no bulbar involvement, and no swallowing complaints.[14] All of the subjects had mild general findings of bulbar involvement and all complained of food catching in the throat at follow-up.

Results of these studies appear to suggest that in the bulbar neurons, there is a slowly progressive deterioration, similar to that observed in the muscles of the limbs. This finding suggests a possible causal relationship between dysphagia progression and PPS progression.[32,33] It can be concluded that although progression of speech and swallowing symptoms is slow, objective measures of swallowing accurately reflect disease progression. Therefore, all phases of the swallow should be reexamined every 3–4 years. Because they used the recommended compensatory swallowing strategies, all subjects who were followed maintained airway safety at their 4-year follow-up study.[33] Therefore, it is recommended that persons with PPS who have complaints seek out a speech-language pathologist who can provide intervention.[17,28]

RECENT SURVEY OF 23 PATIENTS WITH POSTPOLIO SYNDROME

An informal two-page survey was administered to 23 individuals with PPS who attend a support group for families and former patients.[34a] A checklist survey was developed and circulated to all members of the support group inquiring about initial onset, initial symptoms, and changes experienced in the most recent 5 to 10 years. The questions included changes in general weakness, upper and lower extremity function, speech, breathing, swallowing, and eating. There were 10 male and 23 female respondents with ages ranging from 52 to 84 years whose initial illness occurred over the period from 1932 to 1955 and ranged from 20 to 55 years after the initial polio episode. Of the 23 respondents, 21 reported having problems with ambulation, 7 with swallowing, 4 with speech, and 3 with breathing when first affected with polio. All reported that walking assistance was needed, 8 used a cane or walker, 10 were in a wheelchair, and 5 required an electronic scooter for mobility after their initial polio. Balance was difficult for 16, four had problems with upper extremity use such holding objects, and opening jars or lifting and opening doors was difficult for 8 subjects. Changes experienced in the previous 5–10 years indicated exacerbation of problems so that new weakness was reported in the legs or feet in 21, hands or arms in 14, neck and back in 11, speech and voice problems in 12, and difficulty breathing in 11 subjects. Of the 7 subjects who had initial complaints of difficulty swallowing, 5 remained with problems. Seven respondents reported new complaints for a total of 12 of the 23 who had difficulty swallowing. A range of swallowing symptoms was present with "food sticking in the throat" and "trouble swallowing pills" reported in 9 of the 12 with complaints. Swallowing both liquids and solids was difficult for seven subjects and 6 reported that they coughed repeatedly during eating. Reflux was also reported in 7 respondents but may be more related to age alone rather than exacerbation of symptoms. A single respondent thought that choking was worsening and was more prevalent with drinking water. This survey adds to our impression of exacerbation of symptoms and suggests the importance of intervention by speech-language pathologists with expertise in dysphagia.

ROLE OF THE SPEECH-LANGUAGE PATHOLOGIST

Because of the high prevalence of speech, voice, and swallowing complications arising from new changes in oropharyngeal, laryngeal, and esophageal muscle function, referral for evaluation, treatment, and follow-up to a speech-language pathologist is essential. The first step in this process is a complete evaluation of oral-sensory-motor function. This examination lays the foundation for further assessment and is the cornerstone of later therapeutic intervention. The services provided by the speech-language pathologist include screening, clinical assessments, and instrumental voice and swallowing assessments. When swallowing is the primary consideration, services terminate when the patient is nutritionally stable and able to eat with or without special dietary modifications and compensatory strategies.

VOICE ASSESSMENT

Major speech and voice complaints in persons who have had polio and in those with PPS are hypernasality, reduced volume, intermittent aphonia, and hoarseness. These may all have their origin in impaired vocal cord function caused by paralysis of one vocal cord or weakness of other muscles of the larynx. Assessment of voice and vocal cord function may include a fiber optic or nasoendoscopic view of the laryngeal area at rest and during phonation as well as a voice recording. The fiber-optic endoscopic examination (FEES), or nasoendoscopy, is often conducted jointly with an otolaryngologist. The otolaryngologist determines whether structural abnormalities are present that affect voice production or whether surgical intervention is recommended. The speech-language pathologist uses the results of this examination in planning voice therapy.

SWALLOWING ASSESSMENT

A swallowing self-assessment questionnaire should be administered as a first step to determine how the patient perceives his or her ability to swallow. It also guides the clinician in determining how accurate the patient is in explaining his or her complaints.[29] Some of the signs for dysphagia are unintentional weight loss, depression, loss of interest in eating, coughing or choking when eating, food sticking in the throat, difficulty swallowing pills, or indigestion and heartburn. When several of the signs listed in Table 1 are present, the patient should be referred for a more complete clinical swallowing examination that may also include instrumental swallowing assessments (e.g., videofluorography, nasoendoscopy, ultrasound, manometry).

CLINICAL EXAMINATION

The speech-language pathologist conducts a clinical examination of the oropharyngeal and upper aerodigestive structures to examine whether there are abnormal findings that can be associated with PPS.[35] When completed, this examination provides information on the anatomy, symmetry, sensation, strength, and coordination of the lingual, labial, velar, pharyngeal, and facial musculature. This information is used to determine if specific strategies or compensatory maneuvers would be helpful to improve speech, voice, and swallowing. It is important to review the medical history for the effects of medications and any preexisting medical conditions, surgical procedures, and cognitive and psychiatric findings and to interview the patient to affirm reported findings. During the interview, the speech pathologist questions the patient regarding cultural, religious, and socioeconomic issues that may impact function. Mealtime observations are often included in the clinical examination to better assess swallowing. For example, in PPS, the patient would be observed to determine if facial asymmetry was present and how the body was aligned during eating. For patients with PPS, hemiparesis is often present in the oral area. When greater weakness on one side of the body is present, special therapeutic feeding maneuvers may be used effectively.

Oral hygiene and dental condition are other factors included in a clinical examination that impact on speech and swallowing. When hemiparesis exists, cleansing the mouth may be less than optimal, and it has been established that oral bacteria entering the trachea and lungs may be a primary cause of aspiration pneumonia. Thus, persons with PPS must be counseled to observe good oral hygiene.

Table 1. SELF-ASSESSMENT QUESTIONNAIRE FOR DYSPHAGIA

- Do you have difficulty swallowing?
- Do you have pain when you swallow?
- Do you have difficulty chewing hard foods?
- Do you have a dry mouth?
- Do you have excessive saliva or drooling?
- Do you cough or choke before, during, or after swallowing?
- Do you have a feeling that food catches or remains in your throat?
- Do you have mucus dripping into the throat or postnasal drip?
- Does your voice become hoarse after swallowing?
- Do you notice digested particles coming up into your mouth or throat?
- Do you have heartburn or indigestion?
- Do you have difficulty swallowing liquids?
- Do liquids come back up into your nose?
- Do you have difficulty swallowing solids?
- Do you have difficulty swallowing pills?
- Does it take you long to eat?
- Are you embarrassed because of how you eat?
- Have you had episodes of airway obstruction or choking when eating?
- Have you had pneumonia or aspiration pneumonia?

Adapted from Sonies BC, Parent LJ, Morrish K, Baum BJ: Durational aspects of the oral-pharyngeal phase of swallow in normal adults. Dysphagia 3:1–10, 1988; and Sonies BC, Weiffenbach J, Atkinson JC, et al: Clinical examination of motor and sensory functions of the adult oral cavity. Dysphagia 1:178–186, 1987.

INSTRUMENTAL ASSESSMENT OF SWALLOWING

Speech language-pathologists conduct several instrumental procedures to assess safety for oral feeding and to determine if there are swallowing strategies that reduce risk of aspiration. The purpose of these techniques is to examine oral pharyngeal physiology during bolus flow from the oral cavity to the stomach. Each of the procedures has advantages and limitations in safety, ease of administration, comfort, and completeness of information in the output of the image.

Videofluorography

The most complete procedure and the gold standard used to study the swallow is the MBS or VFS (videofluorography) because it images the anatomy of the entire digestive tract and clearly demonstrates bolus flow throughout the tract from mouth to stomach.[22] This procedure is the most appropriate one for diagnosing pharyngeal dysphagia. Its primary limitation is radiation exposure; therefore, caution must be followed during repeated examinations to minimize tissue changes from radiation. Of lesser concern is the unnatural taste and consistency of barium because several commercial products are being developed to improve taste and standardize consistency. During the study, the speech-language pathologist uses different bolus sizes, consistencies, and barium-coated food to examine how the individual swallows. Screening for esophageal dismotility and esophageal or pharyngeal reflux signals referral to a physician for consideration of medical treatment. The speech pathologist is trained to conduct and interpret the results of this study in order to develop an individualized treatment plan to increase adequacy of airway protection, increase nutritional uptake, and increase safety during oral feeding.

Fiberoptic Endoscopic Evaluation or Nasoendoscopy

This examination uses a flexible fiberoptic scope inserted transnasally to the level of the laryngopharynx. One can detect spillage into the valleculae, pyriform sinuses, laryngeal vestibule, and upper trachea before or after the swallow. Residue in the pharynx and risk for later aspiration of ingested material can be determined with FEES. It does not replace the videofluorographic study because the oropharynx cannot be observed with this method. In many cases of polio or PPS, the primary reason for speech or swallowing impairment is weakness or incoordination of the tongue, velum, or oral soft tissues that cannot be seen using this procedure. Therefore, use of FEES is indicated when laryngeal dysfunction is suspected. FEES is performed independently by some speech-language pathologists and in concert with an otolaryngologist in some states and settings.

Ultrasound Imaging

Ultrasound is used by speech-language pathologists to evaluate speech and swallowing.[31,32] Ultrasound is safe, noninvasive, and allows studies to be conducted in the most natural manner using real foods while the patient is seated during eating. Precise movement of the hyoid bone, tongue, and floor of the mouth can be visualized, and the timing of speech and swallowing can be directly assessed. The oral preparation of food and transfer of the bolus into the pharynx is easily defined. Oral structures can be viewed in three dimensions and multiple planes to evaluate progress when continual monitoring is required. It has been found to be helpful for polio because it easily images the activity of the tongue and floor muscles of the mouth and can detect lingual compensations or lingual asymmetry that can be used for biofeedback in the treatment of both speech and swallowing.

Although some other instrumental procedures can be used to study the aerodigestive tract, such as manometry and scintigraphy, these are medical procedures and not generally conducted for purposes of determining behavioral treatment.

The most common findings relative to swallowing difficulty in postpolio in each of the phases of swallowing (i.e., oral preparatory, oral, pharyngeal, esophageal) can be seen in Table 2. Among these are delayed pharyngeal response, residue in the valleculae and pyriform sinuses, and impaired hyoid motion. Taken together, they signal risk for laryngeal penetration and possible aspiration after the swallow.

Table 2. COMMON SWALLOWING FINDINGS IN POSTPOLIO PATIENTS FROM INSTRUMENTAL STUDIES

Oral Preparatory Phase
- Tongue weakness
- Tongue incoordination
- Lingual hemiparesis
- Lingual residue
- Palatal residue

Oral Phase
- Tongue weakness
- Tongue hemiparesis
- Palatal asymmetry
- Reduced velar elevation
- Lingual pumping
- Extra swallowing gestures
- Multiple swallows needed to clear mouth
- Delays in initiating a swallow
- Bolus dripping into valleculae before onset of swallow
- Nasal regurgitation (infrequent)

Pharyngeal Phase
- Delayed pharyngeal response
- Unilateral pooling of the bolus in valleculae
- Unilateral pooling of bolus in pyriform sinus
- Pooling on the side of the major body weakness
- Laryngeal penetration or aspiration
- Incomplete laryngeal closure
- Impaired hyoid motion
- Epiglottic tilting

Esophageal Phase
- Hiatal hernia
- Gastroesophageal reflux
- Esophageal spasm
- Zenker's diverticula

TREATMENT PROVIDED BY THE SPEECH-LANGUAGE PATHOLOGIST

SPEECH AND VOICE TREATMENT

Methods of voice treatment include those that improve volume, reduce hoarseness, reduce nasality, and stimulate vocal fold adduction. Most of the voice retraining techniques use recorded spectral displays, computerized programs, and biofeedback techniques to display when voice quality is within an acceptable range. Self-monitoring and self-evaluation of taped recordings are often used for increasing volume, and specific techniques that improve breath support and pitch are also effective.

SWALLOWING TREATMENT

Swallowing treatment should be initiated to facilitate safe oral feeding needed to sustain adequate health and nutrition. Treatment can be divided into two broad categories: *direct* (food is used) and *indirect* (no food used) swallowing treatment . During the VFS examination, several direct strategies are implemented to determine if they improve the quality and safety of the swallow. These strategies are directly determined from the symptoms of dysphagia seen on VFS and are attempted during the study to determine their usefulness. If they reduce the risk of aspiration and improve the safety of the swallow, they should be incorporated into the therapeutic sessions.

Direct Treatment Strategies

The speech pathologist administers direct swallowing treatment to patients who are able to take food orally but are inconsistent in protecting the airway or have reduced oral motor control, asymmetry, or muscle weakness. Various head and body postures based on VFS findings are used to redirect the bolus and eliminate pharyngeal residue. They include lowering, elevating, and rotating the head and chin.[22] During direct treatment, all food or liquid is presented while therapeutic risk-reduction strategies are used. Direct therapy techniques can also include oral range of motion, lingual resistance, bolus control, vocal fold adduction, laryngeal elevation, tongue base maneuvers, and specific sensory stimulation (i.e., thermal-tactile) for swallowing. Other sensory stimulation techniques may use taste, temperature, texture, and pressure applied to the tongue, lips, velum, pharynx, and external face to stimulate a swallow. If lip seal is weak or mastication and jaw mobility are impaired, other compensations can be used.

Additional swallowing maneuvers can be used to remediate specific problems that impede swallowing.[22] These maneuvers are used to improve vocal fold closure and pharyngeal delays (i.e., supraglottic swallow), close the airway (i.e., super-supraglottic swallow), improve motion of the tongue base (i.e., effortful swallow), and extend opening of the upper esophageal sphincter (i.e., Mendelsohn maneuver).

A variety of biofeedback techniques that include EMG, ultrasound, and laryngeal stimulation can be used to improve swallowing and provide input regarding the patient's ability to reach a target pattern or simulate a profile of a swallow. Whereas ultrasound provides immediate visual input on the way the oral structures coordinate, the other techniques use sensors affixed to the throat that give a line tracing of activity.

For patients with PPS or polio, any of these techniques may be beneficial. However, the most helpful techniques attempt to accommodate for tongue weakness and unilateral pharyngeal or laryngeal muscle weakness.

Dietary modifications are another common direct compensatory technique. Evidence suggests that in neurologic conditions, it is more difficult to swallow liquids; therefore, the use of thickened liquids is often beneficial. The speech pathologist works with the dietitian and the family to determine specific dietary modifications. The speech pathologist then implements these modifications into the overall treatment.

Indirect Treatment Strategies

Some patients with severe dysphagia are unable to clear the airway using a volitional protective cough to clear the material from the laryngeal area. For these patients, food is ill advised and indirect treatment should be initiated. Saliva, tiny drops of water, or lemon-flavored drops of water may be used to stimulate saliva and lubricate the oral cavity as a precursor to indirect therapy. Even intubated non-oral feeders can receive indirect swallow therapy to teach compensatory maneuvers before food is introduced. For patients with severe limitations, a suck–swallow motion may be used or direct tactile stimulation to the lips, tongue, and pharynx may be necessary. Some patients benefit from practicing on an empty straw, and others benefit from stimulation using a cold laryngeal mirror or ices. Therapeutic feeding of small amounts of purees may be used when the patient does not have sufficient strength for oral eating. The speech pathologist works with the patient during the transition from indirect to direct feeding.

Most patients with PPS are able to benefit from direct treatment strategies, and in our experience, few are non-oral feeders.

Summary

Speech-language pathologists who have experience with swallowing can use a variety of instrumental procedures to examine the safety and physiology of the swallow; among the most common procedures are videofluoroscopy, FEES, and ultrasound. Other procedures used in cooperation with a physician are manometry and scintigraphy, an esophagram, and endoscopy. Speech pathologists look for signs and symptoms based on a combination of the clinical and instrumental examination to match symptoms with treatment. Signs of dysphagia most common in polio are "choking" on food and a feeling that "food catches" in the throat. When these are noted, in-depth evaluation procedures should be conducted. When considering which treatment strategies are most helpful in patients with PPS, direct procedures of dietary and postural modifications along with indirect oral stimulation procedures appear most helpful. In general, repeated oral motor exercises that can cause fatigue to the oral pharyngeal system are not recommended in those with PPS. Surgical procedures such as myotomy have not proven totally successful, and unless dysphagia is so severe that nutrition cannot be maintained, placement of a percutaneous endoscopic gastrostomy (PEG) is not recommended.

CONCLUSION

Polio survivors are at increased risk for developing oral pharyngeal muscle weakness that can impact on swallowing and speech production. Swallowing changes constitute a major risk and must be monitored to ensure that the airway is protected and that proper nutrition is maintained. Speech-language pathologists are trained to evaluate and treat speech and swallowing impairment and can use a variety of techniques to improve functioning. Because swallowing is a complex problem, the cooperative efforts of radiologists, gastroenterologists, and otolaryngologists are often required in the diagnostic process. Dietitians are also part of the effort to maintain proper nutrition and work cooperatively with speech-language pathologists. Treatment of the behavioral and physiological aspects of swallowing is the domain of speech-language pathologists. Patients with polio and PPS should be monitored periodically for signs of dysphagia, because they are often unaware of change because of continual use of compensations and lack of understanding of danger signs for aspiration.

References

1. Baugh RF: Otolaryngology manifestation of post polio syndrome. J Natl Med Assoc 85:689–691, 1993.
2. Benini L, Sembenini C, Bulighin GM, et al: Achalasia: A possible late cause of postpolio dysphagia. Dig Dis Sci 41:516–518, 1996.
3. Buchholz D: Dysphagia in post-polio patients. Arch Phys Med Rehabil 69:634–636, 1988.
4. Buchholz DW: Postpolio dysphagia [editorial; comment]. Dysphagia 9:99–100, 1994.
5. Buchholz D, Jones B: Dysphagia occurring after polio. Otolaryngol Head Neck Surg 104:333–338, 1991.
6. Buchholz DW, Jones B: Post-polio dysphagia: Alarm or caution? [editorial]. Orthopedics 14:1303–1305, 1991.
7. Coelho CA, Ferrante R: Dysphagia in postpolio sequelae: Report of three cases. Chung Hua I Hsueh Tsa Chih 43:208–212, 1989.
8. Coelho CA, Ferrante R: Incidence and nature of dysphagia in polio survivors. Arch Phys Med Rehabil 72:1071–1075, 1991.
9. Dalakas M (ed): The Post-Polio Syndrome as an Evolved Clinical Entity. New York, New York Academy of Sciences, 1995.
10. Dantas RO, Meneghelli UG: Achalasia occurring years after acute poliomyelitis. Arch Gastroenterol 30(2–3):58–61, 1993.
11. Dowhaniuk M, Schentag CT: Dysphagia in individuals with no history of bulbar polio. Ann NY Acad Sci 753:405–407, 1995.
12. Driscoll BP, Gracco C, Coelho C, et al: Laryngeal function in postpolio patients. Laryngoscope. 105:35–41, 1995.
13. Garfinkle TJ, Kimmelman CP: Neurologic disorders: amyotrophic lateral sclerosis, myasthenia gravis, multiple sclerosis, and poliomyelitis. JPEN J Parenter Enteral Nutr 6:457–459, 1982.
14. Ivanyi B, Phoa SS, de Visser M: Dysphagia in postpolio patients: A videofluorographic follow-up study. Dysphagia 9:96–98, 1994.
15. Ivanyi B, Nollet F, Redekop WK, et al: Late onset polio sequelae. Arch Phys Med Rehabil 80:687–690, 1999.

16. Jones B, Buchholz DW, Ravich WJ, Donner MW: Swallowing dysfunction in the post-polio syndrome: A cinefluorographic study. AJR Am J Roentgenol 158:283–286, 1992.
17. Jubelt B, Agre J: Characteristics and management of postpolio syndrome. JAMA 284:412–414, 2000.
18. Jubelt B, Cashman NR: Neurological manifestations of the post-polio syndrome. Crit Rev Neurobiol 3:199–220, 1987.
19. Jubelt B, Drucker J: Post-polio syndrome: an update. Semin Neurol 13:283–290, 1993.
20. Kilman WJ, Goyal RK: Disorders of pharyngeal and upper esophageal sphincter motor function. Am J Otolaryngol 3:204–212, 1982.
21. LeCompte CM: Post polio syndrome: An update for the primary health care provider. Nurse Pract 22:133–136, 139, 142–136 passim, 1997.
22. Logemann JL: Evaluation and Treatment of Swallowing Disorders, 2nd ed. Austin, Texas, Pro-Ed, 1998.
23. Mamel JJ: Protracted postpoliomyelitis dysphagia managed with enteral feeding and cricopharyngeal myotomy. Birth Defect Orig Artic Ser 23:55–62, 1987.
24. Munsat TL: Dysphagia in the post-polio syndrome. Poliomyelitis—new problems with an old disease [editorial; comment] [see comments]. N Engl J Med 325:1107–1109, 1991.
25. Ramlow J, Alexander M, LaPorte R, et al: Epidemiology of the post-polio syndrome. Am Epidemiol 136:769–786, 1992.
26. Robinson LR, Hillel AD, Waugh PF: New laryngeal muscle weakness in post-polio syndrome. Laryngoscope 108:732–734, 1988.
27. Schneider S, Ernst U, Duker J, Lucking CH: [Post-polio syndrome with isolated dysphagia]. Nervenarzt 65:560–562, 1994.
28. Silbergleit AK, Waring WP, Sullivan MJ, Maynard FM: Evaluation, treatment, and follow-up results of post polio patients with dysphagia. N Engl J Med 324:1162–1167, 1991.
29. Sonies B: Long-term effects of post-polio on oral-motor and swallowing function. In Halstead L, Grimby G (eds): Post-Polio Syndrome. Philadelphia, Hanley & Belfus, 1995, pp 124–140.
30. Sonies BC: Dysphagia and post-polio syndrome: Past, present, and future. Semin Neurol 16:365–370, 1996.
31. Sonies BC, Chi-Fishman G, Miller J: Ultrasound imaging and swallowing. In Jones B (ed): Normal and Abnormal Swallowing, 2nd ed. New York, Springer-Verlag, 2002.
32. Sonies BC, Dalakas MC: Dysphagia in patients with the post-polio syndrome [see comments]. N Engl J Med 324:1206–1207, 1991.
32a. Sonies BC: Oropharyngeal dysphagia in the elderly. Geriatr Clin North Am 8:569–577, 1992.
33. Sonies BC, Dalakas MC: Progression of oral-motor and swallowing symptoms in the post-polio syndrome. Ann N Y Acad Sci 753:87–95, 1995.
34. Sonies BC, Parent LJ, Morrish K, Baum BJ: Durational aspects of the oral-pharyngeal phase of swallow in normal adults. Dysphagia 3:1–10, 1988.
34a. Sonies BC, Spermeuli M: Postpolio Questionnaire [unpublished survey], 2003.
35. Sonies BC, Weiffenbach J, Atkinson JC, et al: Clinical examination of motor and sensory functions of the adult oral cavity. Dysphagia 1:178–186, 1987.
36. Windebank AJ, Litchy WJ, Danube JR, et al: Late effects of paralytic poliomyelitis in Olmsted County, Minnesota. Neurology 41:501–507, 1991.
37. Wong RK, Maydonovitch CL: Achalasia. In Castll DO (ed): The Esophagus, 2nd ed. New York, Little, Brown, 1995, pp 219–246.

Exercise in the Treatment of Postpolio Syndrome

James C. Agre, MD, PhD

A number of reports have documented that many polio survivors are complaining of new musculoskeletal and neuromuscular symptoms.[1-11] New fatigue, weakness, and difficulties with walking and stair climbing are frequent complaints (Table 1).[5,6,8,9] Cosgrove et al. indicated that decreasing endurance was the single most common complaint in polio survivors.[4] Berlly et al. reported that two thirds of postpolio subjects complained of increasing loss of strength during exercise, a heavy sensation of the muscles, or both.[7] It appears that some of the new problems faced by polio survivors may be related to declining neuromuscular function, which includes decreasing muscle strength and endurance as well as increasing difficulty with fatigue. A concern has been raised as to whether or not exercise or excessive activity may lead to the onset or progression of new or increasing weakness or fatigue in postpolio individuals.

Reasonable criteria for the diagnosis of postpolio syndrome (PPS) have been proposed by Halstead[12] and include the following: (1) prior paralytic polio confirmed by history, physical examination, and electromyography; (2) a period of neurologic recovery followed by an extended interval of functional stability usually lasting 20 or more years; (3) gradual or abrupt onset of nondisuse weakness in previously affected or unaffected muscles, which may be accompanied by other new health problems such as excessive fatigue, muscle pain, joint pain, decreased endurance, decreased function, atrophy, and so forth; and (4) exclusion of medical, orthopedic, and neurologic conditions that might cause the new health problems. These criteria are based on the assumption that the pathologic process involves some motor unit dysfunction with a variable contribution from musculoskeletal overuse. For this reason, Halstead has stated that nondisuse weakness is considered a necessary finding to make the diagnosis of PPS: "Ideally, then, the diagnosis of post-polio syndrome should only be made after a trial of closely supervised exercise to exclude the possibility of disuse weakness."[12] In actuality, however, this suggestion has not been followed. To the author's

Table 1. NEW HEALTH AND ACTIVITIES OF DAILY LIVING
COMPLAINTS IN POSTPOLIO INDIVIDUALS

SYMPTOM	STUDY			
	HALSTEAD & ROSSI[8] ($N = 539$), %	HALSTEAD AND ROSSI[5] ($N = 132$), %	AGRE ET AL.[6] ($N = 79$), %	LONNBERG[9] ($N = 3607$), %
New Health Complaints				
Fatigue	87	89	86	62
Weakness				
Previously affected muscles	87	69	80	54
Previously unaffected muscles	77	50	53	33
Muscle pain	80	71	86	39
Joint pain	79	71	77	51
Cold intolerance	—	29	56	42
Atrophy	—	28	39	—
New ADL Complaints				
Walking	85	64	—	52
Stair climbing	83	61	67	54
Dressing	62	17	16	17

ADL = activities of daily living.

knowledge, none of the studies cited in the scientific and medical literature have followed this specific recommendation. Additionally, each published study may have used somewhat different criteria (often not specifically stated in the article) for the definition of PPS.

Physical exercise is known to be very important to the health and well-being of people.[13–15] This has been known to mankind since at least the time of the ancient Greeks. Whereas regular exercise is known to have a number of beneficial effects, inactivity is known to be associated with a number of adverse effects. Beneficial physiologic effects of regular exercise include reduced heart rate and blood pressure (BP) at rest and during submaximal exercise, morphological changes in skeletal and cardiac muscle, improved muscular strength, increased muscular endurance, improved physical work capacity, enhanced cardiovascular efficiency, and improved aerobic capacity.[13–15] Beneficial psychological adaptations are not as easily quantifiable but include reduced muscular tension; better sense of well-being; improvement in sleep; and aids in motivation to improve other health habits such as dietary changes, weight reduction, and smoking cessation.[13–15] In contrast, limitation in activity level has a number of deleterious effects, including increased resting heart rate and BP at rest and during submaximal exercise, reduced muscular strength, reduced muscular endurance, reduced physical work capacity, diminished cardiovascular efficiency, reduced aerobic capacity, and increased incidence of lipid and lipoprotein abnormalities.[13–15] Several years ago Agre et al. reported an increase in total cholesterol in male and female post-polio patients and a reduction in high-density lipoprotein cholesterol in male post-polio patients.[15a] Although not proven in the study (because it was simply a descriptive study), reduction in physical activity in these patients may have been a factor in their lipid and lipoprotein abnormalities. Excessive activity and overexercise can also lead to problems. It is well known in the sports medicine literature that excessive activity may result in overuse injuries. Thus, the exercise program for any individual, able-bodied or disabled, must strike the correct balance between exercise and appropriate rest and recovery time. This balance is different for each individual.

At the present time, no universal statement can be made regarding specific exercises that will benefit all postpolio individuals. It is doubtful that such will ever be the case. When recommending a therapeutic exercise program for a postpolio individual, one needs to take into consideration the patient's particular clinical situation in order for the program to benefit the patient and not lead to overuse problems. This can be quite challenging for clinicians because every patient is unique. The initial acute poliomyelitis illness affected each patient differently. In each patient, the pattern of muscle weakness is different. For reasons as yet unknown, some muscles were relatively spared and others were severely affected; also, the involvement was often asymmetrical. Thus, in a given patient, some muscles in a limb could have been severely affected by the initial poliomyelitis illness and should be protected from exercise, but other muscles may not be able to receive sufficient exercise so that the severely affected muscles can be protected from overuse. The same principle is true when considering joint pathology. Significant degenerative joint disease is likely to be found in joints in the vicinity of severely weakened muscles. Exercise that might be beneficial to the muscles may lead to further pain from arthritis or arthralgia. When prescribing an exercise program for a specific postpolio individual, it is imperative to take all of the above into consideration and derive an exercise program that will maximally benefit that individual without leading to increased fatigue or muscle or joint pain. This can be very difficult and, in practice, requires a well-considered exercise program and careful evaluation and follow-up of the postpolio patient participating in the program.

This chapter summarizes the evidence cited in the literature linking exercise or activity to the onset or progression of PPS and the maintenance of strength and well-being in postpolio patients.

EVIDENCE LINKING EXERCISE OR ACTIVITY TO THE ONSET AND PROGRESSION OF POSTPOLIO SYNDROME

Previously published reports have identified various predictive factors for the development of PPS.[16–18] In addition to other factors cited, these predictive factors have included a greater severity of the acute poliomyelitis illness,[5,16,19–22] a greater functional recovery after the acute paralytic illness, and a lower residual disability level at the time of presentation to the postpolio clinic[21] and level of physical activity or recent increase in physical activity.[21–30]

SEVERITY OF ACUTE POLIOMYELITIS ILLNESS

A number of studies have reported an association between a greater severity of the acute poliomyelitis illness and the development of PPS.[5,16,18–22] Two of these reports are epidemiologic studies,[18,19] three are clinical reports,[5,16,21] and one is a longitudinal (observational) study in which postpolio individuals were divided into stable and unstable (acknowledging progressive loss of strength) groups.[22] Based on the present hypothesis for the pathogenesis of PPS, the severity of the acute paralytic poliomyelitis illness is an approximate measure of the initial destruction of anterior horn cells. Recovery of strength in the subacute phase is by terminal motor unit reorganization, resulting in significantly enlarged motor units, and by muscle hypertrophy of the myofibrils with exercise. Over time, however, the significantly enlarged motor units may be at risk for deterioration. There is both electrophysiologic and histologic evidence for ongoing denervation and reinnervation of the surviving motor units.[3,31–33] There is also evidence for loss or deterioration of the very large motor units in postpolio individuals over time.[34] Grimby et al. reported the findings of an 8-year longitudinal evaluation of 21 postpolio individuals.[34] Over this period of time, knee extension strength declined by 9% to 15%; endurance decreased; capillarization (i.e., number of blood capillaries per muscle fiber) declined by 15%; and median macro electromyogram (EMG) amplitude increased in 20 legs but decreased in eight of nine legs in which median macro EMG amplitude was 20 times or more greater than normal at the onset of the study. This study demonstrated evidence of ongoing denervation or reinnervation as well as a failing capacity to maintain very large motor units. The break point appeared to be when the median macro EMG amplitude reached a size of 20 times normal. From a theoretical standpoint, individuals who had a more severe acute paralytic poliomyelitis illness and had very large, and probably fragile, motor units would be at greater risk to develop PPS as a result of greater than expected loss in muscle strength through the loss or deterioration of the surviving motor units. It is certainly possible that excessive activity or exercise in these individuals could overstress and ultimately lead to the deterioration or death of the largest, and most fragile, motor units. This process would result in functional decline and the onset of PPS.

GREATER FUNCTIONAL RECOVERY AND LOWER RESIDUAL DISABILITY

Klingman et al. reported an association between the development of PPS and a lower level of residual disability and a greater functional recovery after the acute paralytic illness.[21] This was a retrospective study in which the records of 288 patients with a history of polio were reviewed. Records from 57 patients with PPS (those complaining of declining muscle strength with no other explanation found for the decline) were selected and compared with records of 49 postpolio patients without a history of progressive weakness. Initial weakness was scored on a 6-point scale (1 point given for involvement for each limb, 1 for the back, and 1 for respiratory dysfunction). Those individuals with the most widespread acute involvement were considered to be the most severely affected. Residual disability was indexed by a 5-point scale (0 = no functional disability; 1 = mild disability without need for braces; 2 = moderate disability but ambulatory with braces; 3 = severe disability and used a wheelchair exclusively for mobility; and 4 = total disability and bedridden). Functional recovery was calculated as the arithmetic difference between the initial severity (i.e., initial weakness score) and residual disability scores. The level of residual disability was negatively correlated with the development of PPS and the degree of functional recovery was directly correlated with the development of PPS.

These two reported findings certainly make sense with what is found in postpolio patients in the clinical setting. Individuals who had a more severe acute paralytic illness and resultant greater residual disability (especially those with residual disability scores of 3 or 4, as in this study) would be less likely to have further significant deterioration in function related to the floor effect of the scale. On the other hand, individuals with the greatest functional recovery (i.e., those with the most widespread initial involvement and least residual disability, especially those with no *apparent* functional disability or only *apparent* mild disability, as per the scales used in this study) are at the great risk for the development of postpolio-related problems.

A retrospective clinical study of 104 postpolio patients seen in a postpolio clinic reported by Waring and colleagues[35] provides credibility to this concept. They reported that only 19 patients (18%) were using an orthotic device at the time of the clinical evaluation. After the clinical evaluation, they recommended a number of things to each patient specific to the patient's particular problems. This included a prescription for new orthotic devices for 37 patients (36%). Most of these patients had used orthotic devices in the distant past but then discarded them. Thus, these individuals probably had a significant acute paralysis or paresis and then probably experienced greater functional recovery. After their clinical evaluations, all subjects were sent a questionnaire to complete; 81 patients (78%) returned the questionnaire. Results from the 81 returned questionnaires indicated that patients noted statistically significant ($P < 0.05$) improvements in the ability to walk, perceived walking safety, and reduced knee and overall pain. In the 32 patients who received new orthotic devices and returned the questionnaire, 19 of them reported using the orthotic device daily; 13 patients only used them sporadically. Comparing the data from these two groups showed that those who used their orthotic devices daily rather than only sporadically had statistically significant ($P < 0.05$) improvements in fatigue, weakness, ability to walk, perceived walking safety, and knee pain. This study suggested that the use of appropriate assistive devices can significantly reduce the energy cost for ambulation in postpolio individuals as well as reduce pain and increase the perception of safety while ambulating.

In another clinical study, Luna-Reyes and colleagues demonstrated that the energy cost of ambulation can be reduced by two thirds with the use of proper orthotic devices.[36] Peach and Olejnik have shown that appropriate changes in an individual's activities, use of assistive devices, or both can be very helpful for individuals inclined to make appropriate changes.[37] In this study, the investigators reported that the individuals who were willing to make appropriate changes in their activity, use orthotic devices, and so forth had significant improvement in their clinical situation, but individuals who were unwilling or unable to make such changes continued to have problems or had increasing problems at the time of follow-up. The findings of the Kling-man et al.[21] study does support the hypothesis that overextended, enlarged motor units may be predisposed to premature dysfunction or degeneration; however, there may be other explanations for a postpolio individual's new complaints of dysfunction. Excessive activity in postpolio individuals can, theoretically, lead to further dysfunction and the onset of PPS.

LEVEL OF PHYSICAL ACTIVITY

Early Reports

A number of clinical papers from many years ago have reported that exercise can have detrimental effects in postpolio individuals (Table 2). In 1915, Lovett anecdotally reported that within 1 year of their acute paralytic poliomyelitis illness, four postpolio individuals had increasing muscle weakness associated with an increase in activity.[23] No details were provided, but he warned that overuse of severely affected muscles could lead to a decrease in strength from which the patient might not recover.

In 1953, Hyman anecdotally reported on the case of a 10-year-old girl with acute poliomyelitis who had only antigravity strength of her calf, ankle, and foot muscles.[24] Unbeknownst to the treating physician, the patient's parents had encouraged her to

Table 2. EARLY REPORTS OF DETRIMENTAL EFFECTS OF ACTIVITY OR EXERCISE IN POSTPOLIO INDIVIDUALS					
STUDY	PATIENTS, N	TIME RANGE AFTER ACUTE POLIO	AGE OR AGE RANGE	EXERCISE OR ACTIVITY	RESULTS
Lovett[23]	4	All within 1 year	Not specified; two young men and two children	Anecdotal reports; details not given	Strength decreased with excessive activity
Hyman[24]	1	During acute hospitaliza-tion	10 years	Anecdotal report; details not given	Severe relapse in strength with activity
Mitchell[25]	1	< 1 year	27 years	Anecdotal report; details not given	Severe relapse in strength with activity; slow im-provement with rest
Knowlton and Bennett[26]	4	2–23 years	16–34 years	Anecdotal reports; details not given	Strength decreased with exces-sive activity

exercise as much as possible in the early convalescent phase in a effort to speed up her recovery. The exercise led to a severe relapse, resulting in total paralysis of those muscles. Some slight improvement was reported within 2 months after the patient ceased her unwise exercise.

In 1953, Mitchell anecdotally reported on the possible danger of fatiguing exercise in a polio patient in the early stages of recovery.[25] He described a 27-year-old man who experienced a severe relapse in strength from overactivity in the 2 weeks after discharge from the hospital. In 1957, Knowlton and Bennett anecdotally reported that four individuals experienced significant strength decline as a result of overactivity.[26] These cases occurred 2 to 23 years after the acute paralytic poliomyelitis illness. The activities that lead to the overwork weakness included athletics, business load, army duty, and housework. Knowlton and Bennett concluded that there is a definite hazard to voluntary skeletal muscle from overwork.[26] They believed that this arose from the fact that subjective fatigue, in the face of high motivation, is not a reliable safeguard against overwork. They recommended that, in supervised exercise, the supervisor must be alert to the objective signs of fatigue and should watch the day-to-day performance carefully in order to detect these problems early.

More Recent Studies

Results of more recent studies suggest that excessive activity may be a contributing factor that could lead to overuse and possibly to progressive dysfunction in postpolio patients.[2,27–30,38,39] Two studies were kinesiologic studies assessing the EMG activity of lower limb musculature during ambulation. Perry et al. studied 34 patients with PPS and reported that the average subject overused two muscle groups.[28] It was postulated that the overuse was contributing to the problems in these patients. In the other study by Borg et al., it is shown that the tibialis anterior muscle in some postpolio subjects was maximally recruited during ambulation.[29] It was suggested that ambulation in these subjects could lead to muscle overuse, which could lead to overuse fatigue.

Two clinical studies have reported finding an increase in the serum creatine kinase (CK) concentration in patients with PPS.[38,39] Although an increase in serum CK is found after excessive activity and can indicate muscle damage, the significance of this finding is unknown. Nelson reported that the incidence of an elevated CK concentration was not different between those postpolio patients with PPS and those without the syndrome.[39] Also, the elevation in CK concentration did not correlate with new or residual weakness.

Willen and Grimby assessed pain, physical activity, and disability in 32 consecutive postpolio individuals seen in a postpolio clinic.[27] Pain was commonly reported to be present during physical activity. Physical activity was associated with muscle pain in 25 of 32 (78%) patients and joint pain in 22 of 32 (69%) individuals. Pain intensity (as measured by the visual analogue scale) was positively correlated with level of physical exertion. Individuals who spontaneously chose a walking speed close to their maximum speed were more prone to experience pain in their daily life. The most common reasons given for pain were physical activity during leisure time in 16 (50%), occupational work in 10 (31%), and exposure to cold in 9 (28%) of the 32 patients. In the lower limbs, cramping pain was the most common pain characteristic followed by aching pain. Aching pain was the most common pain experienced in the upper limbs. Pain was not found to be correlated with muscle weakness, which means that an individual does not necessarily experience more pain with more pronounced muscle weakness. On the contrary, it might indicate that those who are less affected by muscle weakness experience more pain, which could be a direct result of a more active lifestyle. CK concentration was elevated in 13 of 32 (41%) individuals. No correlation, however, was found between the CK concentration and either the experience of pain or the overall activity as measured by the Physical Activity Scale for the Elderly. This study concluded that postpolio individuals who experience pain associated with activities of daily living should modify their level of physical activity.

In a study of neuromuscular function comparing 34 postpolio individuals with complaints of progressive decline in strength (i.e., unstable postpolio subjects) to 16 stable postpolio individuals and 41 control (nonpolio) individuals, Agre and Rodriquez reported that the unstable postpolio group had a statistically significant ($P < 0.05$) deficit in strength recovery in 10-minute period of time after exhausting exercise; the stable postpolio group recovered strength in a similar pattern to the control subjects ($P > 0.05$).[22] This finding was postulated to be caused by excessive local muscle fatigue in these individuals.

In a follow-up study, Agre et al. evaluated the subjective time for complete strength recovery in a subgroup of the above cohort (25 unstable postpolio patients, 16 stable postpolio patients, and 25 control subjects.)[30] This study also demonstrated a statistically significant ($P < 0.05$) difference between unstable and stable postpolio subjects. The stable postpolio individuals reported complete strength recovery in the same period of time as the control subjects (average recovery of strength within 1 day after exhausting activity, $P > 0.05$). The unstable postpolio group, however, reported a much greater period of time required for complete strength recovery (average recovery of strength in 2.5 days after exhausting activity, $P < 0.05$ compared with both stable postpolio and to control subjects). Both of these studies provide evidence that unstable postpolio individuals (i.e., those noting a decline in muscle strength) may be more vulnerable to exhausting activity or exercise. It would seem to be most reasonable to recommend that such individuals should modify their level of daily activity to avoid excessive fatigue.

SUMMARY

The summary for evidence linking either exercise or activity to the onset and progression of PPS is found in Table 3. A number of actors have been found to be associated with PPS. Several of these factors could possibly be related to the onset or the progression of PPS many years after the acute paralytic poliomyelitis illness. Some of these possible factors in the literature have included severity of the acute illness, greater functional recovery and lower residual disability, and level of current physical activity. Each of these factors is reviewed here.

Table 3. SUMMARY OF THE EVIDENCE LINKING EXERCISE OR ACTIVITY TO THE ONSET OR PROGRESSION OF POSTPOLIO SYNDROME

TYPE OF STUDY	REFERENCES	COMMENTS
Case reports	Hyman,[24] Mitchell[25]	Anecdotal reports; indeterminate with no specific data provided
Case series	Lovett,[23] Knowlton and Bennett[26]	Anecdotal reports; indeterminate with no specific data provided
Uncontrolled observational studies	Ramlow et al.,[18] Windebank et al.[19]	Epidemiologic studies; report that severity of acute paralytic poliomyelitis illness is a risk factor for development of PPS, but no data provided to link exercise to the development of PPS
	Trojan et al.[16]	Clinical report with no specific data provided to link exercise to the development of PPS
	Halstead and Rossi,[5] Klingman et al.[21]	Retrospective chart reviews; reported that severity of acute paralytic poliomyelitis illness is a risk factor for the development of PPS, but no data provided to link exercise to the development of PPS
	Perry et al.,[28] Berg et al.[29]	Kinesiologic studies demonstrate that some postpolio individuals over-use or near maximally recruit lower limb muscles during ambulation, but no data provided to link exercise to the development of PPS
	Waring et al.,[38] Nelson[39]	Clinical studies report that the concentration of creatine kinase is increased in some postpolio individuals, but no data provided to link exercise to the development of PPS
	Willen and Grimby[27]	Clinical study reporting that activity was associated with pain and the postpolio patients whose self-chosen ambulatory velocity was near their maximal velocity were most prone to pain, but no data to link exercise to the development of PPS
Controlled observational studies	Agre and Rodriquez[22]	Controlled, but not randomly selected, postpolio volunteers; study reported that patients with PPS were more severely affected by the acute paralytic poliomyelitis illness, were weaker, and had deficits in strength recovery after exhausting activity, but no data to link exercise to the development of PPS
Controlled clinical trials		None found in the literature

Studies linking the severity of the acute poliomyelitis illness with activity include two epidemiologic studies[18,19] three retrospective clinical reports,[5,16,21] and one controlled (but not randomly selected) observational study.[22] All of these studies have shown that individuals most severely affected initially tended to be the patients with the more significant problems associated with the late effects of poliomyelitis. However, no studies have shown conclusive data with regard to causation or progression of PPS. Those most severely affected initially had the greatest loss of motor neurons. Many of these individuals had significant recovery of strength after their acute illness related to terminal motor unit reorganization. After decades, however, these very large motor units may be a greater risk for dysfunction or death, and this could result in functional decline in these individuals. Excessive activity in these individuals, from a theoretical standpoint, could exacerbate this process.

Klingman et al. linked greater functional recovery and lower residual disability to patients with PPS.[21] This was a retrospective chart review study in which patients with complaints of progressive decline in strength (and no apparent cause for this decline from chart review) were compared with patients without complaints of progressive decline in strength. What was not learned from this study, however, was how many of these individuals were simply being too active for their own particular clinical circumstances and becoming excessively fatigued, how many of these individuals were not using appropriate assistive devices, and so forth. These other factors can definitely lead to significant problems in postpolio individuals. The reported association from this study between functional recovery and lower residual disability and the onset of PPS, however, does not imply causation.

Several studies have also associated the level of physical activity with patients with PPS or functional difficulties. Four of these studies were anecdotal reports of patients who were excessively active.[23–26] Three reports were of patients shortly after their acute illness,[23–25] but one report was in individuals 2–23 years after their acute illness.[26] None of these anecdotal reports conclusively demonstrates a causality for the development of PPS. Two studies were kinesiologic studies demonstrating that a number of postpolio individuals overuse muscles while ambulating.[28,29] This could certainly lead to overuse problems in these individuals, but the data do not confirm a causation for the development or progression of PPS. Willen and Grimby reported an association between physical activity and pain.[27] The subjects who were most active had the greatest amount of pain. Also, those patients, who spontaneously chose to walk at near maximal velocity, were the patients most prone to pain. This is definite evidence for overuse in these individuals, but does not confirm a causative effect of exercise upon the development or progression of PPS.

In a controlled observational study, Agre et al. reported that patients with PPS (compared with those without PPS) were initially more severely affected by poliomyelitis, were weaker at the time of the evaluation, had a significant deficit in strength recovery after exhausting exercise, and required a greater length of time to fully recover from exhausting exercise.[22,30] These data do not prove causation for the development or progression of PPS, but they may indicate that problems of excessive muscle fatigue or difficulty in recovery of muscle strength after activity may be related to overuse and excessive local muscle fatigue in these individuals.

Although none of the studies published to date has conclusively demonstrated that exercise causes the development or progression of PPS, it is certainly possible that excessive activity or exercise in some of these individuals could overstress and ultimately lead to the deterioration or death of the largest—and most fragile—motor units. However, as previously discussed no specific data in the literature corroborate this hypothesis. It is known, however, that excessive activity or exercise can lead to overuse problems, but this is not a unique problem of polio survivors. A review of the literature reveals that very little is known about the risk of overuse causing persistent muscular dysfunction, either through damage or destruction of the largest, and probably most fragile, surviving motor units or through damage to the muscle itself. The risk for development of PPS in postpolio individuals with exercise at the present time remains an unproven hypothesis. It should also be kept in mind, from the myriad of information from the area of exercise physiology, that inactivity definitely leads to progressive muscular weakness and loss of muscular as well as cardiovascular endurance. It would certainly be deemed wise, however, to recommend that postpolio individuals avoid excessive activity, which can certainly lead to increased fatigue, muscle pain, or joint pain. A balance between activity and rest is, at the present time, the best advice for postpolio individuals. However, this is also prudent advice for all individuals, not just for postpolio individuals.

EVIDENCE LINKING EXERCISE AND ACTIVITY TO THE MAINTENANCE OF STRENGTH AND WELL-BEING IN POSTPOLIO INDIVIDUALS

Many studies in the refereed literature document the benefits of exercise in selected postpolio individuals. This information, however, must also be tempered with information about possible risks associated with exercise. We know very little at the present time of the risk of overuse and whether or not it can lead to permanent muscle damage or deterioration or destruction of the surviving motor units in polio survivors. Such studies would be, from a scientific standpoint, very difficult to perform, and from an ethical point of view, impossible to perform. The exercise studies reviewed here are divided into exercises specifically for muscle strengthening alone, exercises for general endurance or aerobic conditioning (but may also include muscle strengthening exercise), aquatic exercise, and one study of modified aerobic exercise on movement energetics.

MUSCLE STRENGTHENING EXERCISE

Early Strengthening Exercise Studies (1940s–1960s)

Results of the early muscle strengthening exercise studies on postpolio patients are found in Table 4. In 1948, DeLorme et al. studied the effect of exercise on the quadriceps femoris (knee extensor muscles) in 19 postpolio patients between the ages

Table 4. EARLY STUDIES OF BENEFICIAL EFFECTS OF EXERCISE ON MUSCLE STRENGTH IN POSTPOLIO INDIVIDUALS					
STUDY	PATIENTS, N	TIME RANGE AFTER ACUTE POLIO	AGE RANGE	EXERCISE OR ACTIVITY	RESULTS
DeLorme et al.[40]	19	1–49 years	18–50 years	Two separate dynamic exercises; 60 reps in total per session; 4 sessions per week; up to 4 months	Mean strength increase of almost 100%
Gurewitch[41]	13	Early after polio, details not given	1–37 years	Similar to DeLorme, et al., but details not given	Strength improved, but details not given
Mueller and Beckmann[42]	4	6–15 years	Details not given	Three 6-second static maximal contractions daily for 10 weeks	Mean strength increased 37%

of 18 and 50 years.[40] The exercise was initiated between 1 and 49 years after their acute paralytic poliomyelitis illness. Eight of the subjects had bilateral involvement, and 11 had unilateral involvement of the quadriceps muscles. Thus, a total of 27 quadriceps muscle groups were studied. Exercise was performed once daily, 4 days per week, for up to 4 months. Two different exercises were performed. One exercise was performed against gravity or with gravity assistance, depending on the strength of the muscle. If the muscle had sufficient strength to completely extend the knee in the sitting position (antigravity strength or greater), the exercise was performed with the subject in the seated position with a weight placed on the foot. If the muscle was too weak to perform that exercise, the exercise was performed with gravity assistance. In this instance, the subject was placed in a prone position on an exercise table, and knee extension was performed with weights, but with gravity assistance. The second exercise that all subjects performed was a combined hip and knee extension exercise against resistance with the subject in the sitting position. For each of the two exercises, the subjects performed three sets of 10 repetitions with a rest break of about 1 minute between sets. The resistance (weight) was gradually increased throughout the exercise program. As a result of the exercise program, muscle strength was found, on the average, to nearly double. Also, all but three of the quadriceps muscles showed an overall increase in work capacity. Most of the subjects also reported that they were able to perform ordinary activities with less effort and less fatigue.

In 1950, Gurewitsch,[41] using techniques similar to DeLorme and colleagues,[40] evaluated the effect of exercise in 13 patients (age range, 1–37 years; average age, 18 years) soon after their acute paralytic poliomyelitis illness. Although specific data were not reported, Gurewitsch concluded that the muscles strengthened with this technique improved more than muscles strengthened with less intensive exercise. No specific details were provided in this paper.

In 1966, Mueller and Beckmann reported on the effect of isometric exercise in four boys with paresis caused by acute poliomyelitis.[42] Exercise was performed 6–15 years after the acute paralytic poliomyelitis illness. Subjects performed three 6-second maximal static muscle contractions daily with a 2-minute rest break between contractions over a 10-week period. Exercise was performed in a total of two legs, two arms, six hands, and 12 fingers in these four subjects. After the 10-week exercise program, strength increased by an average of 37%.

More Recent Strengthening Exercise Studies (1980s to present)

The results of the more recent muscle strengthening exercise are found in Table 5. In 1987, Feldman and Soskolne reported on the effects of a nonfatiguing exercise program in postpolio individuals.[43] Six patients with PPS (age range and gender not specified) participated in an exercise program three times a week in a physical therapy gymnasium for at least 24 weeks. The exercise was performed on a total of 32 muscle groups in the six patients, and the exercise consisted of nonfatiguing weightlifting. The initial weight that the subject lifted in the exercise program was at 50% of the five RM (the five-repetition maximum [RM]; i.e., the maximal amount of weight that the subject could lift five times and no more). The number of repetitions that the subject lifted was gradually increased, being careful to avoid fatigue. When the subject could successfully lift the weight 30 times, the weight was increased and the number of repetitions was decreased. Again, the subject gradually increased the number of repetitions. Each time that 30 repetitions were reached, the weight was increased and the number of repetitions was decreased. This exercise program resulted in an increase in strength in 14 muscles, no change in strength in 17 muscles, and decreased strength in 1 muscle. It was reported that the subject with the strength decline was under severe emotional strain, which may have been a factor in the strength decline.

In 1987, Einarsson and Grimby[44] and Einarsson[45] reported on the effects of a standardized exercise program on quadriceps femoris strength. Twelve subjects (five men and seven woman; age range, 41 to 63 years) participated in the program, nine of whom had PPS. Subjects exercised three times per week for 6 weeks in the research laboratory on a special dynamometer. All subjects had at least grade 3+ (antigravity plus) strength on manual muscle testing. Subjects performed three sets of static and isokinetic muscle strengthening exercises. Each set of exercise consisted of eight 4-second bouts of exercise alternating between isokinetic and static exercise. Each bout of exercise was followed by 10 seconds of rest. Subjects rested for 5 minutes between sets of exercise. After 6 weeks of exercise, isokinetic strength (at an angular velocity of 60°/sec) statistically significantly ($P < 0.05$) increased by 16%, and static strength statistically significantly ($P < 0.05$) increased by 17%. No apparent muscle damage

Table 5. MORE RECENT STUDIES ON EFFECTS OF EXERCISE ON MUSCLE STRENGTH IN POSTPOLIO INDIVIDUALS

STUDY	PATIENTS, N	TIME RANGE AFTER ACUTE POLIO	AGE OR AGE RANGE	EXERCISE OR ACTIVITY	RESULTS
Feldman and Soskolne[43]	6	Details not given	Details not given	Nonfatiguing weight lifting; < 30 reps per session; 3 sessions per week; at least 24 weeks	Strength increased in 14 muscles; remained the same in 17 muscles; decreased in 1 muscle
Einarsson and Grimby,[44] Einarsson[45]	12	24–61 years	41–63 years	Three sets of static and isokinetic exercise; 3 sessions per week for 6 weeks	16–17% increase in muscle strength; no muscle pathology; 9/12 had increased feeling of well-being
Fillyaw et al.[46]	17	Mean time, 43 years	Mean age, 51 years	Three sets of 10 reps at 50%, 75%, and 100% of 10 RM every other day for up to 2 years	Mean increase of 78% in 10 RM, mean increase in static strength of 8.4%
Spector et al.[47]	6	33–55 years	Mean age, 53 years; range, 40–60 years	Three sets of PRE of knee and elbow extensors; 20, 15, and 10 reps per set; three sessions per week for 9 weeks	Increases in 3 RM of leg press (41%), knee extension (61%), arm press (54%), arm extension (71%); no change in CK or muscle histopathology

(continued)

| | | **TIME RANGE AFTER** | | **EXERCISE** | |
STUDY	PATIENTS, N	**ACUTE POLIO**	AGE OR AGE RANGE	**OR ACTIVITY**	RESULTS
Agre et al.[48]	12	36–49 years	35–60 years	6 to 10 dynamic and static contractions with ankle weights every other day for 12 weeks	Mean increase in amount of weight lifted of > 60%, no change in CK or EMG variables
Agre et al.[50]	7	Mean time since polio, 43 years	Mean age, 51 years; range, 43–62 years	Three sets of 4 maximal 5-second static contractions, 2 days per week, three sets of 12 leg lifts with weights (PRE) 2 days per week for 12 weeks	Mean increase in weight lifted (47%), isokinetic torque (15%), static torque (36%), endurance (21%), work capacity (18%); no change in CK or EMG variables

Table 5. MORE RECENT STUDIES ON EFFECTS OF EXERCISE ON MUSCLE STRENGTH IN POSTPOLIO INDIVIDUALS (CONT.)

occurred as a result of the exercise because muscles biopsies after the study were similar to those beforehand. Strength 6–12 months later did not decline, apparently a result of an increase in ordinary daily activities. Questionnaire data obtained 5–12 months after the completion of the exercise program showed that 9 of the 12 subjects noted an increased feeling of well-being after the program.

In 1991, Fillyaw et al. reported the effect of long-term nonfatiguing exercise in 17 patients (14 women, 3 men; mean age, 51 years) with PPS with grade 3 (antigravity) strength or greater on manual muscle testing.[46] Subjects exercised the quadriceps femoris or biceps humerus muscle group every other day for 1 to 2 years. The exercise consisted of three sets of 10 repetitions with 50%, 75%, and 100% of the 10 RM.

Subjects rested for 5 minutes between exercise sets. Every 2 weeks, the 10 RM was evaluated. Maximum torque was reported to statistically significantly ($P < 0.05$) increase by an average of 8.4% in the exercised muscles compared with control muscles, in which no change in strength was found. The 10 RM increased in 16 of the 17 subjects, and the average increase was statistically significant (78%, $P < 0.05$).

In 1996, Spector et al. reported the effect of a 9-week progressive resistive exercise program in 6 patients (5 men, 1 woman; mean age, 53 years) with postpolio muscular atrophy (i.e., self-report of new weakness).[47] Progressive resistive exercise was performed in one knee extensor and both elbow extensor muscles in all subjects except one subject, who had flaccid paralysis of both elbow extensors from the acute poliomyelitis illness. This individual only exercised one knee extensor muscle. Exercise was performed three times per week on nonconsecutive days for 9 weeks. Subjects completed three sets of 20, 15, and then 10 repetitions of unilateral knee extension and bilateral elbow extension exercise during each exercise session. Initial resistance level was set at approximately 75% of the 3 RM (i.e., the maximum resistance that the subject could perform three—and only 3—repetitions). Upper and lower body exercise was alternated to minimize fatigue, with a rest interval of 90 seconds between sets on a particular machine and 3 minutes between exercises. After 9 weeks of exercise, statistically significant ($P < 0.05$) strength gains were found in all trained muscles. The 3 RM for leg press had a mean increase of 41%; for knee extension, 61%; for arm press, 54%; and for arm extension, 71%. Neither knee extension nor static elbow extension demonstrated any significant increase in strength ($P > 0.05$) when measured dynametrically. The cross-sectional area of the quadriceps femoris and triceps muscles did not significantly ($P > 0.05$) change after the exercise program. The serum CK concentration did not significantly ($P > 0.05$) change during the exercise program. Additionally, no destructive histopathological changes were noted in repeat muscle biopsies, and no consistent changes in muscle fiber size or fiber type percentages were observed after the completion of the exercise.

In 1996, Agre et al. reported the effect of a supervised 12-week nonfatiguing quadriceps femoris muscle strengthening exercise program.[48] Twelve subjects (7 women, 5 men; age range, 36–60 years) with PPS and at least grade 3+ (antigravity plus) strength on manual muscle testing volunteered for the study. Every other day at home, subjects performed 6 to 10 extension exercises with a sandbag weight attached to the ankle. In the sitting position, the subject slowly fully extended the knee and held it for 5 seconds; then they slowly lowered the weight and rested. One repetition was performed every 30 seconds. After six repetitions, subjects reported their rating of perceived exertion (RPE)[49] in the exercised muscle. If the RPE was less than "very hard," the subject continued until the RPE reached a rating of "very hard" or until 10 repetitions were performed. The weight was increased whenever the subject could perform 10 repetitions without reaching an RPE of "very hard." After 12 weeks of exercise, the amount of weight that the subject could lift statistically significantly ($P < 0.05$) increased by more than 60% on the average, but static strength, as measured dynametrically, did not statistically significantly ($P > 0.05$) change. No statistically significant ($P > 0.05$) change was found in the concentration of serum CK throughout the exercise program. No statistically significant ($P > 0.05$) change was found in the amount of jitter or blocking on EMG evaluation. No subject experienced problems with the exercise program. After the exercise program, subjects completed questionnaires. Increased strength in the muscle exercised was reported by 10 of 12 subjects, increased endurance in 8 of 12 subjects, increased work capacity in 9 of 12 subjects, improved recovery of strength after activity in 6 of 12 subjects, improved walking ability in 6 of 12 subjects, and improved stair climbing in 5 of 10 subjects. (Two subjects did not climb stairs before or after the study.)

In 1997, Agre et al. reported on the effect of a supervised 12-week home exercise program on 7 subjects with PPS (mean age 51 years) and at least grade 3+ (antigravity) strength on manual muscle testing.[50] These subjects were recruited from the 12 subjects in the previous study.[48] (Five of those subjects did not volunteer; one subject had moved from the area, and four did not have time to participate because of schedule conflicts.) Exercise was performed at home 4 days per week. On Mondays and Thursdays, subjects performed three sets of four maximal static contractions of the quadriceps femoris muscles held for 5 seconds each. The subject rested for 10 seconds between each repetition and for 1 minute between each of the three sets. On Tuesdays and Fridays, subjects performed three sets of knee extension exercise in the sitting position with a weight on the ankle. For each set of exercise, the subject slowly fully extended and then immediately lowered the weight over a 5-second interval with no rest between the 12 repetitions of the set. The subject rested for 1 minute after the completion of each set. After the third set, the subject rated the RPE.[47] If the RPE was less than a rating of "very, very hard," the ankle weight was increased at the next exercise session. After 12 weeks of exercise, statistically significant ($P < 0.05$) changes were found in the following variables: the weight lifted during the exercise program (47 % increase), isokinetic peak torque (15% increase), static peak torque (36% increase), local muscle endurance (21% increase), and static muscle work capacity (18% increase). No statistically significant ($P > 0.05$) changes were found in the following electromyography variables: fiber density, jitter, blocking, or macro EMG amplitude. Also, no statistically significant ($P > 0.05$) change was found in the serum CK concentration.

GENERAL ENDURANCE OR AEROBIC CONDITIONING EXERCISE

Beneficial effects of aerobic conditioning exercise or general conditioning exercise are summarized in Table 6. Postpolio patients have been reported to be severely deconditioned from a cardiorespiratory standpoint. The average maximal metabolic capacity of a group of postpolio individuals was only 5.6 metabolic equivalents ([MET]; 1 MET equals the energy expenditure at complete rest).[51] This level of aerobic power is similar to that of individuals shortly after sustaining an acute myocardial infarction.[51]

In 1989, Jones et al.[52] evaluated the response to a 16-week, three-times-per-week aerobic exercise program in a group of 37 postpolio subjects (age range, 30–60 years). Sixteen subjects volunteered for the exercise program, and 21 subjects served as control subjects. Exercise subjects exercised on bicycle ergometers using lower limb mus-

Table 6. EFFECTS OF AEROBIC OR GENERAL CONDITIONING EXERCISE

STUDY	PATIENTS, N	TIME RANGE AFTER ACUTE POLIO	AGE OR AGE RANGE	EXERCISE OR ACTIVITY	RESULTS
Jones et al.[52]	37	Details not given	30–60 years	Lower limb, cycle ergometry; 15–30 minutes per session at resting HR plus 70–75% of HR reserve; three sessions per week for 16 weeks	Exercise group power improved 18%; peak VO_2 improved 15%
Kriz et al.[53]	20	11–45 years	30–59 years	Upper limb cycle ergometry, 20 minutes per session at resting HR plus 70–75% of HR reserve; three sessions per week for 16 weeks	Exercise group power improved 12%; peak VO_2 improved 19%
Ernstoff et al.[54]	12	28–44 years	39–46 years	Combination of submaximal endurance and strength training; 1 hour per session; 2 sessions per week for 20 weeks	Peak performance improved on cycle ergometer; HR at submaximal workload decreased; some muscle groups had increased strength

culature. Exercise was performed at a target heart rate of resting heart rate plus 70–75% of heart rate reserve (the difference between resting and maximal heart rate). In an attempt to avoid excessive fatigue, exercise was performed in bouts of 2–5 minutes per bout with 1-minute rest breaks between bouts. Patients were instructed to exercise for a total of 15–30 minutes per session. In most subjects, the exercise was initiated at a lower intensity and duration. Over the first few weeks, the exercise intensity and duration were gradually increased. After 16 weeks of exercise, the exercise subjects had statistically significant ($P < 0.05$) increases in peak oxygen utilization (average increase, 15%) and work power (average increase, 18%); the control subjects had no statistically significant ($P > 0.05$) change in either of those variables. No untoward responses to exercise were noted in any of the exercise subjects. Subjectively, the exercise subjects reported a decrease in fatigue while performing daily activities and an increase in strength in lower limb musculature.

In 1992, Kriz et al. evaluated the response to upper limb aerobic exercise.[53] Exercise was performed three times per week for 16 weeks. Twenty postpolio subjects participated in the study and were randomly assigned to exercise (two women and eight men; mean age, 46 years) and control (eight women and two men; mean age, 41 years). Exercise was performed with arm ergometers with a target heart rate of resting heart rate plus 70–75% of heart rate reserve. Subjects exercised for a total exercise time of 20 minutes per session, exercising in bouts of 2–5 minutes with 1-minute rest breaks between bouts. The exercise group had statistically significant ($P < 0.05$) increases in peak oxygen utilization (average increase, 19%) and work power (average increase, 12%). The control group had no statistically significant ($P > 0.05$) change in either of those variables.

In 1996, Ernstoff et al. reported on the effects of endurance training.[54] Seventeen postpolio patients volunteered for the study. Twelve subjects completed the study, but five did not. (Two subjects dropped from the study because they found the exercise program too difficult, one changed jobs, one became ill unrelated to the study, and one was lost to follow-up.) Eight of the 12 subjects who completed the study had PPS as defined by Halstead and Rossi.[5] Exercise was performed twice weekly for 22 weeks for a total of 40 sessions (group training was discontinued for 2 weeks over a holiday break) in a gymnasium with guidance of a physical therapist. Each exercise session lasted for 60 minutes and consisted of 5 minutes of general warm-up followed by low-resistance, high-repetition exercises for all major muscle groups in both upper and lower extremities as well as the trunk. After 1 month of training, 5 minutes of exercise on a bicycle ergometer was included at approximately 60–80% of maximal heart rate. The amount of time on the bicycle remained at 5 minutes at each session. A 5-minute cool-down period followed at the end of each session. At the completion of the exercise program, muscle strength statistically significantly ($P < 0.05$) increased in a few muscle groups as measured by a hand-held dynamometer (elbow extension, 12%; wrist extension, 13%; and hip abduction, 40%). Static and isokinetic measurements of muscle strength with a Kin-Com dynamometer, however, did not show any statistically significant ($P > 0.05$) change in strength. Exercise on a bicycle dynamometer at a submaximal work load of 70 W showed a statistically significant ($P < 0.05$) reduction in heart rate (mean reduction in heart rate of 6 beats per minute [BPM]) and a statistically significant ($P < 0.05$) increase in maximal heart rate after the training program. Muscle biopsies revealed no statistically significant ($P > 0.05$)

change in cross-sectional area in any of the muscle fiber types after the training program, and computed tomography scan showed no statistically significant ($P > 0.05$) change in thigh muscle area. The predominant complaints related to the exercise program were minor musculoskeletal discomfort of the lower limbs in three subjects. One other subject complained of progressive muscular fatigue during the exercise sessions. It was concluded that the training program could be performed without major complications and resulted in an increase in muscle strength in some muscle groups and in work performance with respect to heart rate at submaximal work load.

AQUATIC EXERCISE

Beneficial effects of aquatic exercise are summarized in Table 7. Two studies have reported the effects of a water exercise program in postpolio patients.[55,56] In 1994, Prins et al. assessed the effect of aquatic exercise in 16 postpolio patients.[55] Subjects were randomly assigned to exercise and control groups. Nine subjects performed exercise, and 7 were control subjects; however, complete data were available on 4 of the control subjects. Exercise was performed three time per week for 8 weeks in a swimming pool. Exercise sessions ranged from 45 to 70 minutes per session. The exercise regimen for each subject was determined individually before commencement of the program based on the subject's strength and swimming experience. In addition to swimming and isolated use of the legs using a kickboard, the exercise subjects also performed a series of arm and leg exercises in the water using fins and hand paddles. Each subject's progress was monitored throughout the exercise program, and exercise was gradually progressed. After the 8-week exercise program in only the exercise subjects, statistically significant ($P < 0.05$) increases in muscle strength were found in some of the upper limb muscle groups and statistically significant ($P < 0.05$) increases in range of motion (ROM) were found in some upper limb motions. Control subjects had no statistically significant ($P > 0.05$) changes in muscle strength or ROM at the completion of the study. No subject complained of any adverse effects from study participation.

In 1999, Willen reported on the effect of dynamic water exercise in postpolio patients.[56] This was one of three studies she performed for her doctoral dissertation. The first study was a report of pain experienced by postpolio patients and included 67 seen at the postpolio clinic in Goteborg, Sweden. Twenty-eight of those subjects participated in the exercise study. Fifteen of those subjects volunteered for the exercise group (13 had PPS) and 13, who did not have time to participate in the exercise study, volunteered to be control subjects (12 had PPS). Exercise was performed twice per week for 5 months. Exercises were led by a physical therapist and lasted 40 minutes per session. The exercise was designed to train general physical fitness, including resistance and endurance activities, balance, stretching, and relaxation. Heart rate was recorded with a heart rate monitor in three individuals chosen at random to obtain information regarding the intensity of the program. This was done after a few weeks of training after the individuals were familiar with the exercise program. Heart rate monitoring of the three individuals showed that heart rate at times was very close to

Table 7. EFFECTS OF AQUATIC EXERCISE

STUDY	PATIENTS, N	TIME RANGE AFTER ACUTE POLIO	AGE OR AGE RANGE	EXERCISE OR ACTIVITY	RESULTS
Prins et al.[55]	13	36–51 years	39–69 years	Swimming and aquatic strengthening exercise; 45–70 minutes per session; three sessions per week for 8 weeks	Several muscle groups with increased strength; some joints with increased ROM
Willen[56]	28	On average, > 40 years, details not given	Mean age, 50 years	General fitness, stretching, endurance, strengthening, balance, relaxation; 40 minutes per session; two per week for 5 months	Reduced HR at submaximal workload and reduced pain in exercise group only; 11/15 in exercise group had increased sense of well-being

HR = heart rate; ROM = range of motion.

peak heart rate, indicating that on some occasions, they were exerting themselves at close to peak effort. After the exercise program, there was no statistically significant ($P > 0.05$) increase in peak exercise, oxygen uptake, or heart rate on a bicycle ergometer in either group. Heart rate in the exercise group, however, at a submaximal level of exertion (the heart rate at the work level before the peak work level at the time of the initial evaluation, which could have been different for each subject) was statistically significantly ($P < 0.05$) reduced after the exercise program (mean reduction of 9 bpm); there was no significant change in the control group (mean increase of 2 bpm). Muscle strength did not statistically significantly ($P > 0.05$) change after the study compared with beforehand in either group. No change in pain was reported by either of the two groups using the visual analogue scale; however, the pain dimension in the Nottingham Health Profile showed statistically significantly ($P < 0.05$) lower distress after training in the exercise group compared with the control group (median value decreased from 37 at the initial evaluation to 18 after the exercise program in the exercise group compared with slight increase from 41 to 46 in the control group at the comparable times). Walking speed did not statistically significantly ($P > 0.05$) change after training, although a majority of individuals in the exercise group did increase their maximal walking speed. After the exercise program, 11 of the 15 subjects reported an increased feeling of well being, 6 of 15 reported pain relief, and 9 of 15 reported increased physical fitness.

MODIFIED AEROBIC EXERCISE AND AMBULATORY EFFICIENCY

Dean and Ross evaluated the effect of a modified aerobic exercise program on movement energetics in postpolio individuals.[57] Twenty postpolio subjects were recruited into the study, and every third subject was assigned to the exercise group. Thirteen subjects were assigned to the control group (10 women and 3 men; mean age, 47 years), and 7 subjects were assigned to the experimental group (5 women and 2 men; mean age, 49 years). The experimental group participated in a 6-week exercise training program for 30–40 minutes, three times per week. The program consisted of treadmill walking at 55–70% of age-predicted maximum heart rate; however, exercise intensity was modified to minimize discomfort, pain, and fatigue. After the 6 weeks of training, no statistically significant ($P > 0.05$) change was noted in the aerobic fitness of the exercise subjects; however, walking duration and movement economy were statistically significantly ($P < 0.05$) improved in the experimental group but not in the control group ($P > 0.05$). It was concluded that the modified aerobic training may play a role in enhancing endurance and reducing fatigue in postpolio individuals by improving the efficiency of movement.

EFFECT OF REST BREAKS DURING LOCAL MUSCLE ACTIVITY ON FATIGUE AND STRENGTH RECOVERY

In 1991, Agre and Rodriquez studied the effect of intermittent activity on muscle fatigue and strength recovery after activity in seven patients with PPS.[58] All patients were evaluated in a muscle physiology laboratory on three separate occasions with at least 1 week between evaluations. At the first visit, static strength of the quadriceps femoris muscles was determined. After a 5-minute rest, the patients statically contracted the quadriceps muscles at 40% of maximal torque for as long as possible until they could not longer maintain the torque output at 40% of the maximum torque. All patients received verbal encouragement to continue as long as possible. During this endurance test subjects reported their RPE[49] at regular intervals. Change in the median frequency of the power spectrum of the surface EMG was also continuously monitored as an electrophysiologic measure of local muscle fatigue.[59–61] Thirty seconds after the patient completed the endurance test, a maximal static contraction of the quadriceps muscle was again performed to determine strength recovery (percent of pre-endurance test torque). The tension time index (TTI) was determined as the product of the torque (in Newton meters) and time (in seconds). At the second visit, essentially the same procedure was performed except that the endurance test was divided into four equal intervals with a 2-minute rest between intervals; the TTI was the same as during the first visit. At the third visit, a similar procedure was followed as in the first two visits except that the endurance test was then divided into 20-second intervals with 2-minute rest breaks between intervals and continued until the RPE exceeded a level of "very hard" or when 6-minutes of exercise had been performed (about three times the duration of the endurance test performed at the time of the first visit).

The results of this study showed a statistically significant ($P < 0.05$) decrease in both the subjective and physiologically measured variables associated with local muscle fatigue at the completion of the endurance test at the time of the second and third visits compared with the first visit. Relative recovery of muscle strength was statistically significantly ($P < 0.05$) better at the time of the second and third visits compared with the first visit. The mean TTI at the time of the third was 337% of that found at the time of the first visit. This study demonstrated that postpolio individuals could perform similar amounts of work with less local muscle fatigue and greater strength recovery when the work was divided into intervals of work and rest and exhaustion was avoided. This study also demonstrated that postpolio individuals could perform much greater work with less local muscle fatigue and greater strength recovery when they stop to rest at intervals and avoid exhausting exercise.

SUMMARY

A summary for evidence demonstrating the effectiveness of exercise in selected postpolio patients is found in Table 8. Ample evidence suggests that exercise can be helpful in some postpolio individuals. The caveat for exercise appears to be one of balance: the exercise or activity needs to be balanced with appropriate rest (so as not to lead to excessive fatigue or muscle or joint pain). Also, clinical judgement is needed. Although the literature demonstrates the effectiveness of exercise in selected postpolio individuals, not all individuals will benefit from it. For some individuals, exercise is more than they can tolerate. For these individuals, simply the performance of activities of daily living with appropriate rest breaks (and use of appropriate assistive aids) is the maximum that they can comfortably and safely perform. Exercise beyond that level of activity may simply lead to overuse problems.

CONCLUSION

The evidence cited in the peer-reviewed literature is inadequate to either accept or reject a casual relationship between exercise and the development or progression of the PPS symptoms of weakness or fatigue. Excessive activity can definitely lead to overuse problems in any individual. This may lead to increasing complaints of fatiguability, weakness, or joint pain.

The peer-reviewed literature does demonstrate that exercise can be beneficial in selected individuals with PPS. The caveat is that not all patients benefit from it. Some have increasing difficulties and problems because the exercise exceeds the individual's tolerance for activity. The exercise in postpolio individuals should be carefully monitored. It also appears prudent that, when a postpolio individual exercises, he or she should avoid activity that leads to excessive fatigue, muscle pain, or joint pain.

Table 8. SUMMARY OF THE EVIDENCE FOR THE EFFECTIVENESS OF EXERCISE IN INDIVIDUALS WITH POSTPOLIO SYNDROME

TYPE OF STUDY	REFERENCES	COMMENTS
Case series	Mueller and Beckmann,[42] Feldman and Soskolne[43]	Two case series with four and six subjects; respectively, demonstrating improved strength or no change in strength in most muscles undergoing exercise; one muscle (of 32 muscles studied) had decreased strength in the Feldman and Soskolne study[43]
Uncontrolled exercise studies	DeLorme et al,[40] Gurewitch,[41] Einarsson and Grimby,[44] Einarsson,[45] Fillyaw et al,[46] Spector et al,[47] Agre et al,[48] Agre et al,[50] Ernstoff et al.[54]	Clinical studies performed without control groups evaluating the pre-exercise to post-exercise function; all studies reported improvement in muscle strength and one that also trained for endurance, showed an improvement in cardiovascular fitness[54]
Controlled observational studies		None found in the literature
Controlled clinical trials	Jones et al,[52] Kriz et al,[53] Prins et al,[55] Willen,[56]	Controlled clinical studies; three studies[52,55,56] divided subjects into exercise and control nonrandomly (subjects volunteered for one group or the other); another one study reported that subjects were randomly divided into exercise and control groups;[53] all studies reported improvements in physiologic function

References

1. Halstead LS, Wiechers DO (eds): Late Effects of Poliomyelitis. Miami, Symposia Foundation. 1985.
2. Codd MB, Mulder DW, Kurland LT, et al: Poliomyelitis in Rochester, Minnesota, 1935–1955; epidemiology and long-term sequelae: A preliminary report. In Halstead LS, Wiechers DO (eds): Late Effects of Poliomyelitis. Miami, Symposia Foundation, 1985, pp 121–134.
3. Dalakas MB, Elder G, Hallat M, et al: A long-term follow-up study of patients with postpoliomyelitis neuromuscular symptoms. N Engl J Med 314:959–963, 1986.
4. Cosgrove JL, Alexander MA, Kitts EL, et al: Late effects of poliomyelitis. Arch Phys Med Rehabil 68:4–7, 1987.
5. Halstead LS, Rossi CD: Post-polio syndrome: clinical experience with 132 consecutive outpatients. In Halstead LS, Wiechers DO (eds): Research and Clinical Aspects of the Late Effects of Poliomyelitis. White Plains, NY, March of Dimes Birth Defects Foundation, 1987, pp 13–26.
6. Agre JC, Rodriquez AA, Sperling KB: Symptoms and clinical impressions of patients seen in a post-polio clinic. Arch Phys Med Rehabil 70:367–370, 1989.

7. Berlly MH, Strausser WW, Hall KM. Fatigue in post-polio syndrome. Arch Phys Med Rehabil 72:115–118, 1991.
8. Halstead LS, Rossi CD: New problems in old polio patients: Results of a survey of 539 polio survivors. Orthopedics 8:845–850, 1991.
9. Lonnberg F: Late onset polio sequelae in Denmark. Scand J Rehabil Med 28(suppl):7–15, 1993.
10. Ivanyi B, Nollet F, Redekop WK, et al: Late onset polio sequelae, disabilities and handicaps in a population based cohort of the 1956 poliomyelitis outbreak in the Netherlands. Arch Phys Med Rehabil 80:687–690, 1999.
11. Nollet F, Beelen A, Prins MH, de Visser M, et al: Disability and functional assessment in former polio patients with and without postpolio syndrome. Arch Phys Med Rehabil 80:136–143, 1999.
12. Halstead LS: Post-polio syndrome: Definition of an elusive concept. In Munsat TL (ed): Post-polio Syndrome. Boston, Butterworth-Heinemann, 1991, pp 23–28.
13. Leon LS, Blackburn H: The relationship of physical activity to coronary heart disease and life expectancy. Ann NY Acad Sci 301:561–578, 1977.
14. Paffenbarger RS, Hyde RT: Exercise in the prevention of coronary heart disease. Prev Med 13:3–22, 1984.
15. Serfass RC, Gerberich SG: Exercise for optimal health: Strategies and motivational considerations. Prev Med 13:79–99, 1984.
15a. Agre JC, Rodriquez AA, Sperling KB: Plasma lipid and lipoprotein concentrations in post-polio patients. Arch Phys Med Rehabil 71:393–394, 1990.
16. Trojan DA, Cashman NR, Shapiro S, et al: Predictive factors for post-poliomyelitis syndrome. Arch Phys Med Rehabil 75:770–777, 1994.
17. Trojan DA, Cashman NR: Current Trends in Post-Poliomyelitis Syndrome. New York, Milestone Medical Communications, 1996.
18. Ramlow J, Alexander M, LaPorte R, et al: Epidemiology of the post-polio syndrome. Am J Epidemiol 136:769–786, 1992.
19. Windebank AJ, Daube JR, Litchy WJ, et al: Late sequelae of paralytic poliomyelitis in Olmsted County, Minnesota. In Halstead LS, Wiechers DO (eds): Research and Clinical Aspects of the Late Effects of Poliomyelitis. White Plains, NY, March of Dimes Birth Defects Foundation, 1987, pp 27–38.
20. Windebank AJ, Litchy WJ, Daube JR, et al: Late effects of poliomyelitis in Olmsted County, Minnesota. Neurology 41:501–507, 1991.
21. Klingman J, Chui H, Corgiat M, Perry J: Functional recovery: A major risk factor for the development of postpoliomyelitis muscular atrophy. Arch Neurol 45:645–647, 1988.
22. Agre JC, Rodriquez AA: Neuromuscular function: Comparison of symptomatic and asymptomatic polio subjects to control subjects. Arch Phys Med Rehabil 71:545–551, 1990.
23. Lovett RW: The treatment of infantile paralysis: preliminary report, based on a study of the Vermont epidemic of 1914. JAMA 64:2118–2123, 1915.
24. Hyman G: Poliomyelitis. Lancet 1:852, 1953.
25. Mitchell GP: Poliomyelitis and exercise. Lancet 2:90–91, 1953.
26. Knowlton GC, Bennett RL: Overwork. Arch Phys Med Rehabil 38:18–20, 1957.
27. Willen C, Grimby G: Pain, physical activity, and disability in individuals with late effects of polio. Arch Phys Med Rehabil 79:915–919, 1998.
28. Perry J, Barnes G, Gronley JK: The post-polio syndrome: An overuse phenomenon. Clin Orth Rel Res 233:145–162, 1988.
29. Borg K, Borg J, Edstrom L, Grimby L: Effects of excessive use of remaining muscle fibers in prior polio and LV lesion. Muscle Nerve 11:1219–1230, 1988.

30. Agre JC, Rodriquez AA, Franke TM: Subjective recovery time after exhausting muscular activity in post-polio and control subjects. Am J Phys Med Rehabil 77:140–144, 1998.

31. Wiechers DO, Hubbell SL: Late changes in the motor unit after acute poliomyelitis. Muscle Nerve 4:524–528, 1981.

32. Wiechers DO: Pathophysiology and late changes of the motor unit after poliomyelitis. In Halstead LS, Wiechers DO (eds): Late Effects of Poliomyelitis. Miami, Symposia Foundation, 1985, pp 91–94.

33. Cashman NR, Maselli R, Wollmann RL, et al: Late denervation in patients with antecedent paralytic poliomyelitis. N Engl J Med 317:7–12, 1987.

34. Grimby G, Stalberg E, Sandberg A, Sunnerhagen KS: A 8-year longitudinal study of muscle strength, muscle fiber size, and dynamic electromyogram in individuals with late polio. Muscle Nerve 21:1428–1437, 1998.

35. Waring WP, Maynard F, Grady W, et al: Influence of appropriate lower extremity orthotic management on ambulation, pain, and fatigue in a postpolio population. Arch Phys Med Rehabil 70:371–375, 1989.

36. Luna-Reyes OB, Reyes TM, So FY, et al: Energy cost of ambulation in healthy and disabled Filipino children. Arch Phys Med Rehabil 69:946–949, 1988.

37. Peach P, Olejnik S: Effect of treatment and non-compliance on post-polio sequelae. Orthopedics 14:1199–1203, 1991.

38. Waring WP, Davidoff G, Werner R: Serum creatine kinase in the post-polio population. Am J Phys Med Rehabil 68:86–90, 1989.

39. Nelson KR: Creatine kinase and fibrillation potentials in patients with late sequelae of polio. Muscle Nerve 13:722–725, 1990.

40. DeLorme TL, Schwab RS, Watkins AL: The response of the quadriceps femoris to progressive resistance exercise in polio myelitic patients. J Bone Joint Surg 30:834–847, 1948.

41. Gurewitsch AD: Intensive graduated exercises in early infantile paralysis. Arch Phys Med Rehabil 31:213–218, 1950.

42. Mueller EA, Beckmann H: Die trainierbarkeit von kindern mit gelaehmten muskeln durch isometrishe knotraktionen. Z Othop 102:139–145, 1966.

43. Feldman RM, Soskolne CL: The use of non-fatiguing strengthening exercises in post-polio syndrome. In Halstead LS, Wiechers DO (eds): Research and Clinical Aspects of the Late Effects of Poliomyelitis. White Plains, NY, March of Dimes Birth Defects Foundation, 1987, pp 335–341.

44. Einarsson G, Grimby G: Strengthening exercise program in post-polio subjects. In Halstead LS, Wiechers DO (eds): Research and Clinical Aspects of the Late Effects of Poliomyelitis. White Plains, NY, March of Dimes Birth Defects Foundation, 1987, pp 275–283.

45. Einarsson G: Muscle conditioning in late poliomyelitis. Arch Phys Med Rehabil 72:11–14, 1991.

46. Fillyaw MJ, Badger GJ, Goodwin GD, et al: The effects of long-term non-fatiguing resistance exercise in subjects with post-polio syndrome. Orthopedics 14:1253–1256, 1991.

47. Spector SA, Gordon PL, Feuerstein IM, et al: Strength gains without muscle injury after strength training in patients with postpolio muscular atrophy. Muscle Nerve 19:1282–1290, 1996.

48. Agre JC, Rodriquez AA, Franke TM, et al: Low-intensity, alternate-day exercise improves muscle performance without apparent adverse affect in post-polio patients. Am J Phys Med Rehabil 75:50–58, 1996.

49. Borg GAV: Perceived exertions: a note on "history" and methods. Med Sci Sports Exerc 5:90–93, 1973.

50. Agre JC, Rodriquez AA, Franke TM: Strength, endurance, and work capacity after muscle strengthening exercise in postpolio subjects. Arch Phys Med Rehabil 78:681–686, 1997.
51. Owen RR, Jones DR: Polio residuals clinic: Conditioning exercise program. Orthopedics 8:882–883, 1985.
52. Jones DR, Speier J, Canine K, et al: Cardiorespiratory responses to aerobic training by patients with post-poliomyelitis sequelae. JAMA 261:3255–3258, 1989.
53. Kriz JL, Jones DR, Speier JL, et al: Cardiorespiratory responses to upper extremity aerobic training by post-polio subjects. Arch Phys Med Rehabil 73:49–54, 1992.
54. Ernstoff B, Wetterqvist H, Kvist H, Grimby G: Endurance training effect on individuals with postpoliomyelitis. Arch Phys Med Rehabil 77:843–848, 1996.
55. Prins JH, Hartung H, Merritt DJ, et al: Effect of aquatic exercise training in persons with poliomyelitis disability. Sports Med Train Rehab 5:29–39, 1994.
56. Willen C: Physical Performance and the Effects of Dynamic Exercise in Water in Individuals with Late Polio [thesis]. Goteborg, Sweden, Department of Rehabilitation Medicine, Institute for Community Medicine, Goteborg University, 1999.
57. Dean E, Ross J: Effect of modified aerobic training on movement energetics in polio survivors. Orthopedics 14:1243–1246, 1991.
58. Agre JC, Rodriquez AA: Intermittent isometric activity: Its effect on muscle fatigue in postpolio patients. Arch Phys Med Rehabil 72:971–975, 1991.
59. Lindstrom L, Magnusson R, Petersen I: Muscular fatigue and action potential conduction velocity changes studied with frequency analysis of EMG signals. Electromyography 10:341–356, 1970.
60. Komi PV, Tesch P: EMG frequency spectrum during dynamic contractions in man. Eur J Appl Physiol 42:41–50, 1979.
61. DeLuca CJ: Myoelectrical manifestations of localized muscular fatigue in humans. Crit Rev Biomed Eng 11:251–279, 1985.

Physical Therapy in the Management of Chronic Poliomyelitis and Postpolio Syndrome

Elizabeth Dean, PT, PhD, and Marijke Dallimore, PT

A novel template for physical therapy including exercise in the management of chronic poliomyelitis, with or without postpolio syndrome (PPS) is described based on a critical analysis and synthesis of the literature. This template addresses the limitations of translating research findings from group data to the individual patient in the clinical situation. In part, these limitations can explain inconsistencies in findings across studies and in individual responses to treatment.

As described in Chapter 1, establishing a diagnosis of PPS is based on a detailed history and physical examination and even then may not be definitive. The symptoms of PPS are nonspecific, and in the absence of any specific tests, the diagnosis is largely one of exclusion. PPS is composed of one or more of the following complaints: new fatigue, weakness and muscle atrophy, muscle and joint pain, dysphagia, respiratory problems, reduced endurance, sleep disturbance, cold intolerance, and cognitive problems. The onset of new disability resulting from these symptoms significantly interferes with basic activities of daily living, including ambulation and movement, and lifting and carrying,[8] resulting in the patients seeking or being referred to physical therapy services. Many polio survivors have accommodated to varying degrees of fatigue, discomfort, pain, and dyspnea. Although adaptive over the years, this accommodation has necessitated that patients now relearn how to use these sensations as the basis for defining thresholds for activity and exercise and for rest and sleep.

Patients with chronic poliomyelitis are complex and challenging to manage and, inevitably, time consuming. Effective management extends beyond isolating a single complaint and treating that complaint in isolation. Patients with chronic poliomyelitis with or without PPS present with multisystem involvement that includes musculoskeletal, cardiopulmonary, and neurologic complications. In addition, the cohort of patients with poliomyelitis is older and often deconditioned (see Dean[25] for review of the negative effects of inactivity); therefore, symptoms can be confounded by one or more of the following:

cardiac and circulatory conditions, pulmonary conditions, hypertension and stroke, osteoarthritis, fibromyalgia, hypothyroidism, and diabetes. These conditions, most of which have a significant lifestyle component, need to be effectively controlled before rehabilitation or concurrent with it. In this way, symptoms associated with PPS can be better isolated and treated. This approach maximizes the patients' physiologic reserve capacity and thereby the summative and multiplicative effects of an eclectic treatment program.

TEMPLATE OF PHYSICAL THERAPY MANAGEMENT

The template for physical therapy management is presented in Table 1. Its overall effectiveness is contingent upon a close working relationship with other health care professionals. The prescription of specific physical therapy interventions is based on a detailed

---

Table 1. PRINCIPLE-BASED TEMPLATE FOR PHYSICAL THERAPY MANAGEMENT OF PATIENTS WITH CHRONIC POLIOMYELITIS WITH AND WITHOUT PPS

Communication
Incorporate an interdisciplinary team-based approach
Foster an effective therapeutic relationship
Listen and provide emotional support
Empower the patient with knowledge about PPS and skills to self-monitor and modify the treatment regimen
Facilitate learning by individualizing the educational plan and material and the mode of delivery
Facilitate adherence to recommendations
Screen for language and literacy barriers

History, Assessment, and Problem Definition
Perform history and multisystem assessment (at least two sessions)
Isolate symptoms of PPS and identify factors that confound their presentation
Review medications to determine positive and negative effects on function
Assess lifestyle factors:
    Physical activity level and exercise, nutritional status and weight, smoking history, alcohol consumption, sleep and rest, and stress
Prioritize lifestyle modification plan
Prioritize problem list (team), short- and long-term plan and treatment outcomes

Treatment Intervention Plan
Optimize health and well-being (team)
Optimize medication regimen (team) and monitor response; exploit noninvasive physical therapy to reduce unnecessary or ineffective medications and side effects
Manage comorbidities (team): serially or concurrently
Manage oxygen transport deficits, including those associated with sleep disturbance, and choking and swallowing dysfunction
Focus treatments on the underlying problems of the prioritized problem list
Select and prescribe physical therapy interventions (see Table 2): Serially or concurrently
Monitor and follow-up patient's adherence to recommendations and response to treatment interventions
Modify treatment commensurate with changes in status
Modify health plan commensurate with changes in status
Schedule follow-up and provide mechanism for the patient to contact the team

history and clinical examination. At least two sessions are needed to ensure the validity and reliability of the clinical picture and to resolve inconsistencies. Clinical decision making involves prioritizing interventions, defining their parameters, and establishing whether interventions are instituted concurrently or serially. The sequence and timing of the interventions that are instituted serially must be established. The specific interventions that can be integrated in the overall physical therapy management of chronic poliomyelitis or PPS are shown in Table 2. After a brief description of contemporary physical therapy practice and the format of this review, the specific findings from the analysis of the literature related to physical therapy interventions are outlined.

CONTEMPORARY PHYSICAL THERAPY PRACTICE AND OUTCOMES

Contemporary physical therapy focuses on the process of disablement, or the impact of the patient's condition on function, rather than a primary emphasis on treating the signs

Table 2. INTERVENTIONS RELATED TO THE PHYSICAL THERAPY MANAGEMENT OF CHRONIC POLIOMYELITIS WITH OR WITHOUT PPS
Communication
Patient-centered, team-based therapeutic relationship
Individualized patient education
Foster compliance and adherence to recommendations
Interventions to optimize oxygen transport and reduce risk of catastrophic events
Respiratory prophylaxis
Management of choking and swallowing dysfunction
Smoking cessation
Correction of disordered sleep
Thoracic orthotic support
Noninvasive mechanical ventilation
Supplemental oxygen
Breathing control and coughing maneuvers
Suctioning
Nutrition and weight control
Quality of nutrition to meet metabolic and energetic demands
Weight control (prescription of weight control or weight reduction)
Therapeutic exercise prescription
Stretching
Specific functional training
Aerobic conditioning
Exercise to improve movement economy
Postural alignment and re-education
Strength training
Fatigue management and energy conservation
Work simplification and pacing
Prescriptive rest and sleep to be maximally restorative
Aids, devices, equipment, and orthoses
Manual therapy, including mobilization and manipulation
Electrotherapy modalities
Physical agents and mechanical modalities
Acupuncture and its variants

and symptoms of disease.[49] Assessment is based on an analysis of the patient's general health as well as problems at the levels of impairment, functional limitation, and disability. Contemporary physical therapists are health care practitioners who focus primarily on evidence-based, noninvasive interventions in which education and exercise are fundamental components. Treatment outcomes are directly related to function, health status, and quality of life as well as impairments.

Noninvasive physical therapy includes education related to lifestyle and health behaviors in addition to self-management skills, therapeutic exercise, fatigue management, aids and devices, and the application of physical modalities and adjuncts. To maximize the effectiveness of physical therapy, recommendations, and health education, the cognitive status and learning style of the patient provide the basis for the format and delivery of the education component of treatment.

FORMAT OF THIS REVIEW

Systematic reviews and meta-analyses have become commonly accepted tools to assess best practices for a range of conditions. These approaches, however, are limited in the evaluation of best practices related to chronic poliomyelitis and PPS for several reasons:

- Studies are limited by inadequate definition of the sample of patients studied *vis a vis* an established definitive diagnosis of PPS versus chronic poliomyelitis without late onset symptoms.
- Patients are typically older adults who are physically deconditioned.
- The clinical picture is confounded by comorbidities with variable descriptions regarding their control.
- Patients may be taking medications that mask or exacerbate symptoms.
- The symptoms associated with PPS are nonspecific and subjective, making objective assessment and measurement difficult.
- Physical therapy management is eclectic, which makes isolation of variables and study of their interrelationships difficult.
- Comparable interventions are applied differently or have different prescriptive parameters across studies and patients, making comparisons among studies difficult.
- Because multiple interventions are used, there is a paucity of sufficient studies, let alone well-controlled studies, on any one intervention.
- The relationship between impairment measures and health status and quality of life is weak.
- The natural history of PPS has a progressive component, so a reduced rate of deterioration is a valid outcome. This outcome is difficult to capture in scientific studies.
- Even if there is no change in symptoms, a reduced need for medications is a valid treatment outcome; however, this may go unrecognized.

Because of these limitations, a template of best physical therapy practice is presented here based on a critical analysis and synthesis of theoretical, observational, and experimental studies related to the physical therapy management of patients with chronic poliomyelitis and PPS. Articles published in peer-reviewed journals and accessed through Medline, Cumulative Index of the Nursing and Allied Health Library (CINAHL), and the Cochrane Library (evidence-based practice data base) are included.

PHYSICAL THERAPY–RELATED INTERVENTIONS

Clinical decision making in the physical therapy management of patients with PPS is based on a detailed history of the initial onset of the disease and the onset of new late-onset problems, a multisystem assessment with supporting test results related both to PPS and comorbidity, and assessment of lifestyle behaviors and psychosocial status. Tests and measures of particular interest to the physical therapist include vital signs, electrocardiographic studies, muscle strength, endurance and fatigue profile based on manual muscle testing or myometry, range of motion, limb length, balance, posture and gait analysis, basic spirometry, oximetry, and an exercise test when possible.[24] These may be complemented by electromyography and nerve conduction studies. Subjective visual analog scales and the modified Borg scale are essential in the evaluation and in treatment prescription, because patients' complaints of fatigue, weakness, pain, and dyspnea are subjective. Thus, these scales are used to define the upper limits of activity and exercise in conjunction with objective measures and to define a threshold for instituting and defining the parameters of rest. Old and new deformities, including spinal curvature, are assessed. The patient's mobility aids, equipment, and devices are reviewed for type and appropriateness. An assessment of the patient's learning style and readiness to incorporate recommendations and changes is fundamental to the success of the therapeutic program and achieving its outcomes.

Of particular importance in the musculoskeletal assessment is the differentiation between those muscles that were initially affected by poliomyelitis and those that were not. The report of the patient is not sufficient. The differentiation between disuse of muscle versus overuse is fundamental to the prescription of exercise versus rest or a combination of the two. Direct evaluation of the relationship between exercise and recovery with rest and sleep, in combination with the patient's report, help to make this distinction. Muscles and joints that were unaffected by poliomyelitis can manifest secondary signs and symptoms because of compensatory strain. An analysis of the patient's capacity to recover physiologically with rests and sleep establishes the parameters of an activity and rest program so that physiologic function and endurance are maximized.

Physical therapy intervention ranges from preventive strategies and recommendations alone to the prescription of one or multiple interventions. In some cases, a couple of assessment visits may be all that is needed with provision for follow-up some months later. In complicated cases necessitating serial medical management of comorbidities and eventual concurrent physical therapy interventions, management requiring close supervision and regular follow-up may span several months.

COMMUNICATION

Although not a primary physical therapy intervention, communication is fundamental to the therapeutic relationship and the empowerment of the patient and the patient's long-term adherence to recommendations. A patient-centered, team-based approach in which team members share common goals with the patient is necessary in managing patients with chronic poliomyelitis.[15,91] Patient satisfaction with the therapeutic relationship is associated with the degree of emotional support and understanding received.[66] Patients with chronic poliomyelitis can have difficulty coping with the onset of a second disability resulting from PPS (e.g., chronic stress, anxiety, depression and compulsive type A behavior).[17] Patients with such conditions need to be identified and treated concurrently with physical therapy. In addition, adherence by the patient to a lifelong program is essential to maximize positive long-term outcomes.[15,20,67,90] Following patients more than 2 years, Peach and Olejnik reported a strong long-term relationship between strength and reduction of pain and adherence to recommendations, with a program of orthotic fitting, lifestyle modification, weight reduction, reduction in work hours, and aerobic conditioning.[84] Furthermore, the perception of an individual's capacity to cope and access resources is associated with reduced symptomatic distress.[65] A rich source of information can be obtained from the patient's reports of coping strategies.[76,100]

Depression can impact on the perception of severity of symptoms, learning, and coping strategies.[59] Although not a feature of PPS *per se,* when depression and distress are features of the clinical presentation, the capacity to cope can be affected.[92] Comparable to other chronic conditions, functional capacity may improve when depression is managed. Family support and attitude toward disability are also important variables in maximizing treatment responses.[57] Social support is well known to be fundamental to one's quality of life.[52] Overall, survivors of poliomyelitis report being satisfied with their lives; however, disturbing flashbacks to traumatic experiences at disease onset can be incapacitating.[100]

Some patients with PPS exhibit cognitive changes such as central fatigue, impaired attention and concentration, word finding difficulty,[18] and psychosocial distress.[93] These changes need to be considered in individualizing the format and delivery of patient education and determining a patient's capacity to comply with recommendations.

INTERVENTIONS TO OPTIMIZE OXYGEN TRANSPORT AND REDUCE THE RISK OF CATASTROPHIC EVENTS

Because impairment of oxygen transport constitutes significant risk with respect to morbidity and mortality,[70] and that physical therapy imposes demands on oxygen delivery, optimizing cardiorespiratory status is a priority. Impairments affecting the oxygen transport pathway can result from central neurologic insults, as well as the peripheral effects of chronic poliomyelitis on respiratory and chest wall musculature and spinal deformity.[68] A detailed analysis of the patient's oxygen demands and capacity to supply oxygen to working muscle and other tissues is conducted. In addition to its effects on the musculoskeletal system (i.e., muscles, joints, and postural alignment), chronic poliomyelitis can affect lung function; the position of the heart in the thoracic cavity (hence, pumping efficiency); and although not well documented, potentially autonomic function.

Cardiorespiratory impairments that have been reported and require management include hypercapnia,[72] restrictive lung pathology with hypoventilation,[38] and respiratory muscle weakness.[14,29,38] Exercise testing can be a useful tool to unmask ventilatory deficits that are not apparent at rest.[63,99] Patients with severe pulmonary compromise who are reliant on accessory muscle use to breathe may not be able to tolerate upper extremity exercise without worsening their breathing distress. In such patients, the following parameters need to be monitored: heart rate, blood pressure (BP), breathing pattern, arterial saturation, and perceived exertion and dyspnea.

Various noninvasive interventions can be prescribed for polio survivors with respiratory symptoms. Marked pulmonary compromise combined with impaired cough is an indication for breathing control and coughing maneuvers. With training, patients can learn to stack breaths with deep insufflation, thereby increasing cough force and effectiveness.[58] Some patients with tracheostomies suction themselves to remove pulmonary secretions they are unable to clear effectively on their own. These patients are also taught to move and change their body positions frequently coordinated with breathing control and coughing maneuvers to mobilize and remove secretions.[26–28,71] Movement and body positioning exert potent and direct effects on oxygen transport, and these interventions can be exploited by physical therapists in the management of patients with chronic as well as those with acute cardiopulmonary deficits by enhancing lung volumes and flow rates, reducing pulmonary closing volumes, enhancing airway clearance, and optimizing oxygenation.[33] Respiratory muscle training has been reported to have some role in reversing the effects of respiratory muscle weakness.[61] However, comparable to the training of other skeletal muscle in polio survivors, weakness of the respiratory muscles should be discriminated from fatigue; otherwise, resistance muscle training may contribute to deterioration.

Mechanical ventilation, oxygen supplementation, and other adjuncts may be useful. Nocturnal ventilation, for example, may be indicated to address nocturnal respiratory insufficiency and enhance the quality of the patient's night's sleep.[10,11,13,21,22,46,88] Oxygen therapy may be indicated based on blood gases and arterial saturation, but it is not a substitute for mechanical ventilation.[12] Chest wall bracing should be considered cautiously because it can contribute to further pulmonary compromise. Although a chest wall brace may have some role in supporting the chest walls of patients who are too weak and fatigued to effect normal respiratory mechanics without severe dyspnea, it also can contribute to further weakness of the respiratory muscles through disuse.

A predictor of respiratory insufficiency is the presence of the classic "polio belly," which is associated with atrophy of the abdominal muscles.[51,88] Loss of abdominal muscle strength impairs the patient's capacity to cough. The greater the patient's pulmonary compromise, the more detrimental the effects of active and passive smoking. Thus, smoking cessation should be a focus of management to enhance health and functional capacity[45] along with routine flu prophylaxis.

Choking and swallowing dysfunction are consistent with laryngeal pathology[40] and are life threatening. New laryngeal involvement is indicated by slowly progressive dyspnea, dysphagia and hoarseness[40,87]; as well as dysphonia, vocal weakness, and fatigue.[1] Swallowing symptoms are managed with techniques that reduce the risk of choking and aspiration. Recommendations regarding avoiding aggravating foods; taking small bites; chewing well; not drinking, talking, or laughing when eating. Eating in an upright position and avoiding recumbent positions for at least 1 hour after eating can reduce aspiration risk. As a precaution, the patient's family and the patient should be instructed in the Heimlich maneuver to relieve potential inadvertent upper airway obstruction.

Sleep disturbance[17,89] and sleep-disordered breathing[53] are of clinical significance in survivors of poliomyelitis for three reasons. First, sleep disturbance can compromise oxygen transport and predispose the patient to inadequate oxygen saturation and cardiac dysrhythmias while sleeping. Second, impaired sleep leads to daytime fatigue and somnolence, hence reduced functional capacity. Third, sleep deprivation contributes to reduced respiratory muscle endurance.[19] Remedying sleep disturbance is a priority, and in severe cases, it may require remediation before an activity or exercise program is instituted. Sleep studies are indicated if the patient reports excessive daytime sleepiness and respiratory complaints.[89]

A thorough assessment of oxygen transport during activity—and, in some instances, sleep—yields essential information with respect to the patient's capacity to sustain a given level of activity. This information can be used to assess risk when a patient undergoes routine medical and surgical procedures or uses pharmacologic agents that affect oxygen transport. Patients with poliomyelitis—with or without ventilatory complications at onset—may be at increased risk with the administration of muscle relaxants and anesthesia, exposure to a monotonous pattern of tidal ventilation with anesthesia and mechanical ventilation, maintaining a static body position for a prolonged period, and mobility restriction.[24,38] Adverse reactions need to be anticipated during medical and surgical procedures so that alternative interventions can be considered or, if adverse reactions occur, they are detected early and appropriate intervention instituted.

NUTRITION AND WEIGHT CONTROL

Living with a chronic condition, particularly one associated with physical deformity, postural malalignment, and muscle imbalance, impacts on nutritional requirements, both in terms of nutrients to support physiologic wear and tear and repair as well as the associated increased energy cost of ambulation.[39,86,98,104] Performing activities of daily living can be considered as demanding physically and psychologically for polio survivors as sports events being performed by athletes. Similarly, patients need to be appropriately fueled nutritionally to perform daily activities at the highest level of their capacity.

Individuals who are physically challenged often have difficulty maintaining optimal body weight. The loss of muscle mass and bone demineralization caused by restricted mobility reduces correspondingly the ideal weight for that individual to the low end of the body mass index (BMI) range or below. Thus, excessive weight (i.e., BMI > 25) is disproportionately high in this population. Excessive weight increases the energy demands and the mechanical demands of movement, contributing to muscle and joint overuse and strain, which further restricts the patient's activity. Maintaining optimal activity levels is essential for health and fitness and helps patients be independent and meet the needs of daily life. The detrimental effects of excess weight are exacerbated with aging. Monitoring patients' nutritional regimens is aimed at optimizing functional capacity and maintaining an optimal body weight. Because of their physical limitations, survivors of poliomyelitis have difficulty losing weight. Maintaining an optimal body weight is a function of both nutritional intake and energy expenditure, necessitating a judicious activity or exercise prescription when possible.

THERAPEUTIC EXERCISE

Physical therapists prescribe exercise for a range of therapeutic goals. With respect to chronic poliomyelitis with or without PPS, these goals include a combination of specific (e.g., for gait or fall prevention) or general muscle strengthening,[6,7,37,41,47,73,102] aerobic conditioning,[5,32,37,56,64] postural reeducation and movement economy,[32,35,98] flexibility and contracture avoidance,[95] and overall health benefit.[9] Other reasons physical therapists prescribe exercise for patients with chronic poliomyelitis include weight control, BP control, stress management and relaxation, bone health, sleep enhancement, incontinence management, and immunity-boosting and psychological effects. Studies related to exercise that have particular relevance to the template for physical therapy management are described in this chapter.

Physical therapists are particularly concerned with improving a given patient's capacity to perform specific functional activities and therefore exploiting the specificity of training principle. Appropriate exercise tests are selected to obtain baseline measures of pre-exercise program status (see Noonan and Dean[78] for details of selection and interpretation of exercise tests appropriate for the PPS population). Walking is a primary example of a functional activity and is comparatively easy to study. Although Dean and Ross[35] reported that survivors of poliomyelitis exhibit minimal aerobic conditioning with a short-term, low-intensity walking program (1 hour three times a week for 6 weeks), a combination of strength and endurance training (1 hour twice a week for 6 months) was reported by Ernstoff and coworkers[42] to improve muscle strength in selected muscles and aerobic performance, evidenced by a reduced heart rate at submaximal heart rates. Although Dean and Ross[32,35] reported no conventional signs of aerobic conditioning in their sample, patients walked longer with reduced complaint of fatigue and discomfort or pain after training. This finding likely reflects improved movement efficiency and reduced musculoskeletal strain. Improved movement efficiency is associated with reduced energy demands and thus, may reduce fatigue. The apparent lack of aerobic response to exercise suggests that the exercise stimulus was insufficient to elicit these effects. Consistent with what might be predicted, the gait of patients with PPS is less stable than control subjects, and leg weakness is an important determinant of unstable gait and falls.[54,69]

With the propensity for lower extremity involvement in PPS, Kriz and colleagues investigated the benefit of upper extremity aerobic training by 10 individuals with PPS.[64] They undertook a 16-week program, three times a week, for 20 minutes a session. The intensity was set at 70–75% of heart rate reserve plus resting heart rate. After the training, the experimental subjects showed improved aerobic capacity and muscle strength compared with the control group. The improvement was considered comparable to able-bodied individuals. The researchers concluded that a moderately intense aerobic upper extremity program was effective and safe for individuals with PPS.

Often patients with PPS are deconditioned aerobically,[34,56,77] further complicating their presentation. However, the results of conventional exercise tests in people with neurologic disorders have to be viewed cautiously. Conducting valid tests of aerobic capacity is difficult because of inconsistencies in the procedures, and the termination point is usually attributable to fatigue or pain rather than aerobic limitation.[36,78] Despite this limitation, one study recommended modified peripheral muscle endurance training for individuals with weak leg muscles and low oxygen uptake and general aerobic fitness training for those with good leg muscle strength.[101] To circumvent this methodologic issue, Noonan and coworkers examined submaximal indices of aerobic capacity and validated their use as predictors of functional capacity based on self-reports in patients with PPS.[79] Recommendations for exercise testing in patients with varying abilities, assuring validity and reliability, have been described by Noonan and Dean.[78] The goals of the test need to be established beforehand so that the appropriate test is selected. In most cases, submaximal tests can provide the information needed to address treatment goals without the risk of a maximal test on already strained muscles, ligaments, and joints and without the increased probability of producing invalid or unreliable test results.

The literature on stretching is scant. There are reports that increasing flexibility can minimize muscle and joint injury,[2] and it is advised after a short period of low-intensity warm-up exercise, which may not be possible in persons with severe physical disabilities. In patient populations, stretching is recommended to maintain the integrity of the muscle and to avoid unwanted contractures. In some cases, contractures are desirable where joints have been surgically fused to provide greater stability. In these instances, stretching is contraindicated.

Exercise capacity is limited in patients with PPS for many reasons. The limiters need to be identified so that exercise can be prescribed based on a consideration of physiologic reserve capacity, which can be compromised by muscle and joint overuse in patients with PPS.[2,24] Thus, to prescribe therapeutic exercise, muscle weakness secondary to muscle disuse versus overuse needs to be discriminated, and this needs to be determined for the various muscle groups. Creatine kinase, a muscle injury marker, has been reported to increase progressively with ambulation in some patients which is consistent with musculoskeletal strain.[97]

The goal of exercise prescription for patients with PPS is to obtain an optimal therapeutic functional outcome while avoiding overuse and further deterioration. Activity and exercise are prescribed to avoid undue fatigue and muscle and joint pain and prolonged recovery of muscle strength. Thus, prescribing exercise for polio survivors is best based on subjective parameters such as thresholds defined on visual analog scales for fatigue, weakness, pain, and dyspnea or a combination rather than on such conventional objective parameters as heart rate and BP.[31,35] Based on the patient's electrodiagnostic findings and symptoms, Halstead and colleagues[50] recommended exploiting the stronger and unaffected muscles in an exercise program while resting, bracing affected and atrophied muscles. With a conservative approach tailored specifically to each patient, the goal is to reverse, delay, prevent, or mitigate the new problems. However, an exercise program needs to be instituted in combination with a nutritional program and modification of other lifestyle factors, including smoking, to accentuate the beneficial effects of the program and limit adverse effects.

Progressive deterioration in strength of survivors of poliomyelitis exceeds that of healthy control subjects,[62] and this effect is marked in the knee extensors.[77] Increased recovery time from exhaustive isometric muscular exercise is greater in patients with unstable PPS than in stable or control subjects.[5]

Early studies on exercise prescription for patients with PPS described improved muscle strength in selective muscle groups with nonfatiguing strengthening exercises.[43,44] Although there is physiologic justification for low-intensity, resistance exercise in the presence of muscle disuse versus overuse, prescribing the initial starting weight is difficult.

When the first anecdotal reports of patients experiencing new problems emerged in the late 1970s and early 1980s, physiologic and clinical studies reported that traditional resistive muscle training was contraindicated for denervated muscle because of the potential for increased muscle weakness and further functional deterioration.[57] This was exemplified in a case report by Gross and Schuch.[48] The 59-year-old patient underwent "an aggressive, six-week isokinetic exercise program." Contrary to the investigators' conclusion, Dean and colleagues showed that the results of the study supported overuse and deterioration rather than improvement with no adverse effects.[37]

Perry and coworkers examined the relationship between lower extremity strength and gait characteristics in 24 patients with PPS.[85] They emphasized the relative importance of plantar flexion and hip abduction in predicting speed of stride length. Furthermore, these investigators emphasized the essential role of plantar flexor strength in gait. If the plantar flexors are overused and unable to be strengthened, then an orthosis or permanent contracture needs to substitute.

Nordgren and colleagues described some limitations of strength assessment and training in individuals with PPS.[80] They reported that in a sample of 11 patients, subjective evaluation of muscle strength was not associated with objective measures of metabolism, magnetic resonance imaging, electromyography (EMG), or muscle strength.

Agre and coworkers examined the effect of a low-intensity, alternate-day, 12-week quadriceps muscle strengthening exercise program on muscle strength and motor unit integrity in 12 patients with PPS.[7] They reported that patients were able to lift more weight after participating in the program and that there were no apparent short-term adverse effects as indicated by change in motor units reflected by EMG, or levels of serum creatine kinase.

Hydro or aquatic therapy was used extensively in the management of patients with subacute poliomyelitis during the epidemic. Although its physiologic effects have not been well studied, aquatic therapy could be prescribed to yield both a strengthening and aerobic response (see Chapter 11). Because of the buoyancy of water, important gravitational effects are forfeited. Limitations of this form of exercise are largely practical ones regarding getting in and out of the pool, pool depth, and temperature. Physical therapists should play a role in the design of facilities for the public to ensure that facilities meet the needs of persons with disabilities.

Although exercise may have an important role for maintaining or restoring bone health in persons with PPS, no studies have been reported examining the role of exercise for this purpose in this population. The more disabled and less physically active the individual, the greater the risk of osteoporosis. In addition, an asymmetrical gait can reduce stability and increase the risk of falls and fractures.[69] Patients with PPS heal and recover more slowly. If medical management of a fracture requires restricted activity, polio-affected muscles atrophy quickly. In addition, the risk of medical and surgical complications is increased.

Individuals with PPS have been reported to experience increased prevalence of urologic symptoms, including bladder disorders, stress incontinence, and erectile dysfunction in men compared with those without PPS. In a study of 242 female and 88 male survivors of poliomyelitis, Johnson and coworkers examined the prevalence of urologic problems that could be attributable to PPS.[55] There may be a role for noninvasive physical therapy management of stress incontinence and sexual dysfunction in this population comparable to the needs of other patient populations with these concerns.

In sum, with respect to therapeutic exercise prescribed by physical therapists for patients with chronic poliomyelitis, the principle of specificity of training need to be exploited as much as possible. However, certain precautions need to be observed in this population, and the prescription should be modified based on the presentation of PPS. Guidelines for resistance strengthening exercise of importance to physical therapists are based on differentiating muscle weakness caused by disuse versus overuse to avoid exacerbating the patient's symptoms. Lower intensities, intermittent exercise schedules, and longer recovery periods are indicated. Guidelines for aerobic exercise include a modified prescription based primarily on subjective (e.g., pain, fatigue, exertion, or dyspnea) rather than objective parameters (e.g., heart rate, electrocardiogram [ECG], BP, breathing pattern, and arterial saturation), intermittent exercise schedule, and prolonged course. Postural alignment is optimized to reduce biomechanical stress and undue energy cost of ambulation. Activity and exercise are balanced with prescribed rest to optimize physiologic recovery. Overall aerobic exercise benefit may be achieved with less risk by exercising stronger uninvolved muscles while weaker involved muscles are braced or rested. All exercise testing and training should include appropriate monitoring of a combination of subjective as well as objective responses to exercise. A primary caveat in the exercise testing and prescription of exercise for survivors of poliomyelitis with PPS is avoidance of overuse. At present, this is best assessed clinically using serial subjective and objectives measures of responses to activity and exercise as well as recovery.

FATIGUE MANAGEMENT AND ENERGY CONSERVATION

One explanation for PPS has been degeneration of distal axonal sprouts of oversized motor units and a declining motor unit pool.[57] Thus, minimizing the physical and mechanical demands on affected and unaffected muscles is a justifiable goal.[37,83] For some individuals, this may be the only intervention needed to increase function. More often, energy conservation is advocated in combination with other strategies as a means of managing fatigue associated with muscle overuse and central fatigue. Lesions of the reticular activating system have been implicated in the etiology of central fatigue[16]; therefore, its management is more elusive.

Sleep (which may be disturbed in survivors of poliomyelitis) and rest are judiciously prescribed to maximize physiologic and psychological recovery, hence daily function.[23,53] Subjective scales such as the visual analog scales for fatigue, weakness, pain, exertion, and dyspnea provide a rational basis for defining thresholds for rest as well as activity and exercise.[31,35] Lack of sleep, reduced growth hormone levels, and fibromyalgia are common concerns in polio survivors that produce symptoms mimicking PPS. Resolution of these problems may completely reverse their symptoms.[94] Profiles of the quality and quantity of a patient's night's sleep and rests yield valuable information regarding the patient's capacity to recover from physical and mental activity.[31] Prescriptive rests may enable the patient to manage fatigue effectively.[81,82] Pacing has been showed to be effective in minimizing muscle aching and cramping,[103] which may be particularly beneficial in patients with unstable signs and symptoms.[5] Balancing work and rest in a prescriptive manner can reduce local muscle fatigue, increase work capacity, and reduce recovery time.[4] Aids and devices can be effectively prescribed to minimize undue physical stress and fatigue.[24] These should be prescribed judiciously because muscle wasting in survivors of poliomyelitis may be exacerbated when exercise stress is removed with resting, pacing, and orthoses. These interventions need to be considered carefully, recognizing that each muscle may differ in the amount of support it needs with respect to rest and exercise stress. These factors must be balanced to ensure that function is not compromised. For example, an orthosis may be prescribed for intermittent use to be worn only when the muscle it supports shows signs of fatigue.

AIDS, DEVICES, EQUIPMENT, AND ORTHOTICS

Aids, devices, equipment (e.g., wheelchairs, walkers, crutches, and chair escalators installed at home), and orthotics may need to be considered for symptom management, muscle and joint protection, and promotion of movement efficiency and reducing undue postural malalignment and energy cost, which can contribute secondarily to further overuse and fatigue. Aids, devices, and orthoses need to be introduced gradually so affected muscles and joints can adapt. Soft tissue appears to be less resilient in polio survivors and requires a longer period to adapt to new orthotics and devices. Orthotic use can contribute to muscle atrophy, so they need to be prescribed on an intermittent schedule to preserve remaining muscle strength as well as rest for the muscle as it fatigues. Even small biomechanical changes effected by the introduction of new orthotics can initially exacerbate the patient's complaints of muscle and joint discomfort. Introduction of a new device too quickly may result in its being abandoned by the patient. Appropriate orthotic use has been associated with improved ability to walk, walking safety, and reduced local and general pain in patients with PPS.[96] Therefore, appropriate fitting and paced introduction of the orthotic in conjunction with education are important to ensure that maximal benefit is derived from its use.

MANUAL THERAPY

Although no studies have been reported on use of manual therapy, including orthopedic mobilization and manipulation, in the management of PPS, they may have a role in the management of comorbidity. However, weak musculature, strained ligaments, and osteoporosis that may be present in an individual with PPS may be contraindications.

ELECTROTHERAPY MODALITIES

Reports on the selective application of electrotherapy modalities for complaints specific to chronic poliomyelitis or PPS are limited. Functional electrical stimulation may have a limited role in strengthening muscle in some patients[2]; however, there is agreement in the field that electrical stimulation produces the best results when a muscle is totally denervated yet has the potential for reinnervation such as in acute poliomyelitis.[30] Pain control modalities may have some benefit; however, they should not replace the need to eliminate the underlying cause or minimize its effects.

PHYSICAL AGENTS AND MECHANICAL MODALITIES

Heat and rest have been reported to relieve symptoms in patients with PPS.[101] With respect to magnetotherapy, static magnetic fields of 300–500 Gauss over a pain trigger point has been reported to provide prompt pain relief.[95] The application of hyperbaric therapy (100% oxygen at 2 atmospheres each day for 1 month and then weekly for 1 year) has been reported in one case of PPS to increase strength, reduce motor unit degeneration, and enhance regeneration of motor units.[74] Pain control modalities may have some benefit; however, they should not replace the need to eliminate the underlying cause or minimize its effects.

ACUPUNCTURE AND ITS VARIANTS

Acupuncture and its variants such as acupressure and acupuncture-like transcutaneous nerve stimulation (TENS) may have a role in pain control for some patients. However, comparable to other modalities, the underlying cause must be addressed and treated if possible.

RESEARCH CONSIDERATIONS AND PRIORITIES

Research priorities for physical therapy management of chronic poliomyelitis with and without PPS are summarized in Table 3. Many of these priorities focus on elucidation of principles of management as opposed to simply symptom-specific interventions, as well as the need to examine the interactive effects of eclectic treatments, which has rarely been a focus of study.

Table 3. PHYSICAL THERAPY RESEARCH PRIORITIES

Pathophysiology
  Further elucidation of risk factors for PPS and their modification
  Refinement of strategies for preventing PPS
  Refinement of objective and subjective measures in the diagnosis of physical
    therapy problems and "condition-specific" outcomes
  Impact of lifestyle behaviors on symptoms and their management
  Wellness and prevention strategies specific to the needs of polio survivors
  Discrimination of fatigued vs. weak muscles (both peripheral and respiratory)
Communication
  Application of adult learning and teaching principles in the health education
    of polio survivors
  Principles of empowering the patient in the therapeutic relationship with the
    health care provider
  Principles for maximizing adherence of patients to therapeutic recommendations
Interventions to optimize oxygen transport and reduce risk of catastrophic events
  Role of noninvasive ventilation and functional capacity
  Evaluation of swallowing strategies to minimize dysphagia
Nutrition and weight control
  Impact of optimal nutrition on enhancing function in chronic poliomyelitis
  Strategies for weight control in patients who are prone to gain weight because
    of inactivity
Therapeutic exercise
  Prescription of functional training as a primary treatment intervention
  Further investigation of the principles for prescription of strength training
  Further investigation of the principles for prescription of aerobic training
  Evaluation of exercise parameters based on minimizing subjective complaints
    rather than objective measures
Fatigue management and energy conservation
  Principles of rest prescription for the fatigued muscle and principles of exercise
    prescription for the weak muscle to avoid contributing to overuse
  Principles for prescribing general activity
  Principles for prescribing restorative rest and sleep
  Principles for balancing rest and sleep and activity and exercise
Aids, devices, equipment, and orthoses
  Principles for prescribing aids and devices
  Principles for prescribing orthotics and maximizing their effects
Manual therapy, including mobilization and manipulation
  Unlikely to need specific manual therapy for the management of chronic polio-
    myelitis with or without PPS; may have a nonspecific role in management of
    comorbidity
Electrotherapy modalities
  Examination of its efficacy in controlling pain
Physical agents and mechanical modalities
  Examination of their efficacy in controlling pain
Acupuncture and its variants
  Examination of its efficacy in controlling pain

Studies examining symptom-specific interventions are limited by many factors, including trials that are conducted on groups. Such studies are predicated on the homogeneity of the group to be able to generalize to the population. However, in reality, one patient is very different from the next. With respect to physical therapy management, the results of these studies cannot be readily translated to the needs of the single survivor of poliomyelitis with a myriad of confounding problems, either related or not related to a history of poliomyelitis, and on a medication regimen that confounds the clinical presentation. Clinical decision making focuses on matching the therapeutic regimen to the specific needs of the patient as a whole as described in the evidence-based template of care presented in this review, including the initial disease involvement and severity, onset of new problems, cognitive status, general health, nutritional status, weight, lung function, comorbidity, response to medications, and lifestyle factors. Because of the multi-pronged approach indicated in the physical therapy management of survivors of poliomyelitis, special attention is given to determining whether interventions are introduced serially or concurrently for maximal benefit. Studies are needed to refine further the prescription of multi-pronged treatment approaches in the management of patients with PPS.

Factors that contribute to the challenges in the clinical management of patients with a history of poliomyelitis also contribute to the enormous challenges of conducting best-practice research in this area. These factors and the paucity of studies with comparable objectives have precluded the opportunity to conduct systematic reviews and meta-analyses based on their stringent inclusion criteria or to extract valid information from their results. Despite their reported robustness, these methodologies will not be able to be conducted or yield valid results without systematic tight experimental controls of the independent and dependent variables in the source studies. For example, valid and reliable clinical measures of muscle strength have been lacking. Hand-held dynamometry has been compelling in the assessment of patients with neurological conditions, including PPS.[60,75] However, reservations have been expressed about its use in the PPS population in favor of a fixed dynamometer.[3] In addition, muscle testing typically requires repeated measures. This methodology can be fatiguing for patients with PPS, which may confound the results and complicate standardization of the procedures. Other methodological concerns in the poliomyelitis population include the elimination of extraneous confounding variables related to diagnosis and care and stringent patient selection with attention to their medication regimens. No two patients with a history of poliomyelitis are identical even when considering the type and level of involvement and presence or absence of late effects, without the additional consideration of age, comorbidity, medications, and lifestyle. Furthermore, treatment is often eclectic; thus, treatment effects are difficult to isolate. These factors are likely to result in variable study outcomes reflecting variable subject responses. Thus, a principle-based approach to the physical therapy management of persons with chronic conditions such as poliomyelitis is a more rational approach than searching for and applying a standardized treatment regimen based on management of individual symptoms.

SUMMARY AND CONCLUSIONS

The literature related to the physical therapy management of the patient with chronic poliomyelitis and PPS confirms that:

- Treatment planning may be more effective overall when it is a component of the interdisciplinary team evaluation and management plan.
- Treatment response can be enhanced when patients perceive that practitioners validate their concerns and listen and that they are in therapeutic relationships in which they feel empowered.
- Treatment response can be enhanced when physical therapy is one component of the patient-focused interdisciplinary team.
- Treatment response is commensurate with degree of adherence to therapeutic recommendations.
- Clinical outcomes can be enhanced when the patient's general health is optimized.
- Respiratory, hemodynamic, and swallowing or choking need to be reviewed and managed as priorities.
- Respiratory compromise can exist in individuals who had no ventilatory involvement at onset of PPS.
- Respiratory support, including nocturnal noninvasive ventilation, can enhance function.
- Maximizing sleep quality enhances function.
- Optimizing nutrition enhances function.
- Coexistent morbidity that can contribute to impaired function (including depression) must be optimally managed, either concurrently or serially in conjunction with ongoing physical therapy.
- Pharmacologic management must be reviewed to minimize adverse effects on function and, when necessary, to reduce symptoms and maximize functional capacity.
- There may be psychological as well as practical explanations as to why patients do not adhere to therapeutic recommendations.
- An eclectic therapeutic regimen that includes education, exercise, fatigue management, use of orthotics, weight loss, and pain control can be highly effective in controlling disabling PPS symptoms when prescribed on an individual basis.
- Weight control alone may be singularly important in ameliorating symptoms.
- Exercise prescription is based preferably on subjective responses such as fatigue, weakness, pain, dyspnea, or a combination, rather than conventional heart rate measures, using visual analog scales.
- Lower-intensity, short-duration, intermittent activity or exercise rather than higher-intensity, longer-duration continuous exercise performed within subjective limits of tolerable fatigue, weakness, and pain, can translate into a greater volume of work or exercise being performed over a given period of time without adverse responses.

> Improving postural alignment and reducing the energy cost of ambulation may reduce fatigue, reduce biomechanical strain, and increase function.

> Clinical decision making includes decisions regarding capitalizing on the summative and multiplicative effects of combining treatments by sequencing and introducing them at judicious times.

> Treatments are directed toward prevention or worsening of PPS as well as symptom reduction.

> The effect of physical therapy interventions in the management of patients with PPS is challenging to study using the traditional impairment biomedical model because of the variability of the type and severity of the condition, muscle groups affected, limbs affected, patients' interpretations of the impact of their conditions on their lives, associated deformity, coexistent morbidity, use of medications, and psychological overlay.

The physical therapy prognosis for patients with chronic poliomyelitis with or without PPS can be favorable with a principle-based template of care. The principles of practice are categorized into those related to the interdisciplinary team, effectiveness of the therapeutic relationship, and individually determined learning and teaching strategies; effective control of comorbidities; optimization of lifestyle related to health and wellness; management of oxygen transport deficits and dysphagia; prescription of physical therapy interventions and determination of whether they are introduced serially or concurrently; appropriate monitoring of the patient's adherence to the recommendations and response to the program; and scheduling of follow-up and provision of a mechanism for the patient to contact the team. Patients with a history of poliomyelitis are complex, necessitating a principle-based, multi-pronged treatment approach over the long term. In this way, the summative and multiplicative effects of combining treatments can be maximized. This template can serve as a prototype for the physical therapy management of patients with other chronic conditions as well.

References

1. Abaza MM, Sataloff RT, Hawkshaw MJ, et al: Laryngeal manifestations of post poliomyelitis syndrome. J Voice 15:291–294, 2001.
2. Agre JC: The role of exercise in the patient with post-polio syndrome. Ann NY Acad Sci 753:321–334, 1995.
3. Agre JC, Herbison GJ: Strength changes over time among polio survivors [letter to the editor]. Arch Phys Med Rehabil 81:1538, 2000.
4. Agre JC, Rodriquez AA: Intermittent isometric activity: its effect on muscle fatigue in postpolio subjects. Arch Phys Med Rehabil 72:971–975, 1991.
5. Agre JC, Rodriquez AA, Franke TM: Subjective recovery time after exhaustive muscular activity in postpolio and control subjects. Am J Phys Med Rehabil 77:140–144, 1998.
6. Agre JC, Rodriquez AA, Franke TM: Strength, endurance, and work capacity after muscle strengthening exercise in postpolio subjects. Arch Phys Med Rehabil 78:681–686, 1997.
7. Agre JC, Rodriquez AA, Franke TM, et al: Low-intensity, alternate-day exercise improves muscle performance without apparent adverse affect in postpolio patients. Am J Phys Med Rehabil 75:50–58, 1996.

8. Ahlstrom G, Karlsson U: Disability and quality of life in individuals with postpolio syndrome. Disabil Rehabil 22:416–422, 2000.
9. Astrand P-O: Exercise physiology and its role in disease prevention and in rehabilitation. Arch Phys Med Rehabil 68:305–309, 1987.
10. Bach JR: Management of post-polio respiratory sequelae. Ann N Y Acad Sci 753:96–102, 1995.
11. Bach JR, Alba AS, Bohatiuk, G, et al: Mouth intermittent positive pressure ventilation in the management of postpolio respiratory insufficiency. Chest 91:859–864, 1987.
12. Bach JR, Rajaraman R, Ballanger F, et al: Neuromuscular ventilatory insufficiency: Effect of home mechanical ventilator use versus oxygen therapy on pneumonia and hospitalization rates. Am J Phys Med Rehabil 77:8–19, 1998.
13. Bach JR, Smith WH, Michaels J, et al: Airway secretion clearance by mechanical exsufflation for post-poliomyelitis ventilator-assisted individuals. Arch Phys Med Rehabil 74; 170–177, 1993.
14. Borg K, Kaijser L: Lung function in patients with prior poliomyelitis. Clin Physiol 10: 201–212, 1990.
15. Boyle CM. Differences between patients' and doctors' interpretation of common medical terms. Br Med J 2:286–289, 1970.
16. Bruno RL, Cohen JM, Galski T, Frick NM: The neuroanatomy of post-polio fatigue. Arch Phys Med Rehabil 75:498–504, 1994.
17. Bruno RL, Frick NM. The psychology of polio as prelude to post-polio sequelae: Behavior modification and psychotherapy. Orthopedics 14:1185–1193, 1991.
18. Bruno RL, Zimmerman JR: Word finding difficulty as a post-polio sequelae. Am J Phys Med Rehabil 79:343–348, 2000.
19. Chen H-I, Tang Y-R: Sleep loss impairs inspiratory muscle endurance. Am Rev Respir Dis 140:907–909, 1989.
20. Creange SJ, Bruno RL: Compliance with treatment for postpolio sequelae. Am J Phys Med Rehabil 76:378–382, 1997.
21. Culebras A: Sleep and neuromuscular disorders. Neurol Clin 14:791–805, 1996.
22. Curran FJ, Colbert AP: Ventilatory management in Duchenne muscular dystrophy and postpoliomyelitis syndrome: twelve years' experience. Arch Phys Med Rehabil 70:180–185, 1989.
23. Dean AC, Graham BA, Dalakas M, Sato S: Sleep apnea in patients with postpolio. Ann Neurol 43:661–664, 1998.
24. Dean E: Clinical decision making in the management of the late sequelae of poliomyelitis. Phys Ther 71:752–761, 1991.
25. Dean E: Bedrest and deconditioning. Neurol Rep 17:6–9, 1993.
26. Dean E: Mobilization and exercise. In Frownfelter D, Dean E (eds): Principles and Practice of Cardiopulmonary Physical Therapy. St. Louis, Mosby, 1996.
27. Dean E: Body positioning. In Frownfelter D, Dean E (eds): Principles and Practice of Cardiopulmonary Physical Therapy. St. Louis, Mosby, 1996.
28. Dean E: Late sequelae of poliomyelitis. In Frownfelter D, Dean E (eds): Clinical Case Study Guide to Accompany Principles and Practice of Cardiopulmonary Physical Therapy. St. Louis, Mosby, 1996.
29. Dean E: Oxygen transport deficits in systemic disease and implications for physical therapy. Phys Ther 77:187–202, 1997.
30. Dean E, Agboatwalla M, Dallimore M, et al: Poliomyelitis (part II): Revised principles of management. Physiother 81:23–28, 1995.
31. Dean E, Dallimore M: Activity rest profiles: A basis for fatigue management in patients

with the late sequelae of poliomyelitis. Proceeding of Canadian Physiotherapy Association Congress, Victoria, BC, 1996.

32. Dean E, Ross J: Modified aerobic walking program: effect on patients with postpolio syndrome symptoms. Arch Phys Med Rehabil 69:1033–1038, 1988.

33. Dean E, Ross J: Oxygen transport: the basis for contemporary cardiopulmonary physical therapy and its optimization with body positioning and mobilization. Phys Ther Prac 1:34–44, 1992.

34. Dean E, Ross J: Movement energetics of individuals with a history of poliomyelitis. Arch Phys Med Rehabil 74:478–483, 1993.

35. Dean E, Ross J: Effect of modified aerobic training on movement energetics in polio survivors. Orthopedics 14:1243–1246, 1995.

36. Dean E, Ross J, Bartz J, Purves S: Improving the validity of clinical exercise testing: the relationship between practice and performance. Arch Phys Med Rehabil 70:599–604, 1989.

37. Dean E, Ross J, MacIntyre D: A rejoinder to "Exercise Programs for Patients with Post-Polio Syndrome: A case report": A short communication. Phys Ther 69:695–699, 1989.

38. Dean E, Ross J, Road JD, et al: Pulmonary function in individuals with a history of poliomyelitis. Chest 100:118–123, 1991.

39. Dontas AS, Moschandreas J, Kafatos A: Physical activity and nutrition in older adults. Public Health Nutr 2:429–436, 1999.

40. Driscoll BP, Gracco C, Coelho C, et al: Laryngeal function in postpolio patients. Laryngoscope 105:35–41, 1995.

41. Einarsson G: Muscle conditioning in late poliomyelitis. Arch Phys Med Rehabil 72:11–14, 1991.

42. Ernstoff B, Wetterqvist H, Kvist H, Brimby G: Endurance training effect on individuals with postpoliomyelitis. Arch Phys Med Rehabil 77:843–848, 1996.

43. Feldman RM, Soskolne CL: The use of nonfatiguing strengthening exercises in post-polio syndrome. In Halstead LS, Wiechers DO (eds): Research and Clinical Aspects of the Late Effects of Poliomyelitis. White Plains, NY, March of Dimes Birth Defects Foundation, 1987, pp 335–341.

44. Fillyaw MJ, Badger GJ, Goodwin GD, et al: The effects of long-term non-fatiguing resistance exercise in subjects with post-polio syndrome. Orthopedics 14:1553–1556, 1995.

45. Glantz SA, Parmley WW: Passive smoking and heart disease. Mechanisms and risk. JAMA 273:1047–1053, 1995.

46. Goldstein RS, Molotia N, Skrastins R, et al: Assisting ventilation in respiratory failure by negative pressure ventilation and by rocking bed. Chest 82:470–474, 1987.

47. Grimby F, Stalberg E: Dynamic changes in muscle structure and electrophysiology in late polio with aspect on muscular trainability. Scand J Rehabil Med 30(suppl):33–44, 1994.

48. Gross MT, Schuch CP: Exercise programs for patients with post-polio syndrome: A case report. Phys Ther 69:72–76, 1989.

49. Guide to Physical Therapist Practice, 2nd ed. Washington, DC, American Physical Therapy Association, 2001.

50. Halstead LS, Gawne AC, Pham BT: National Rehabilitation Hospital limb classification for exercise, research, and clinical trials in post-polio patients. Ann NY Acad Sci 53:343–353, 1995.

51. Hamilton EA, Nichols PJR, Tait GBW: Late onset of respiratory insufficiency after poliomyelitis Ann Phys Med 10:223–229, 1970.

52. Hollingsworth L, Didelot MJ, Levington C: Post-polio syndrome: Psychological adjustment to disability. Issues Ment Health Nurs 23:135–156, 2002.

53. Hsu AA, Staats BA: "Postpolio" sequelae and sleep-related disordered breathing. Mayo Clin Proc 73:216–224, 1998.
54. Hurmuzlu Y, Basdogan C, Stoianovici D: Kinematics and dynamic stability of the locomotion of post-polio patients. J Biomech Eng 118:405–411, 1996.
55. Johnson VY, Hubbard D, Vordermark JS: Urologic manifestations of postpolio syndrome. J Wound Ostomy Continence Nurs 23:218–223, 1996.
56. Jones DR, Speier J, Canine K, et al: Cardiorespiratory responses to aerobic training by patients with postpoliomyelitis sequelae. JAMA 261:3255–3258, 1989.
57. Jubelt B, Cashman NR: Neurological manifestations of the post-polio syndrome. Crit Rev Neurobiol 3:199–220, 1987.
58. Kang SW, Bach JR: Maximum insufflation capacity. Chest 118:61–65, 2000.
59. Kemp BJ, Adams BM, Campbell ML: Depression and life satisfaction in aging polio survivors versus age-matched controls: Relation to post-polio syndrome, family functioning and attitude toward disability. Arch Phys Med Rehabil 78:187–192, 1997.
60. Kilmer DD, McCrory MA, Wright NC, et al: Hand-held dynamometry reliability in persons with neuropathic weakness. Arch Phys Med Rehabil 78:1364–1368, 1997.
61. Klefbeck B, Lagerstrand L, Mattsson E: Inspiratory muscle training in patients with prior polio who use part-time assisted ventilation. Arch Phys Med Rehabil 81:1065–1071, 2002.
62. Klein MG, Whyte J, Keenan MA, et al: Changes in strength over time among polio survivors. Arch Phys Med Rehabil 81:1538–1539, 2000.
63. Knobil K, Becker FS, Harper P, et al: Dyspnea in a patient years after severe poliomyelitis: The role of cardiopulmonary exercise testing. Chest 105:777–781, 1994.
64. Kriz JL, Jones DR, Speier JL, et al: Cardiorespiratory responses to upper extremity aerobic training by postpolio subjects. Arch Phys Med Rehabil 73:49–54, 1992.
65. Kuehn AF, Winters RK: A study of symptom distress, health locus of control, and coping resources of aging post-polio survivors. Image J Nurs Sch 6:325–331, 1994.
66. Ley P: Communicating with Patients. London, Croom Helm, 1988.
67. Ley P, Morris LA: Psychological aspects of written information for patients. In Rachman S (ed): Contributions to Medical Psychology. Oxford, Pergamon Press, 1984.
68. Lin MC, Chen WJ, Cheng Pt, et al: Pulmonary function and spinal characteristics: Their relationships in persons with idiopathic and postpoliomyelitis scoliosis. Arch Phys Med Rehabil 82:335–341, 2000.
69. Lord SR, Allen GM, Williams P, Gandevia SC: Risk of falling: Predictors based on reduced strength in persons previously affected by polio. Arch Phys Med Rehabil 83:757–763, 2002.
70. Mahgoub A, Cohen R, Rossoff LJ: Weakness, daytime somnolence, cough, and respiratory distress in a 77-year-old man with a history of polio. Chest 120:659–661, 2001.
71. Massery M: The patient with neuromuscular and musculoskeletal dysfunction. In Frownfelter D, Dean E (eds): Principles and Practice of Cardiopulmonary Physical Therapy. St. Louis, Mosby, 1996.
72. Midgren B: Lung function and clinical outcome in postpolio patients: A prospective cohort study during 11 years. Eur Respir J 10:146–149, 1997.
73. Milner-Brown HS: Muscle strengthening in a post-polio subject through a high-resistance weight-training program. Arch Phys Med Rehabil 74:1165–1167, 1993.
74. Nakajima M, Kuwabara S, Uchino F, Hirayama K: Enhanced regeneration of terminal axons after hyperbaric oxygen therapy in a patient resembling progressive postpoliomyelitis muscular atrophy. Rinsho Shinkeigaku 34:48–51, 1994.
75. Nollett F, Beelen A: Strength assessment in postpolio syndrome: Validity of a hand-held dynamometer in detecting changes. Arch Phys Med Rehabil 80:1316–1323, 1999.
76. Nollett F, Beelen A, Prins MH, et al: Disability and functional assessment in former polio

patients with and without postpolio syndrome. Arch Phys Med Rehabil 80:136–143, 1999.

77. Nollet F, Beelen A, Sargeant AJ, et al: Submaximal exercise capacity and maximal power output in polio subjects. Arch Phys Med Rehabil 12:1678–1685, 2001.

78. Noonan V, Dean E: Submaximal exercise testing: Clinical application and interpretation. Phys Ther 80:782–807, 2000.

79. Noonan V, Dean E, Dallimore M: The relationship between self-reports and objective measures of disability in patients with late sequelae of poliomyelitis: A validation study. Arch Phys Med Rehabil 81:1422–1427, 2000.

80. Nordgren B, Falck B, Stalberg E, et al: Postpolio muscular dysfunction: Relationships between muscle energy metabolism, subjective symptoms, magnetic resonance imaging, electromyography, and muscle strength. Muscle Nerve 20:1341–1351, 1997.

81. Packer TL, Martins I, Krefting L, Brouwer B: Activity and post-polio fatigue. Orthopedics 14:1223–1226, 1995.

82. Packer TL, Sauriol A, Brouwer B: Fatigue secondary to chronic illness: Postpolio syndrome, chronic fatigue syndrome, and multiple sclerosis. Arch Phys Med Rehabil 75:1122–1126, 1994.

83. Peach PE: Overwork weakness with evidence of muscle damage in a patient with residual paralysis from polio. Arch Phys Med Rehabil 71:248–250, 1990.

84. Peach PE, Olejnik S: Effect of treatment and noncompliance on post-polio sequelae. Orthopedics 14:1199–1203, 1991.

85. Perry J, Mulroy SJ, Renwick SE: The relationship of lower extremity strength and gait parameters in patients with post-polio syndrome. Arch Phys Med Rehabil 74:165–169, 1993.

86. Rimmer JH, Braddock D: Health promotion for people with physical, cognitive and sensory disabilities: An emerging national priority. Am J Health Promot 16:220–224, 2002.

87. Robinson LR, Hillel AD, Waugh PF: New laryngeal muscle weakness in post-polio syndrome. Laryngoscope 108:732–734, 1998.

88. Saltzstein RJ, Melvin JL: Abdominal distention as an indication of post-polio ventilatory insufficiency. Am J Phys Med Rehabil 67:85–86, 1988.

89. Steljes DG, Kryger MH, Kirk BW, Millar TW: Sleep in postpolio syndrome. Chest 98:133–140, 1990.

90. Stice KA, Cunningham CA: Pulmonary rehabilitation with respiratory complications of postpolio syndrome. Rehabil Nurs 20:37–42, 1995.

91. Stranghelle JK, Festvag LV: Postpolio syndrome: A 5-year follow-up. Spinal Cord 35:503–508, 1997.

92. Tate D, Kirsch N, Maynard F, et al: Coping with the late effects: Differences between depressed and nondepressed polio survivors. Am J Phys Med Rehabil 73:27–35, 1994.

93. Thoren-Jonsson AL, Hedbery M, Grimby G: Distress in everyday life in people with poliomyelitis sequelae. J Rehabil Med 33:119–127, 2001.

94. Trojan DA, Cashman NR: Pathophysiology and diagnosis of post-polio syndrome. NeuroRehabilitation 8:83–92, 1997.

95. Vallbona C, Hazlewood CF, Jurida G: Response of pain to static magnetic fields in postpolio patients: A double-blind pilot study. Arch Phys Med Rehabil 78:1200–1203, 1997.

96. Waring WP, Maynard FG, Grady W, et al: Influence of appropriate lower extremity orthotic management on ambulation, pain, and fatigue in a postpolio population. Arch Phys Med Rehabil 70:371–375, 1989.

97. Waring WP, McLaurin TM: Correlation of creatine kinase and gait measurement in the postpolio population. Arch Phys Med Rehabil 73:37–39, 1992.

98. Waters RL, Hislop HJ, Perry J, Antonelli D: Energetics: Application to the study and management of locomotor disorders. Orthop Clin North Am 9:351–362, 1978.
99. Weinberg J, Borg J, Bevegard S, Sinderby C: Respiratory responses to exercise in post-polio patients with severe inspiratory muscle dysfunction. Arch Phys Med Rehabil 80: 1095–1100, 1998.
100. Wenneberg S, Ahlstrom G: Illness narratives of persons with post polio syndrome. J Adv Nurs 31:354–361, 2000.
101. Widar M, Ahlstrom G: Experiences and consequences of pain in persons with post-polio. J Advanced Nursing 28:606–613, 1998.
102. Willen C, Cider A, Sunnerhagen KS: Physical performance in individuals with the late effects of polio. Scand J Rehabil Med 31:244–249, 1999.
103. Willen C, Grimby G: Pain, physical activity, and disability in individuals with late effects of polio. Arch Phys Med Rehabil 79:915–919, 1998.
104. Woo J: Relationships among diet, physical activity and other lifestyle factors and debilitating diseases in the elderly. Eur J Clin Nutr 54(suppl 3):143–147, 2000.

Aquatic Therapy for Polio Survivors

Kathryn A. Smith, BS, MPT

For centuries, the aquatic environment has been used therapeutically as well as to promote wellness.[5,48] During the polio epidemics in the first half of the 20th century, despite the fear of the transmission of polio through public pools, much knowledge was gained about the treatment of patients in the water. The rehabilitative benefits of the water for polio patients were discovered in Warm Springs, Georgia, when a boy with poliomyelitis accidentally fell into the water from his wheelchair. He discovered use of his lower extremities, which were thought to be completely paralyzed. This prompted continued aquatic exercise sessions and swimming for the child. The boy made marked gains in strength and mobility as he progressed from wheelchair mobility to independent ambulation with a cane and without lower extremity bracing.[38,48]

The therapeutic use of the water for the rehabilitation of polio patients flourished at Warm Springs and other rehabilitation hospitals throughout the United States as other polio patients, including Warm Springs' most famous client, Franklin Delano Roosevelt, experienced increased strength, mobility, function, and recreational opportunities through rehabilitation programs that incorporated aquatic therapy treatments.[29,38,48] These treatments were typically performed in warm pools with an emphasis on stretching and strengthening (Figs. 1 and 2).[29] However, gait and functional training were also performed in the therapeutic pools during the polio era (Figs. 3 and 4).[29,36]

Today, although more comprehensive and scientific knowledge exists to substantiate the use of aquatic therapy,[5] there are still insufficiencies in the literature.[34] However, numerous anecdotal reports have supported the use of the aquatic environment as a valuable treatment tool for neurorehabilitation.[2,15,21,23,25,29,30,34,38] Aquatic therapy is believed to have many physical and psychological benefits.[5,8,9,21,29] Additionally, for some individuals with disabilities, the water may be a more suitable environment for exercise than land.[19,21,33,47] Willen et al. studied 15 individuals with late effects of poliomyelitis using a program of non-swimming dynamic exercises performed in a heated pool and found decreased exercise heart rate, decreased resting heart rate, decreased pain, and increased perception of well-being and physical fitness compared with non-exercising control subjects.[46]

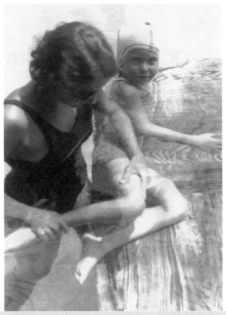

Figure 1. Stretching exercises performed at Warm Springs Institute for Rehabilitation, Warm Springs, GA, in the 1940s.

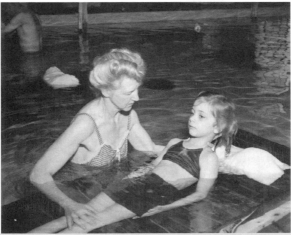

Figure 2. Strengthening exercises performed at Warm Springs Institute for Rehabilitation, Warm Springs, GA, in the 1940s.

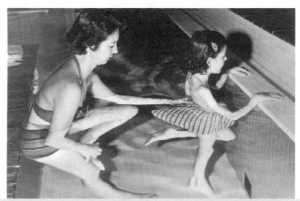

Figure 3. Gait training performed at Warm Springs Institute for Rehabilitation, Warm Springs, GA, in the 1940s.

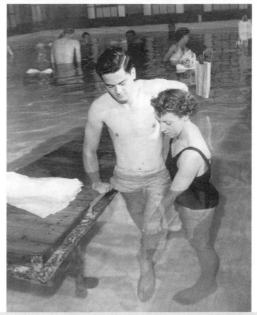

Figure 4. Gait training performed at Warm Springs Institute for Rehabilitation, Warm Springs, GA, in the 1940s.

PRECAUTIONS AND INDICATIONS

The water has unique effects on the systems of the body. Therefore, before a patient begins aquatic therapy treatments or any type of aquatic exercise program, the patient's therapist must consider the possible effects of immersion in relation to any health concerns; communicate risks to the patient; and when needed, perform appropriate medical management. For polio survivors, this usually requires that evaluation and treatments initially be performed by a licensed therapy professional with specialized training in aquatic therapy and knowledge of problems associated with polio and postpolio syndrome (PPS).[25]

The goal of aquatic therapy is to progress the patient to a higher functional level in his or her land mobility skills or activities of daily living (ADLs).[25,38,42] Therefore, the therapist's initial evaluation of the patient should be a land-based evaluation. The evaluation should determine medical history, impairments, functional problems, functional goals, and plan of treatment, including appropriateness for participation in aquatic therapy. This is followed by an in-pool evaluation to determine the individual's response to the aquatic environment, response to aquatic treatment techniques, and safety in the water. It should be noted that even individuals with severe disability, significant medical histories, and more complicated medical problems can often participate in aquatic therapy if they have access to a facility that will accommodate their needs. For these clients, it is essential to enlist the skilled services of a licensed therapy professional, such as a physical, occupational, or recreation therapist, with training in provision of aquatic therapy and a thorough understanding of the physiologic responses of the body to immersion.[5]

The cardiac, renal, and respiratory systems are taxed to a greater degree when a person is submerged in the water. When an individual enters the water, fluid centralization occurs. Fluid centralization is the shunting of fluid from the extremities to the thoracic area. This increases central blood volume by 60% (or 0.7 L), with one third of this volume taken up by the heart and two thirds by the great vessels of the lungs.[1,2] Cardiac volume is also increased by 27–30%, which results in increased stroke volume and blood flow to the organs.[2,37] In an attempt to maintain cardiac output, the heart rate drops somewhat. However, despite this reflexive decrease in heart rate, blood pressure (BP) and cardiac output still are generally increased. For this reason, clients with vascular or cardiac complications should be screened and monitored carefully and should begin aquatic therapy or aquatic exercise only under the direct supervision of a medical professional.[21] Acute congestive heart failure is a contraindication to aquatic therapy.[10,32]

The renal system is also greatly affected by immersion. Creatinine clearance, sodium and potassium excretion, and urine output are all increased with immersion.[2] These changes begin immediately with immersion, peak at about 2 hours, and are increased with greater depth of immersion or with colder water temperatures.[2] Individuals with severe renal dysfunction may not be appropriate candidates for participation in aquatic therapy or exercise. This should be determined based on the severity of the disease, the proposed treatment techniques to be used, and the depth and temperature of the water. Diabetes and urinary incontinence are generally considered precautions, not contraindications, for aquatic therapy. Individuals with these conditions can generally participate if appropriate medical management and patient education are performed. However, the licensed medical professional familiar with the patient must make this determination.

Lung volumes are decreased when an individual enters the water to the level of the thorax.[2] Decreased lung volumes are caused by the hydrostatic pressure of the water pushing in on the thorax and the increased blood volume to the lungs.[2] Still, even patients with significantly decreased lung volumes may be able to participate in aquatic therapy with appropriate management and supervision.[16] We generally advise that oxygen saturation is monitored for individuals on external oxygen or with severe respiratory dysfunction. Patients with weakness or paralysis in the muscles of respiration, as is common with polio patients, may have increased awareness of the hydrostatic pressure of the water's pushing in on the thoracic area. This may or may not be associated with increased difficulty of breathing, even when oxygen saturation levels remain stable. For most patients, this is a sensation they grow accustomed to, and their participation is not affected. Still, therapists may choose to decrease the amount of submersion of the patient's thorax by adjusting the depth at which aquatic therapy is performed or by applying therapy procedures that maintain the client floating in a supine position to increase client comfort.

In addition to the aforementioned contraindications and precautions to aquatic therapy, there are other precautions that may affect participation in aquatic activity with some individuals in the age ranges associated with polio and PPS. These include, but are not limited to, decreased sensation, incontinence, gastrostomy, colostomy, and containable open wounds.[10,16] Individuals with these conditions can typically participate in aquatic therapy with appropriate medical management and patient education. For example, patients can be instructed in the application of a bio-occlusive dressing to contain wounds, gastrostomy, or colostomy sites. It is also important to note that an aquatic program may be logistically difficult for a patient to participate in and, if not done in an appropriate facility, may place the patient at undue risk for falls.

PROPERTIES OF WATER

In addition to understanding the physical changes that occur with immersion and medical management of the various precautions to aquatic activity, the therapist providing aquatic treatments must have a thorough understanding of the properties of water.[5,15,42] Water possesses many unique properties that make it an appropriate—and often the most desirable—environment in which to treat polio patients. The properties of water include density, specific gravity, hydrostatic pressure, buoyancy, specific heat, viscosity, turbulence, and refraction. Frequently, these properties can be enhanced through the use of equipment, facility design, or therapist handling. Furthermore, because the properties of water are inherent to the water itself, there are often multiple therapeutic benefits working simultaneously to address the patient's problems. It is essential for practitioners to fully understand these properties in order to maximize the benefit of the aquatic therapy session for the patient.

DENSITY AND SPECIFIC GRAVITY

The properties of density and specific gravity are used to physically describe and define a substance. *Density* is defined as mass per unit volume. *Specific gravity* is defined as the ratio of the density of a substance to the density of water and, therefore, the specific gravity of water is equal to one by definition. Specific gravity less than one is required for floatation. Lean body tissues have a specific gravity of 1.1, and body fat has a specific gravity of 0.90.[38] Average specific gravity of the human body with air in the lungs is 0.974.[20] However, a person's individual body type and composition must be considered. A higher percentage of lean body tissue increases a person's specific gravity and inhibits floatation; conversely, a higher percentage of adipose tissue lowers specific gravity and increases floatation.

Furthermore, the composition and muscle tone of each body segment must be considered because each segment has its own specific gravity, density, and propensity to float. Spastic extremities tend to have increased density and specific gravity, causing them to sink. Extremities that are flaccid tend to have decreased density and specific gravity with associated tendency to float. It is important for therapists to consider these changes in extremity composition for appropriate setup of patients for aquatic therapy. Setup also depends on the treatment selected. For example, floating a patient in a supine posture is commonly used for aquatic therapeutic exercise, as will be described later. If a patient has unilateral muscle tone changes, as is observed in many polio survivors, the density on one side of the body is different than on the other side of the body. This causes rotation of the body toward the side of increased density. Therefore, additional floatation equipment may be added to the side of increased density to prevent rotation. Furthermore, water temperature, therapist handling, patient posture, speed of movement, and vestibular stimulation may alter muscle tone and can be varied by the therapist.[38]

Additionally, polio patients may have more difficulty maintaining an upright standing position in the pool because of the alteration of muscle tone of the extremities or trunk, causing destabilization. This may be therapeutic because it may enable the practice of balance reactions necessary to regain balance.[18] However, if the treatment performed requires stability, as with many therapeutic exercises, the therapist may alter the setup by adjusting his or her handling, water depth, equipment, or upper extremity support.

HYDROSTATIC PRESSURE

Another property of water is hydrostatic pressure. The *hydrostatic pressure* of water is exerted equally in all directions around any given point in the water.[38] This provides external support to assist in maintaining balance and increase independence for therapeutic exercise and the practice of functional mobility skills.[21] Lord et al. report that older adults and those with disability show decreased body sway with aquatic exercise intervention.[26] Furthermore, older adults who have participated in aquatic exercise demonstrate better balance as measured by the Berg Balance Scale and Timed Up and Go than the general older adult population.[28] As previously discussed, hydrostatic pressure causes increased work of breathing because of the resulting decrease in lung volumes and decrease in the pressure gradient of respiration. Johnson and colleagues propose that this increased resistance to breathing can be used to strengthen weak respiratory muscles.[22]

Although hydrostatic pressure is exerted equally around any given point in the water, the pressure increases with increased fluid depth at a rate of 22.4 mmHg/ft.

Therefore, at 4 feet of water depth, the water exerts pressure of 88.9 mm Hg, exceeding normal diastolic BP.[38] This gradient pressure may help alleviate lower extremity edema, which is common in individuals with low muscle tone. Bookspan and Paolone proposed that water's ability to counter venous pooling in the extremities may be caused by mechanisms other than hydrostatic pressure.[4]

Additionally, the gradient force established by the hydrostatic pressure of water provides an increased force at the bottom of a floating object than exists on the part of an object more near the surface. This creates a force that pushes the object in an upward direction. This upwardly directed force, known as buoyancy, causes floatation when applied to an object with a specific gravity less than water. Floatation occurs when the weight of the submerged portion of the body is equal to the weight of the displaced water.[38]

BUOYANCY

Buoyancy is used to customize therapeutic exercise. In the water, exercises can be performed in a buoyancy-assisted (BA), buoyancy-supported (BS), or buoyancy-resisted (BR) position (Figs. 5, to 7). BA exercises are performed with an upward direction of movement toward the surface of the water. BS exercises are in a direction parallel to the surface of the water, neutral to the buoyant force. BR exercises are performed in a downward direction opposing the buoyant force.[25,38] Muscles below a fair grade, able to complete the fully available range of motion (ROM) against gravity on land but unable to hold against resistance, should do BA or BS exercises. Muscles stronger than a grade of fair should do BR exercise.[25] By using BA, BS, or BR positioning, therapists can use the water to customize a therapeutic exercise program for polio survivors based on the client's manual muscle test and other evaluation procedures.

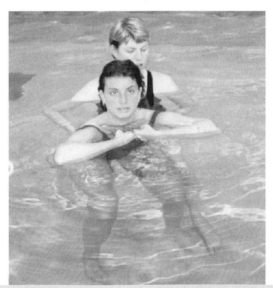

Figure 5.   Buoyancy-supported triceps extension.

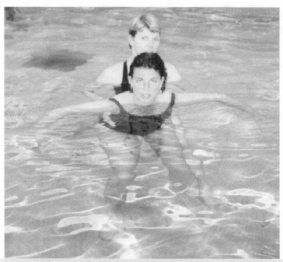

Figure 6. Buoyancy-assisted triceps extension.

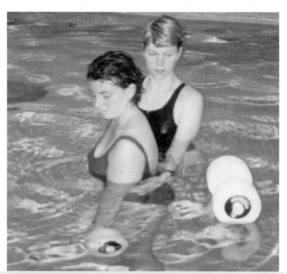

Figure 7. Buoyancy-resisted triceps extension.

Buoyancy is also used therapeutically to enable individuals to practice functional mobility and ADL skills.[18,29] Broach et al.[6,8] and Gehlsen et al.[17] have found aquatic therapy to be an effective means of increasing functional mobility in individuals with weakness caused by neuromuscular disorders. Johnson proposes that the muscular effort used to propel a person's body on land against gravity can instead be channeled into the coordination of purposeful movement when the person is in the water.[22] Some polio survivors cannot practice certain functional tasks, such as ambulation, sit to stand, or upper body dressing independently on land because of severe weakness and the resistive force of gravity that acts on the body. However, if the patient is positioned in the water to enable the force of buoyancy to facilitate the movement, he or she often can perform these and other mobility tasks more independently.[29] This allows for task specific strengthening, muscle re-education, practice of balance reactions necessary for task safety, and increased motivation inherent in completing a meaningful task independently.[18,21,22,29] Therapists can progress the difficulty of the task by moving the patient to gradually more shallow water, decreasing external stabilization, altering the task, or adjusting therapist handling with the goal of progressing the person to land.[29]

Additionally, for polio survivors with severe weakness, the buoyancy of the water assists the individual in lifting the extremity through a greater ROM than may be possible on land.[29] This may assist with improved strengthening by allowing the client to work more independently through a greater ROM. Furthermore, because the individual must sustain the contraction throughout the ROM to progress the movement, it is possible that increased feedback is provided to the neuromuscular system than would be possible with the external support necessary to complete the task on land. It should be noted that because of the addition of the force of buoyancy, muscle activation patterns for gait and other functional tasks could be altered from what they are on land.

Just as the human body has a center of gravity (COG), typically located at the second sacral vertebrae when the body is in the anatomical position, it also has a center of buoyancy (COB), which is typically located midchest.[2] Furthermore, each body segment has its own COG and COB. It is important to note that a person's body frame, body composition, alterations in muscle tone, and amount of submersion in the water may alter the location of these centers. Both the forces of gravity and buoyancy act from these centers on a body submerged in water, and these forces oppose each other.[2] When the centers are aligned vertically in a submerged body, a traction force results, which opens joint spaces.[2] For individuals with arthritis or other compressive disorders of the joints, the water provides an environment in which therapeutic exercises can be performed or functional tasks can be practiced with decreased pain and increased mobility.[18,19,33,41] Aquatic therapy equipment can often be applied to increase the tractioning effect for pain relief during the aquatic exercises. For example, in deep water, floatation can be added at the neck, shoulders, or upper trunk with small weights added to the ankles to provide increased tractioning during vertical activities performed in the water. This activity is contraindicated for any person with instability of the joints. Conflicting opinions exist as to the usefulness of aquatic tractioning performed on a statically floating body for the long-term relief of pain.[9,12]

The interaction of the forces of gravity and buoyancy can also be used to facilitate a more upright sitting or standing posture in individuals with trunk weakness. When the COB and COG are not vertically aligned, a rotational force is created that tends to assist the patient in maintaining an upright posture.[2] Postural dysfunction of a prolonged nature that has resulted in fixed contractures, such as a fixed kyphosis or scoliosis, would most likely not be improved by this facilitation. The effect of the aquatic environment and aquatic therapy on altering further progression of abnormal postures caused by fixed contractures has not been investigated.

SPECIFIC HEAT

The water's property of *specific heat* also has therapeutic value for the polio patient. The specific heat of water is greater than that of the human body. Additionally, water has higher thermal conductivity than bloodless human tissue, and these tissues are good insulators.[2] For these reasons, the temperature of the water is readily transferred to the human body and can alter core body temperature. Temperatures above 90° are used to facilitate relaxation and stretching, decrease pain, and increase mobility (Fig. 8).[38] However, fatigue may be increased with increased water temperature. Also, core body temperature is increased at higher exercise intensities and in individuals with increased body fat.

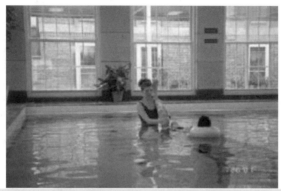

Figure 8.   Passive range of motion to hamstrings on a plinth in a warm pool.

For polio survivors, particularly those with PPS, water temperature between 90° and 92°F is generally recommended, and these patients should begin an aquatic exercise program with a short session, often just 10 minutes of time in the water.[25] The length of the sessions should be gradually increased as the patient demonstrates increased endurance without increased fatigue. Temperatures above 90° are not recommended for individuals participating in high-intensity aerobic workouts in the water because they can cause injury. Water temperatures exceeding 96° are not appropriate for any intensity of aquatic exercise because of the increased stress on the cardiovascular system and the risk of injury. Additionally, temperatures lower than 85° are generally not appropriate for individuals with cold intolerance, which affects some polio survivors.[25]

VISCOSITY

Viscosity is the property of friction in fluids[20] and contributes to the increased independence patients experience in the water. Viscosity slows the momentum of movement, which has several implications for rehabilitation of polio survivors. If loss of balance occurs during aquatic activities, the viscosity of the water slows the fall and increases time for practice of balance reactions. This facilitates motor learning during balance training for fall prevention.[18,22,40]

During therapeutic exercise, water's viscosity prevents the use of momentum to create movement, a common way of "cheating" during land exercise. For example, an individual attempting to perform elbow flexion on land from a standing position may rock his or her trunk in an anterior-posterior manner to create momentum and assist the biceps in completing the movement. During aquatic exercise, the patient must work throughout the entire ROM to complete the exercise because of the viscosity of the water's counteracting the inertial momentum of the movement. However, it is important to note that because viscosity counteracts momentum and that momentum is used in normal gait, the elimination of the momentum force may alter muscle activation patterns for gait. Although no study of muscle activation patterns during water walking has been conducted, alterations in the parameters of walking, including slower cadence, decreased walking speed, and decreased step length, have been noted.[14] However, improvements in ambulation cadence, velocity, single-limb stance time, and step length on land have been documented with aquatic interventions for individuals with hemiplegia by Morris et al.[31] and Taylor et al.[43]

Viscosity is also used therapeutically to grade exercise resistance.[22] Increasing the size, changing the shape, or increasing the speed of the moving extremity or the entire body can increase the viscous force, which is the force required to overcome the viscosity of the water. Applying certain types of therapeutic exercise equipment can alter the size and shape of an extremity or body moving through the water. The application of such equipment increases the work performing functional tasks or therapeutic exercises in the water. The speed of the movement may also be increased or decreased to proportionally increase or decrease the work required to perform the movement.[29] Because of the potential for muscle overuse and difficulties with fatigue experienced by some polio survivors, patients should begin therapeutic exercise programs without the addition of equipment that will increase the viscous force.

TURBULENCE

The *turbulence* of the water the must also be considered and can be altered to adjust the work of performing therapeutic exercises in the water. The turbulence of water increases with either increased velocity of water movement or with increased velocity of an object moving through the water (Fig. 9). For an individual participating in aquatic therapy or water exercise, increased turbulence results in increased work. Turbulence increases the work of moving through the water as well as the work of maintaining a position in the water. Therapists may manually create turbulence, position a client near a pool jet, or involve the patient in group therapy to increase the turbulence of the water, thereby increasing the work of therapeutic exercises or tasks performed in the pool. Turbulence may also be applied to destabilize a patient for balance training. It is recommended that polio survivors begin aquatic therapy or exercise in a pool with minimal turbulence because of the potential for muscle overuse. This may require scheduling aquatic therapy sessions during times of low pool usage.

REFRACTION

Refraction is another property of water that should be considered, especially for those with visual impairment or balance dysfunction. As light hits the surface of the water, a medium in which the velocity of light is less than its velocity through air, the ray of light is bent. This creates a visual illusion of submerged objects' being shorter than they actually are.[2] The altered visual feedback may cause decreased balance in those with visual impairment. Additionally, the reflection of light and objects on the surface of the water can cause further disruption of balance. These alterations in visual feedback may be used therapeutically to decrease reliance on visual feedback in individuals who normally rely on watching their feet for maintaining balance during ambulation. Therapists should explain the alterations in visual feedback to patients before participation in aquatic therapy and use this property of water as a means of encouraging visual scanning of the environment during functional tasks such as walking.

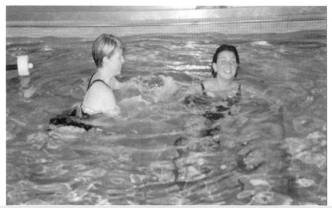

Figure 9. Sitting balance training with turbulence to destabilize.

Not only do the unique properties of water make it an ideal environment for many polio survivors to work toward therapy goals and improved functional abilities, but also therapists specializing in aquatic therapy often have expertise in advanced aquatic therapy techniques that may benefit these patients. Several advanced aquatic therapy techniques have emerged that offer greater variety of aquatic treatment options and the ability to more accurately address patient problems. Several of the techniques more commonly applied with polio survivors, including those with PPS, are described.

ADVANCED AQUATIC THERAPY TECHNIQUES

WATSU

Watsu, short for *water shiatsu,* was developed by Harold Dull at Harbin Hot Springs in California in 1980.[13,27] The technique is based on the principles of Zen shiatsu and uses the properties of water while incorporating stretching, acupressure, rotational movement patterns, rhythmic movements, and bodywork.[13] Watsu was originally developed to benefit the general population.[29] It is also used clinically to decrease pain, increase flexibility, facilitate relaxation, improve tidal volume, provide muscle re-education, improve breathing, and promote general wellness in those with a variety of movement problems common to polio survivors.[27,29,39,44] However, these results have not been verified experimentally.[44] Many clinicians report that Watsu is particularly useful in assisting those patients with decreased joint ROM, muscle guarding, chronic pain, or fatigue (Figs. 10 and 11).[27,29,39]

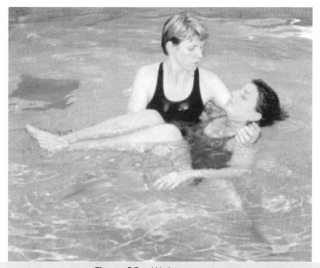

Figure 10. Watsu.

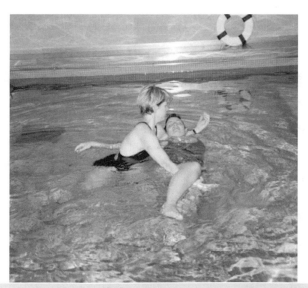

Figure 11. Watsu.

BAD RAGAZ RING METHOD

The development of the Bad Ragaz Ring Method (BRRM), another advanced aquatic therapy technique, began in the 1930s in the hot springs of Bad Ragaz, Switzerland.[29,38] Originally, the method incorporated active ROM exercises performed on fixed treatment boards in the water. In 1957, use of floatation rings developed by Knupfer of Wilbad, Germany, was introduced at Bad Ragaz by Nele Ipsen. The floatation rings, positioned at the neck, hips, and ankles, are used as a means of creating a supine posture with neutral body alignment. In 1967, Bridget Davis and Verena Laggatt, physiotherapists at Bad Ragaz, incorporated the use of Margaret Knott's patterns of proprioceptive neuromuscular facilitation (PNF), a widely used land-based therapy technique.[11,38]

The BRRM setup, hand holds, exercises patterns, and verbal commands are still used widely today to improve strength, ROM, endurance, trunk stability, relaxation, and motor control.[15,29,38] The exercise patterns can be applied passively, isometrically, isotonically, or isokinetically to allow for a high degree of customization based on the pa-

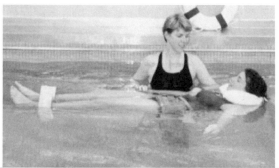

Figure 12. Bad Ragaz ring method: active strengthening for shoulder abduction and adduction.

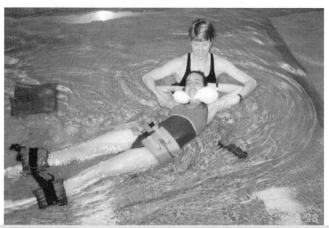

Figure 13. Bad Ragaz ring method: passive stretching to the trunk.

tient's needs (Figs. 12 and 13).[11,38] For polio survivors, this technique may be appropriate to address specific functional mobility problems, areas of joint tightness, specific muscle weakness, or pain associated with chronic movement dysfunction or overuse.

TASK TYPE TRAINING APPROACH

The Task Type Training Approach (TTTA), developed by David M. Morris in 1992, is a set of principles originally designed to guide the aquatic therapy treatment for stroke patients. This approach uses current motor learning principles adapted to rehabilitation performed in the water. It is a task-oriented approach that emphasizes the practice of functional skills, active problem solving, progression to land, and use of the unique properties of water to enable participation at the highest level of independence. Its principles include working in the most shallow water tolerated; practicing functional activities as a whole; systematically removing external stabilization; encouraging stabilizing contractions in upright positions with movement of selected body segments; encouraging quick, reciprocal movement; encouraging active movement; and gradually increasing the difficulty of the task. Although this approach was originally intended for individuals having suffered stroke or traumatic brain injury, it has substantial benefits for polio survivors who desire improved functional mobility. This approach can be applied to facilitate increased strength, endurance, balance and motor learning during the practice of functional mobility and ADL tasks.[29,38]

AI CHI

Development of Ai Chi, an aquatic exercise technique based on Tai Chi, began by Jun Konno, founder of the Aqua Dynamics Institute in Yokohama, Japan.[39] It was brought to the United States in 1993 and presented at the Aquatic Therapy and Rehabilitation Conference. Ruth Sova, founder of Aquatic Exercise Association, further developed the Ai Chi program with Jun Konno.[24]

Ai Chi is quickly gaining popularity as a method of improving balance, flexibility, ROM, coordination, wellness, blood circulation, kinesthetic awareness, metabolism, and mental alertness as well as decreasing stress, anxiety, depression, fatigue, and insomnia. Ai Chi incorporates specific movements in coordinated, repetitive, rhythmic patterns. Proper postural alignment, deep breathing, and relaxation are emphasized.[39] Ai Chi can be provided in a group setting, as an individualized exercise program, or components can be incorporated into other therapeutic exercises.

Recent research promotes the use of Tai Chi as a method of improving balance in older adults.[28] Polio survivors may demonstrate an increased risk of falls above that of the general population because of the physical problems associated with the disease. Furthermore, those with PPS, having progressive fatigue and weakness, are at an even higher risk of falls and related injuries. Theoretically, participation in an Ai Chi program may help decrease this risk of falls and provide a variety of other benefits, as previously mentioned. However, it is essential that instructors or therapists providing such a program be aware of exercise guidelines for polio survivors, also previously mentioned.

THE HALLIWICK METHOD AND SWIM TRAINING

In addition to Watsu, BRRM, TTTA, and Ai Chi, therapists specializing in aquatic therapy may have advanced knowledge and skills in the Halliwick Method or other adapted swim training techniques that can enable polio survivors to participate in swimming as a lifetime recreational activity. [5] Swimming is an excellent form of exercise that improves strength, cardiovascular endurance, trunk stability, respiratory function, joint mobility, physical fitness, motor control, body awareness, coordination and well-being (Fig. 14).[3,7,23,28,35,38] Swimming can provide these benefits with greater ease of movement and decreased loading of the joints.[38] For these reasons, swimming has been used therapeutically for clients with a variety of diagnoses, movement problems, and paralysis.[5,7,16,23,35,38,45,47]

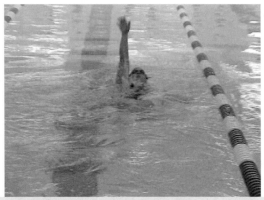

Figure 14.   Swim training of a patient with paraplegia.

However, incorrect technique or excessive repetition of swimming movements may lead to microtrauma of the joints or other injury to the musculoskeletal system. For polio survivors, great care must be taken in recommending particular swim strokes. An understanding of the mechanics of swimming is necessary to avoid recommending swim strokes that will cause increased trauma to joints already experiencing overuse syndromes commonly seen in polio survivors.[15] Additionally, swimming presents the risk of generalized muscle overuse. For these reasons, swim training for polio survivors requires the assistance of individuals with advanced training in swim instruction for those with mobility impairments as well as understanding of the problems commonly associated with polio.

The Halliwick Method was developed by James McMillan, a naval engineer, in London, England, in the 1930s.[29,45] The method is based on the principles of hydrodynamics and human development and was originally designed to teach swimming to children with cerebral palsy.[45] However, the technique has been used with adults and children with a variety of diagnoses for therapeutic rehabilitation of specific movement problems.[29,38] McMillan used his knowledge of engineering, physics, and fluid mechanics as well as enlisting the help of others in the fields of medicine, neurophysiology, physiotherapy, psychology, pedagogy, and sociology in the development of the approach. The approach uses facilitative or inhibitive handling techniques, specific rules of movement that relate to the properties of water, and a specific sequence of training known as the 10-Point Program.[38] The method is used to teach swimming skills to individuals with physical disability as well as to improve physical fitness, strength, joint ROM, balance, motor control, muscle tone, kinesthetic awareness, mental adaptability, body schema, and posture and to decrease fear of the water.[29,38,45]

FINDING AN APPROPRIATE THERAPIST

The availability of aquatic therapy services is increasing rapidly in the United States, and generalized aquatic therapy services are found readily. However, finding a practitioner with training in specific advanced aquatic techniques as well as experience in working with polio survivors is often difficult. Several organizations may be helpful in locating such practitioners. These include, but are not limited to, the American Physical Therapy Association's Aquatic Section, Aquatic Therapy Rehab Institute, Worldwide Aquatic Bodywork Association, Aquatic Resources Network, and International Halliwick Association. Furthermore, contacting local hospitals or clinics with programs specifically for polio survivors as well as polio support groups may be helpful.

In addition to locating a therapist who has had continuing education in the advanced aquatic techniques, the discipline of the therapist should be considered. Physical, occupational, recreation, speech, and massage therapists as well as therapy assistants in each discipline may pursue continuing education in advanced aquatic techniques. Therefore, identifying which discipline is most appropriate for the treatment of the patient's problems and functional limitations is essential.

Some professionals without medical training may have knowledge of the advanced techniques previously discussed. For example, Watsu and Ai Chi, having been originally created for use with a well population, may be provided by individuals not licensed to perform medically based therapy services. However, it is important for polio survivors that all exercises and advanced aquatic techniques be initiated by a professional with a license to provide skilled, medically based therapy services because of the risk of overworking and the common presence of additional complicating medical diagnoses present in polio survivors.

REQUIREMENTS OF THE FACILITY

In addition to understanding the treatment guidelines for working with polio survivors, the physiologic responses of the body to immersion, the properties of water and how they can be used clinically, and advanced aquatic therapy techniques, therapists providing aquatic therapy services to polio survivors must consider issues related to the pool facility. Each patient's facility needs differ, but, in general, the following features should be available at the pool facility to accommodate the needs of the general population of polio survivors.

The pool should have close, accessible parking with short walking distance to the facility entrance, dressing room, and pool itself to prevent overexertion caused by long walking distances.[25] All doors to the facility, dressing rooms, restrooms, and pool should be automated and accessible to all types of manual and electric wheelchairs and scooters. The dressing room changing areas, showers, and toilets should also be accessible to clients with all types of mobility equipment and should have handrails for added safety for ambulating clients. It is ideal to have a private dressing area with changing mat for caregiver-assisted dressing changes, showers, and toileting. The dressing rooms, toilets, showers, and pool deck should have a slip-resistant surface that will not deteriorate with frequent cleaning and pool chemicals.[25] Any braces or equipment normally used for ambulation should be worn for deck ambulation as well but removed just before entering the water. Use of aquatic exercise shoes is often recommended for polio survivors not requiring bracing for ambulation due to increased risk of falls in this group. The pool should have visually distinguishable stairs with bilateral railings for ambulatory clients and a lift or ramp for safe entry of those in wheelchairs (Fig. 15).[25] Some pools may also be accessible for a wheelchair to elevated deck transfer if the individual can perform safe scooting transfers and has the upper body strength and mobility to slowly lower the body into the water (Fig. 16). A certified lifeguard should monitor the pool at all times. The depth of the water should gradually increase without sharp drop-off and allow therapeutic exercise at chest to waist depth. The pool temperature is ideal for the polio survivor at 90–92°.[25] Air temperature should be maintained at 3° higher than the water temperature to minimize humidity and inhalation of pool chemicals, which escape with evaporation.

DISCHARGE PLANNING

It is important for the therapist to discuss any constraints of the environment with the patient before the first pool session. Additionally, the therapist and patient must discuss the discharge plan, including the patient's desire and ability to continue with an aquatic exercise program after discharge, the patient's preference for a group or independent exercise program, facility requirements at the facility at which the patient

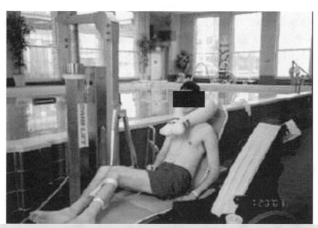

Figure 15.   Hydraulic lift for pool entry.

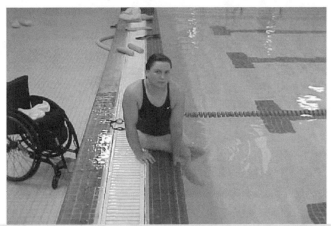

Figure 16.   Transfer from wheelchair to elevated deck for poolside transfer.

will perform the exercise, and any need for assistance by family members or facility personnel.

Many individuals enjoy the fun and socialization offered by a community-based aquatic exercise class (Figs. 17 and 18). Many pools offer such classes under the supervision of a trained instructor. This type of generalized aquatic exercise program can benefit individuals with various neuromuscular disorders.[17] Often a variety of classes are offered to best fit the needs of the participants. The referring therapist should discuss the class format and skill level required to participate with the instructor before patient referral into such a group aquatic class. With the patient's approval, the therapist should also inform the instructor of the needs of the patient and the risks associated with polio and PPS. Written exercises, with illustrations, should be provided to the patient by the therapist before discharge. The patient should be able to incorporate these exercises into the aquatic class program. Initially, this may require one-on-one assistance by the therapist or trained aquatic program staff. The therapist should also provide the class instructor with a copy of the client's exercise program.

Some individuals require continued one-on-one supervision, are unable to find a group class that fits their needs, or prefer to exercise independently. For these individuals, it is beneficial if a transitional rehabilitation program exists for improved transition from therapy to a community aquatic program. Some pools offer such a transitional rehabilitation program under the direction of an exercise physiologist, recreation therapist, or other professional staff. A close working relationship between the aquatic program staff and the referring therapist creates an ideal environment for progressing the patient to independence in an ongoing health and wellness aquatic program. Again, written exercises, with illustrations, should be provided to the patient by the therapist before discharge for continued progress in strengthening and mobility. The therapist should also provide the assigned professional staff member from the transitional rehabilitation program with a copy of the exercise program and any information needed for the client's safe participation.

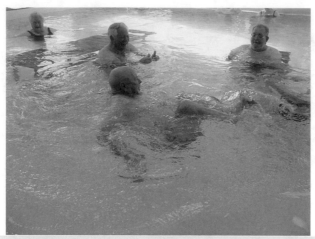

Figure 17. Community supervised open pool session.

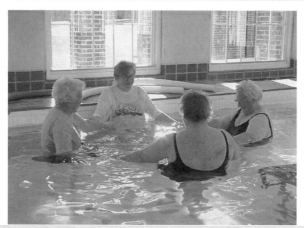

Figure 18. Community aquatic exercise class activity.

CONCLUSION

Professionals working with polio survivors in the aquatic environment should be familiar with the needs particular to this group, the necessity to avoid muscle overuse, and the general guidelines for exercise. Furthermore, a thorough understanding of the physiologic responses of the body to immersion, the risks associated with these changes, and the use of the properties of water is essential. The client's needs and facility requirements must always be considered for both the treatment facility and for facilities that will be used after discharge. Early and thorough discharge planning based on the needs and desires of the patient is essential. Most polio survivors, including those with PPS, can participate in and will benefit from aquatic therapy and transition to individual or group aquatic community exercise programs. Additionally, because of the unique properties of water, the aquatic environment may be the most comfortable, enabling, and beneficial environment in which polio survivors can exercise and work to preserve and gain strength, endurance, and mobility.

References

1. Arborelius M, Balldin UI, Lilja B, Lundgren CE: Hemodynamic changes in man during immersion with the head above water. Aerospace Med 43:593, 1972.
2. Becker BE, Cole AJ: Comprehensive Aquatic Therapy. Woburn, MA, Butterworth Heinemann, 1996, pp 17–72, 143–178.
3. Berger BG, Owen DR: Mood alteration with swimming—swimmers really do feel better. Psychosom Med 45:425–433, 1983.
4. Bookspan J, Paolone AM: Posture apnea interaction during total body cold water immersion [abstract]. Undersea Biomed Res 18(suppl):66, 1991.
5. Broach E, Dattilo J: Aquatic therapy: A viable therapeutic recreation intervention. Ther Rec J 30:213–227, 1996.
6. Broach E, Dattilo J: Effects of aquatic therapy on adults with multiple sclerosis. Ther Rec J 35:141–154, 2001.
7. Broach E, Groff D, Dattilo J: Effects of an aquatic therapy swimming program on adults with spinal cord injuries. Ther Rec J 31:161–173, 1997.
8. Broach E, Groff D, Dattilo J, et al: Effects of aquatic therapy on adults with multiple sclerosis. Ann Ther Rec 7:1–19, 1997/98.
9. Campion MR: Adult Hydrotherapy: A Practical Approach. Oxford, Heinemann Medical Books, 1990.
10. Contraindications and Precautions to Aquatic Therapy. Alexandria, VA, Aquatic Physical Therapy Section of the American Physical Therapy Association, 1998.
11. Cunningham J: Applying the Bad Ragaz method to the orthopedic client. Orthop Phys Ther Clin North Am 3:165–178, 1994.
12. Davis A: Traction on land and in the pool. J Aqua Phys Ther 1:6–7, 1993.
13. Dull H: Watsu: Freeing the Body in Water, 2nd ed. Middletown, CA, Worldwide Aquatic Bodywork Association, 1997.
14. Fowler-Horne A: Walking parameters when walking in water. J Aqua Phys Ther 8:6–9, 2000.
15. Garrett G: A stroke of genius: Rehabil Manage 56–59:128, 1994.
16. Garvey LA: Spinal cord injury and aquatics. Clin Man 11:21–24, 1991.
17. Gehlsen GM, Grigsby SA, Winant DM: Effects of an aquatic fitness program on the muscular strength and endurance of patients with multiple sclerosis. Phys Ther 64:653–657, 1984.
18. Geigle PR, Cheek WL, Jr. Gould ML, et al: Aquatic physical therapy for balance: The interaction of somatosensory and hydrodynamic principles. J Aqua Phys Ther 5:4–10, 1997.
19. Hall J, Skevington SM, Maddison PJ, Chapman K: A randomized and controlled trial of hydrotherapy in rheumatoid arthritis. Arthritis Care Res 9:206–215, 1996.
20. Haralson KM: Therapeutic pool programs. Clin Man 5:10–12, 1986.
21. Hurley R, Turner C: Neurology and aquatic therapy. Clin Man 11:26–29, 1991.
22. Johnson BA, Li Y, Hartman AGC: A case study of upper extremity stroke rehabilitation using aquatic exercise techniques: A motor control and learning perspective. J Aqua Phys Ther 6:12–23, 1998.
23. Johnson CR: Aquatic therapy for an ALS patient. Am J Occup Ther 42:115–120, 1988.
24. Kunno J, Sova R: Ai Chi Flowing Aquatic Energy, DSL, Ltd, 1996.

25. Leonard RB: Pool Exercise: Principles and Guidelines for Polio Survivors. Warm Springs, GA, Roosevelt Warm Springs Institute for Rehabilitation, 1994.
26. Lord S, Mitchell D, Williams P: Effect of water exercise on balance and related factors in older people. Aust Physiother 39:217–222, 1993.
27. Lutz ER: Watsu: Aquatic bodywork. Beginnings (March/Apr): 9–11, 1999.
28. Maginnis ME, Privett JL, Raskas WA, Newton RA: Balance abilities of community dwelling older adults engages in a water exercise program. J Aquat Phys Ther 7:6–12, 1999.
29. Morris DM: Aquatic neurorehabilitation. Neurol Rep 19:22–28, 1995.
30. Morris D: Aquatic rehabilitation for the treatment of neurologic disorders. J Back Musculoskel Rehabil 4:297–308, 1994.
31. Morris D, Buettner TL, White EW: Aquatic community based exercise programs for stroke survivors. J Aqua Phys Ther 4:15–20, 1996.
32. Moschetti M, Cole AJ: Aquatics: Risk management strategies for the therapy pool. J Back Musculoskel Rehabil 4:265–272, 1994.
33. Norton CO, Hobbler K, Welding AB, Jensen GM: Effectiveness of aquatic exercise in the treatment of women with osteoarthritis. J Aquat Phys Ther 5:8–15, 1997.
34. Olsen PJ: Aquatic physical therapy for chronic painful conditions: an outcome study. Aquat Phys Ther Rep 3:12–14, 1995.
35. Pachalski A, Merkarski T: Effect of swimming on increasing cardio-respiratory capacity in paraplegics. Paraplegia 18:190–196, 1980.
36. Ray MB: The implications of hydrotherapy. Arch Phys Med 27:742–749, 1946.
37. Risch WD, Koubenec HJ, Beckmann U, et al: The effect of graded immersion on heart volume, central venous pressure, pulmonary blood distribution and heart rate in man. Pflugers Arch 374:117, 1978.
38. Ruoti RG, Morris DM, Cole AJ: Aquatic Rehabilitation. Philadelphia, Lippincott Williams & Wilkins, 1997.
39. Sadusky J: Delving deeper: Nontraditional techniques expand the scope of aquatic therapy. Rehabil Manage (Dec/Jan): 28–32, 1999.
40. Simmons V, Hansen PD: Effectiveness of water exercise on postural mobility in the well elderly: An experimental study on balance enhancement. J Gerontol A Biol Sci Med Sci 51:233–238, 1996.
41. Styer-Acededo J: Aquatic PT: equipment and clinical decision making. Phys Ther Mag (Jan):43–72, 1995.
42. Styer-Acevedo J, Cirullo JA: Integrating land and aquatic approaches with a functional emphasis. Orth Phys Ther Clin North Am 3:165–178, 1994.
43. Taylor EW, Morris, DM, Shaddear S, et al: The effects of water walking on hemiplegic gait. Aquat Phys Ther Rep 1:10–21, 1992.
44. Vargas LG: The effect of aquatic physical therapy on improving motor function and decreasing pain in a chronic low back pain patient: A retrospective case report. J Aqua Phys Ther 6:6–10, 1998.
45. Vogtle LK, Morris DM, Denton BG: An aquatic program for adults with cerebral palsy living in group homes. Phys Ther Case Rep 1:250–259, 1998.
46. Wille'n C, Sunnerhagen KS, Grimby G: Dynamic water exercise in individuals with late poliomyelitis. Arch Phys Med Rehabil 82:66–72, 2001.
47. Woods DA: Aquatic exercise programs for patients with multiple sclerosis. Clin Kinesiol 46:14–20, 1992.
48. Wynn KE: Lily ponds, Warm Springs, and fortunate accidents: A brief history of aquatic physical therapy. Phys Ther Mag (Dec):44–45, 1994.

Screening and Treatment of the Polio Foot and Ankle

Brent Bernstein, DPM, and Anne C. Gawne, MD

Survivors of poliomyelitis with foot and ankle complaints are encountered commonly in podiatric, rehabilitation, and orthopedic medicine. At the height of the epidemic between 1951 and 1954, more than 50,000 cases of polio per year were reported.[26] In 1952, in the United States 57,879 people were paralyzed, 3145 of whom died. In 1989, a survey by the National Center for Health Statistics estimated that there were more than 640,000 polio survivors in the United States.[27] There are currently millions of polio survivors worldwide, many of whom are suffering from significant disability from the original polio, or postpolio syndrome (PPS).

Acute poliomyelitis is a viral infection of the spinal cord caused by an enterovirus. The virus settles in the anterior horn cell, destroying it and causing a flaccid paralysis, with loss of muscle tone and deep tendon reflexes, leading to muscle atrophy.[31] With time, there is reinnervation and improvement of strength in many muscle groups, but sometimes this can lead to muscle imbalances, such as weak dorsiflexors and stronger plantar flexors. These patients may also have asymmetry in the pattern of involvement, with premature closure of the epiphyses at the knee and metatarsals in the affected limb, leading to a relative leg length or foot size discrepancy if there is unequal involvement in the lower extremities (Fig. 1).[6] Limb length differences are usually no greater than 1.5 inches but may be much greater. Because columns of anterior horn cells innervate muscles, there is variable involvement of muscles in the lower extremities.[30] Some muscles, such as the tibialis anterior or the quadriceps, are more vulnerable to complete paralysis because short columns of anterior horn cells innervate them. The peronei, gastrocnemius, tibialis posterior, and hamstrings are moderately vulnerable to the virus, but the intrinsic muscles of the foot and the long extensors and flexors to the toes are less vulnerable.[17] The polio virus causes a pronounced atrophy of up to 80% of the muscle bulk, flaccidity, hypotonia, and loss of the deep tendon reflexes and autonomic responses. The period of acute paralysis was followed by recovery of some, but not necessarily all, of the muscles. Although polio affects

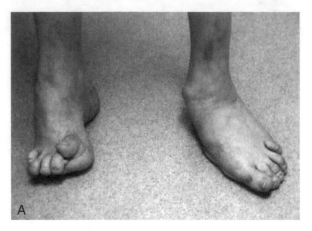

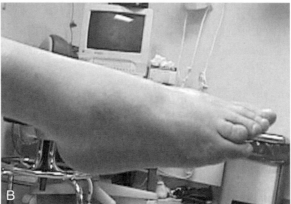

Figure 1. Growth arrest. *A,* Limb length discrepancy with associated typical asymmetric foot deformities, pes planus on long leg and cavus on short leg. *B,* Brachymetatarsia of 4th metatarsal.

only motor nerves (sensory nerve function is spared), these authors have noted anecdotally that approximately 23% of nondiabetic polio survivors have loss of protective cutaneous sensation as measured by the ability to perceive a nylon monofilament on the foot.

During the polio epidemics in the first half of the 20th century, rehabilitation focused on aggressive strengthening of paralyzed muscles. Moist heat and range of motion exercises were also done to prevent deformity. Orthoses were prescribed in order to assist patients with independent ambulation, but a number of surgical procedures were done on the lower extremities to make the limbs functional again (Fig. 2). These included hamstring transfers; release of hip, knee, or ankle contractures; and epiphysiodesis to slow growth of the unaffected leg. Toward the end of the convalescent stage, the final reconstructive procedures were performed to stabilize and realign subluxations and severe deformities including arthrodeses and osteotomies. Despite treatment, it was common for polio survivors to have abnormal forces develop across a joint because of muscle imbalances (Fig. 3). For instance, genu recurvatum develops when there is a weak quadriceps in order to stabilize the knee during the stance phase of gait.[28,33,36] Chronically as the polio survivor ages, residual deformities slowly become established and rigid, and osteoarthritis is common. This leads to pain and further problems.

TREATMENT OF PRIMARY DEFORMITIES

The initial, primary deformities are linked directly to the damage from the poliomyelitis virus (see column 1 in Table 2). Tachdjian studied equinovarus deformities, caused by weak peroneus longus, peroneus brevis, and anterior tibialis, with strong gastrocnemius-soleus and toe flexors.[34] Although this was most commonly treated with an Achilles tenotomy, the procedure did not always solve the problem. Irwin discussed the difficult problem of calcaneous deformity.[16] Langenskiold addressed forefoot supinatus deformity.[23] Many of the classic surgical procedures that all providers of foot and ankle care have performed were developed to treat the onslaught of poliomyelitis survivors. These included tendon transfers such as an anterior transfer of the posterior tibial tendon or flexor digitorum longus to correct drop foot or an equinus deformity leading to a better result than a simple Achilles tenotomy. There were also transfers of the biceps femoris and semitendonosis tendons anteriorly to the patellar tendon to treat genu recurvatum.[32] Fusions were performed such as the triple arthrodesis for a drop foot, tarsometatarsal truncated-wedge arthrodesis for equinovarus and cavus foot deformities,[18] and pantalar fusions for complex deformi-

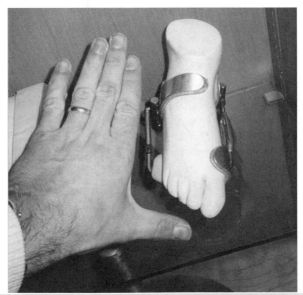

Figure 2. Pediatric brace to prevent varus deformity.

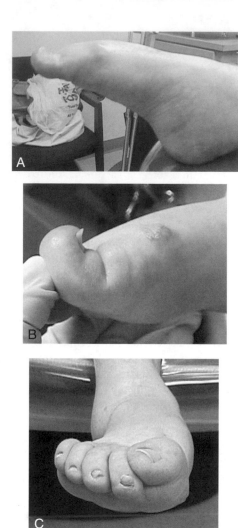

Figure 3. Some primary foot deformities. *A*, Hallux flexus. *B*, Interphalangeal extensus deformity of hallux. *C*, Forefoot valgus. *(Continues)*

ties of the foot and ankle.[15] Osteotomies of the calcaneus for cavus foot was done by Dwyer[8] and combined with plantar soft tissue stripping for cavovarus foot.[7] Metadductus deformity was addressed through multiple metatarsal basal osteotomies as discussed by Berman and Gartland.[3] The classic Robert Jones operation for clawed hallux was commonly performed on polio survivors.[24] Other common foot surgeries included the Green Grice subtalar blocking procedure, the posterior bone block for equinus, the Silver and Dwyer calcaneal osteotomies, and the triple arthrodesis. Leg length differences were treated with procedures such as an epiphysiodesis done on the longer, nonaffected limb. Perry reviewed her experience through the gamut of polio

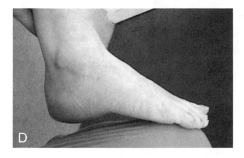

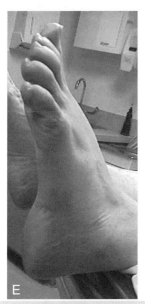

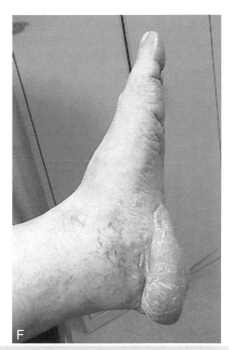

Figure 3. *(Continued)* *D* and *E*, Anterior cavus. *F*, Calcaneus.

procedures of the lower and upper extremities during the 1940s and 1950s and into the present day, including a procedure called the triple tenodesis for stabilization of the recurvatum knee.[29] She also discussed the sometimes deleterious effects of procedures such as the triple and pantalar arthrodesis as knees develop degenerative changes.

SECONDARY OR RESIDUAL DEFORMITIES

Currently in the United States, most physicians encounter patients in the final (residual) stage of polio. In this stage, chronic deformities become established and rigid. Secondary deformities and pathologies develop because of the long-standing biomechanical faults, as shown in Figure 4. In addition, many of these patients may

PATIENT #	CHIEF COMPLAINT BY DIAGNOSES	SECONDARY DIAGNOSES	TREATMENT OFFERED	TREATMENT ELECTED BY PATIENT	GENDER
	Table 1. FOOT CLINIC REGISTRY OF 45 CONSECUTIVE POSTPOLIO PATIENTS, 5/15/01 TO 5/15/02				
1	DJD ankle joint	Equinus Pseudo-equinus	Fusion ankle	Watchful waiting	Female
2	Cavus foot	DJD STJ	Brace adjust	Same	Female
3	Cavus foot	DJD Chopart joint Equinus	Brace adjust	Same	Female
4	Autonomic dysreflexia	Equinovarus	Lifestyle changes	Same	Male
5	Anterior cavus	Callus	Insert adjusted Debridement	Same	Female
6	Equinus	None	TAL MAFO	Same	Female
7	Autonomic dysreflexia	Flaccid paralysis	Lifestyle changes	Same	Female
8	Dropfoot Equinus	Callus	Debridement	Same	Male
9	DJD Lisfranc's joint	Equinovarus	Fusion Lisfranc's and TNJ	Watchful waiting	Female
	DJD TNJ	Metatarsalgia	TNJ		
10	DJD TNJ/CCJ	Old STJ fusion	Fusion TNJ/CCJ	Watchful waiting	Male
11	Equinus Tripping	Hammertoes	Heel lift Toe splints	Same	Female
12	Calcaneous deformity	Callous	Debridement	Same	Female
13	Equinus Pseudoequinus	Triple arthrodesis In varus Loose staple	TAL, hardware out, exostectomy, MAFO	Same	Female
14	Pes planus Plantar fasciitis	None	Insert modified Steroid injection	Same	Female
15	TNJ/CCJ DJD Ankle joint DJD	Old STJ fusion	Watchful waiting	Same	Male
16	Hammertoes Clawtoes	Keratosis	Toe splints Debridement	Same	Female
17	Overcorrected calcaneal osteotomy with valgus RF	Mallet toe	Triple arthrodesis with Ilizarov Fusion DIPJ	Same	Female
18	Cavus	Metatarsalgia	Silicone pad	Same	Male

(continued)

	CHIEF			TREATMENT	
PATIENT #	COMPLAINT BY DIAGNOSES	SECONDARY DIAGNOSES	TREATMENT OFFERED	ELECTED BY PATIENT	GENDER

Table 1. FOOT CLINIC REGISTRY OF 45 CONSECUTIVE POSTPOLIO PATIENTS, 5/15/01 TO 5/15/02 (Continued)

PATIENT #	CHIEF COMPLAINT BY DIAGNOSES	SECONDARY DIAGNOSES	TREATMENT OFFERED	TREATMENT ELECTED BY PATIENT	GENDER
19	Flaccid dropfoot	LLD	Heel lifts MAFO	Same	Female
20	1st MPJ DJD	Old Jones FF valgus	Hemi-joint implant	Patient deferred Sx	Female
21	Diffuse ankle pain with Hx of AJ fusion	Old Jones	KAFO attached to accomodative foot orthotic/ metatarsal pad	Same	Female
	Knee instability	Anterior cavus Capsulitis 2, 3 MPJ			
22	Flail ankle	Failed MAFO, Hx of STJ Fusion	AJ fusion with Ilizarov	Same	Female
23	Anterior cavus with metarsalgia	1st IPJ DJD with cock-up hallux Hammertoes FF valgus	Foot orthotic	Same	Female
24	Cavus	LLD Cock-up hallux	Watchful waiting	Same	Male
25	Swan neck hallux	Equinus FF varus	Silicone pad Heel lift	Same	Female
26	Button scar lesion	Auton. dys.	Insert modified	Insert modified	Female
	Calcaneus deformity	Hammertoes	Hammertoe Sx Debridement	Sx pending Debridement	
27	PTTD	Pes planus	UCBL insert Injection	Same	Female
28	Lisfranc's joint DJD Old triple LLD with inadequate lift	B/L involvement with flaccid paralysis in equinouvarus with KAFO	Defer Sx because B/L Injection, NSAID, magnet, shoe modification, lift, Insert	Patient elected conservative care: injection, medications, shoe lift and bracing	Female

(continued)

	CHIEF			TREATMENT	
PATIENT #	COMPLAINT BY DIAGNOSES	SECONDARY DIAGNOSES	TREATMENT OFFERED	ELECTED BY PATIENT	GENDER
29	Pronated cavus left HAV left Joplin's neuroma Painful scars from Green-Grice, TAL, B/L failed Jones	LLD right Atrophied leg Equinovarus right Swan neck hallux right Keratototic scar right heel s/p button for transfer of peroneus longus	Debridement of heal lesion	Same	Female
30	Neuritis intermediate dorsal cutaneous nerve left s/p DJD ankle joint	Iatrogenic reversed LLD from epiphysiodesis Scars from SPLATT, TAL, Green/Grice, EHL transfer with subsequent plantar flexed 1st metatarsal Lower leg atrophy left	Perineural steroid injections Depth shoe and MAFO	Same	Female
31	Thick toenails	Asymptomatic leg atrophy	Quarterly debridement of toenails	Same	Male
32	Metatarsalgia with paresthesias right, plantarflexed with 1st metatarsal (hx of EHL to FHL transfer)	None	MAFO with cutout under 1st metatarsals	Same	Male
33	PTTD with pronated Left foot	Flexed 4, 5 toes Left leg atrophy with mild dropfoot Tyloma 4th metatarsal head	MAFO with UCBL attached and debridement of tyloma	Same	Female

(continued)

	CHIEF			TREATMENT	
PATIENT #	COMPLAINT BY DIAGNOSES	SECONDARY DIAGNOSES	TREATMENT OFFERED	ELECTED BY PATIENT	GENDER

Table 1. FOOT CLINIC REGISTRY OF 45 CONSECUTIVE POSTPOLIO PATIENTS, 5/15/01 TO 5/15/02 (Continued)

PATIENT #	CHIEF COMPLAINT BY DIAGNOSES	SECONDARY DIAGNOSES	TREATMENT OFFERED	TREATMENT ELECTED BY PATIENT	GENDER
34	Quad and anterior lower compartment leg atrophy with genu recurvatum right	Valgus right foot	KAFO with droplocks and DF assist ankle with attached UCBL	Same	Male
35	Cavus	None	Accomodative foot orthotic	Same	Female
36	LLD right with secondary valgus hindfoot and DJD of subtalar joint	Cavus foot left	Triple arthrodesis right with corticotomy and lengthening of tibia on Ilizarov frame to correct LLD	Same	Male
37	Dropfoot and FF valgus right s/p triple arthrodesis (as adult)	Cocked-up hallux right	None	Same	Male
38	Gorilloform navicular with brace irritation	Dropfoot Quadriceps weakness	KAFO with accomodation of navicular	Same	Female
39	Splayfoot	None	Bunionectomy and osteotomies of 1st and 5th metatarsals	Same	Male
40	Incompletely corrected calcaneocavus s/p triple arthrodesis right	Callus right foot LLD right S/p Jones right	Quarterly debridement of callus Depth shoes and total contact inserts with accomodations	Same	Female
41	No obvious residual polio deformities	DM CVA/walker	Routine foot care linked to DM	Same	Male

(continued)

	CHIEF			TREATMENT	
PATIENT #	COMPLAINT BY DIAGNOSES	SECONDARY DIAGNOSES	TREATMENT OFFERED	ELECTED BY PATIENT	GENDER
42	Rigid varus hind-foot with flaccid ankle left Right flatfoot	Rigid PF 1st metararsal with hallux malleus Overlapping 2nd toe Swan neck 3rd toe Prominent 5th metatarsal base $1^1/_2$ inch LLD	Extra-depth shoes with T strap lat-erally on left and medially on right	Same	Female
43	Dropfoot with genu recur-vatum	Morton's neuroma Joplin's neu-roma s/p sesamoid-ectomy	KAFO Recommend neuroma excisions and implan-tation to muscle	KAFO Watchful waiting on neuromas	Male
44	Left equinovarus with adventitous bursa over lateral malleolus (clubfoot-like severity) not controlled with MAFO; com-plete loss of peroneal strength; post-tibia spared	Hx triple arth-rodesis right and tendon transfers Powerline repairman, so no metal braces tolerated	Posterior tibial tendon transfer to cuboid and percutane-ous achilles tendon trans-fer followed by high top boot and T strap	Same	Male
45	Equinus with dropfoot	Hammertoes with bursitis PIPJs	Rec. TAL, MAFO, arth-roplasties of digits	Pt. elects no treat-ment	Female

AJ = ankle joint; Auton. dys. = autonomic dysreflexia; B/L = bilateral; CCJ = calca-neocuboid joint; CVA = cerebrovascular accident; DIPJ = distal interphalangeal joint; DJD = degenerative joint disease; DM = diabetes mellitus; EHL = extensor hallu-cis longus; FF = forefoot; Hx = history of; KAFO = knee-ankle-foot orthosis; LLD = limb length discrepancy; MAFO = molded ankle foot orthosis; MPJ = metatarso-phalangeal joint; NSAID = nonsteroidal anti-inflammatory drug; PF = plantar flexion; PIPJ = proximal interphalangeal joint; Pt. = patient; PTTD = posterior tibial tendon dys-function; s/p = postoperative status; SPLATT = split anterior tibial tendon; STJ = sub-talar joint; Sx = surgery; TAL = tendo-Achilles lengthening; TNJ = talonavicular joint; TT = tendon transfer; UCBL = University of California Biomechanics Laboratory orthosis.

Table 1. FOOT CLINIC REGISTRY OF 45 CONSECUTIVE POSTPOLIO PATIENTS, 5/15/01 TO 5/15/02 (Continued)

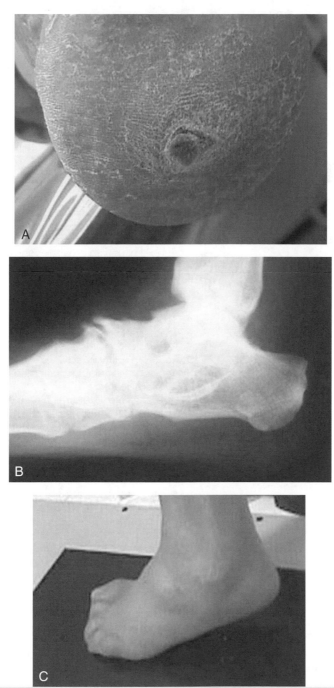

Figure 4. Secondary foot disorders. *A*, Keratotic scar from button technique for old tendon transfer. *B* and *C*, Residual equinus in patient with triple arthrodesis.

be suffering from PPS with the development of new weakness and symptoms decades after the initial acute infection.[13] Affected muscles subsequently show signs of fatigue and pain. Although the initial procedures allowed years of assisted ambulation, secondary disorders are now being diagnosed (see column 2 of Table 2). One of the main causes of this is the added stress to adjacent joints after fusion and stress placed on joints from abnormal biomechanics and leg length differences; this causes pain mainly in the back and lower extremities.[38] In addition, many polio survivors

Table 2. MUSCULOSKELETAL DEFORMITIES

PRIMARY	SECONDARY
Primary gastrocsoleus equinus	Hallux abductovalgus
Primary gastrocnemius equinus	Hallux limitus
Dropfoot	Hallux limitus with previous Jones teno-suspension
Equinus with dropfoot	Hammertoes, mallet toes, swan neck deformities
Flail ankle	Autonomic dysreflexia
Paralytic pes planus	Secondary equinus with weak quadriceps and genu recurvatum
Inversion of foot	Predislocation syndrome of MTP joint
Calcaneus	Recurrent primary equinus
Adducted forefoot	Bony ankle equinus (spurring, talar dome adaptation)
Global cavus	Overcorrected deformities (triple arthrodesis or Dwyer in varus)
Medial column cavus	Flexible or semiflexible flatfoot secondary to equinus or long residual extremity
Anterior cavus	Cavus foot secondary to short residual extremity
Calcaneocavus	Posterior tibial tendon dysfunction
Claw toes	Secondary hallux varus or pan-digital varus
Hallus varus	Loose or broken residual hardware
Hallux extensus	Chronic osteomyelitis
Hallux flexus	Keloids and hypertrophic scars secondary to incisions or button-technique tendon transfers
Limb length discrepancy	Numbness and reflex sympathetic dystrophy
Brachymetatarsia	Degenerative joint disease of joints adjacent to fusions or caused by chronic malalignment
Calf hypertrophy or calf atrophy	Fibromyalgia-like trigger point pain
Clawed hallux	Metatarsalgia
Peripheral neuropathy arterial insufficiency caused by poliomyelitis	Brace ulcers, adventitious bursae, or hyperkeratotic lesions

MTP = metatarsophalangeal.

have deformities in adulthood that were untreated as children or develop additional deformities due to muscle imbalances as they have ambulated over their lifetime. These problems range from orthopedic deformities secondary to long-standing malalignment to vascular and skin disorders. Also, malunions, over-corrections, nonunions, and symptomatic scars are common along with overlengthening or overshortening of limb length discrepancies.

EVALUATION OF FOOT PROBLEMS IN POLIO SURVIVORS

The authors of this chapter sent a survey to 150 polio survivors as part of their monthly mailing in a polio support group newsletter in order to determine the nature and type of foot disorders that they are having and the treatment (if any) they are receiving. Inclusion criteria was a history of paralytic polio followed by recovery. Not all of the patients met the criteria for PPS. The survey asked questions such as if they had foot pain, foot deformity, foot surgery (as a child, adolescent, or adult). The patients were asked to describe the deformity and type of surgery, whether they wore a brace or special shoes, if they used another assistive device for ambulation or mobility, if they suffered from intolerance to cold, and which type of health provider they saw for their foot care.

Eighty-three polio survivors completed the questionnaire, including 45 women and 38 men between the ages of 46 and 82 years (mean age, 64 years). The majority of the respondents (89%) reported that they had foot deformity, ranging from limb length discrepancies, osteoarthritis and hammertoes to cavus feet, equinus, and drop foot, and 70% reported some type of lower extremity surgery, including many types of soft tissue and bone surgery in both childhood and throughout adulthood. Fifty-four percent reported that they had foot pain and 73% experienced a cold extremity. All of the subjects reported that they used some type of appliance, assistive device, special shoe, or brace for ambulation, and all saw an orthotist or pedorthist. Only 8.4% reported currently seeing a podiatrist, but 38% saw a physiatrist. The majority of respondents (88%) were receiving care from their primary care physician.[12] These results correspond well with another survey of biomechanical physicians that also revealed that only a small percentage of postpolio patients received podiatric care, although said care was extremely effective.[4]

After this survey, in order to better understand the severity of foot problems, the authors studied 45 consecutive symptomatic polio survivors referred to a foot clinic from a postpolio clinic. In addition to a full history, questions regarding fatigue as related to walking and sitting tolerance were included, and a detailed pain questionairre was completed. This was followed by a physical examination, with special attention paid to orthopedic and neurologic systems.[17] The lower extremity examination included evaluation of the hip and knee, noting contractures, weakness, and pain on range of motion as well as leg length discrepancies. Bilateral dermal temperature readings, vasculature levels, and transcutaneous oximetry measurements were documented. Protective sensation was tested with a 10-gauge monofilament. Muscle strength by group was evaluated using the Medical Research Council scale of 0 to 5.[14] There was a general inspection and video of stance, mobility, aids, and transfers, followed by routine analysis of plan-

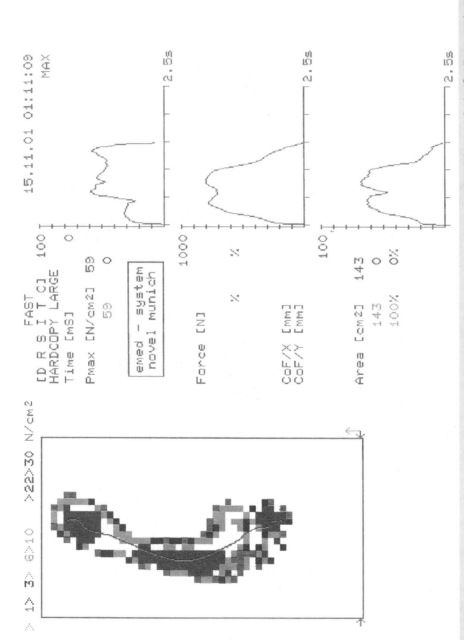

Figure 5. Plantar pressure measurements. A, Heal to toe composite in stride with maximal pressure measurements in cavus foot. *(Continues, next page)*

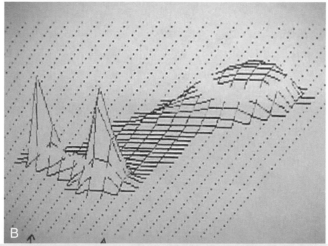

Figure 5. *(Continued)* B, Three-dimensional view of same foot.

tar foot pressures with a piezoelectric pressure pad on an elevated walking platform (Fig. 5). Patients brought in all past and present braces, shoes, and assistive devices, which were inspected for fit, control, and wear. A detailed description of deformities, including the degree of correctability of each, was performed with digital photography. Plain radiographs of the ankle and foot and computed tomography–assisted limb length studies were ordered if a leg length discrepancy was noted (Fig. 6). A synopsis of the examinations of the 45 patients referred to the foot clinic is shown in Table 1, including treatment recommendations and treatment elected by the patients.

Of the 45 subjects studied (30 women and 15 men ages 44 to 84 years with a mean age of 64 years), 98% percent reported that they had foot pain and 89% had foot deformities. Of the latter group, 33% had equinus or equinovarus deformities, 33% had toe deformities, 22% had a cavus or anterior cavus deformity, 22% had metatarsalgia and frontal plane forefoot deformities, 22% had keratosis and bursitis, 20% had degenerative joint disease, and 17% had limb length discrepancies. Interestingly, 22% of participants had evidence of iatrogenic lesions (e.g., scars, neuroma, prominent hardware). Autonomic dysreflexia was present in 6% of subjects. One third of the subjects had dropfoot or flail ankle, and pes planus or posterior tibial tendon dysfunction was present in 16%.

Thirty-seven percent of the patients reported a history of some type of lower extremity surgery, including soft tissue and bone surgery in childhood and throughout adulthood. Treatments offered included orthoses, shoe and heel lifts, new braces (e.g., ankle foot orthoses [AFOs]), adjustments of existing braces, injections, routine debridement of skin lesions, toe splints, and surgery as well as "watchful waiting." Surgery was thought to be potentially beneficial in 31% of the subjects, but only 16% of the subjects studied proceeded with elected to have surgery. Surgical procedures ranged from simple bunionectomies and Achilles tendon lengthenings to tibial lengthenings, complex tendon transfers, and ankle arthrodesis.

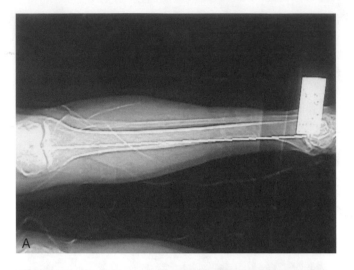

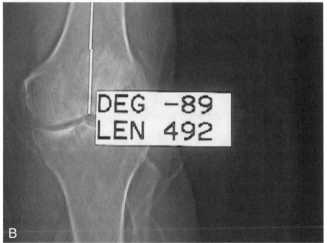

Figure 6. Limb length measurements. *A*, CT scan assisted segmental measurements. *B*, Close-up of measurement.

In a similar study, Keenan evaluated 200 consecutive polio survivors presenting with orthopedic complaints in 1994.[29] The subjects had a mean age of 54 years. Equinus was a very common diagnosis, and the most common treatment was surgery. Of the 200 patients seen, they recommended surgery for 79 (40%); 46 (23%) subjects elected to proceed.

NONSURGICAL TREATMENTS OF POSTPOLIO FOOT DISORDERS

Objectives for nonsurgical treatment of foot disorders in this patient population include (1) accommodation of rigid conditions and toe deformities; (2) offweighting to provide shock absorption and cushioning of bony prominences and contracted digits; (3) control of flexible conditions and rigid deformities to allow a stable plantigrade foot that will help prevent strain on soft tissues and joints and allow better fit of shoe wear; (4) pharmacologic reduction of pain; (5) patient education on proper shoe wear, orthotic use, skin care, and temperature regulation; (6) improvement of gait; (7) prevention of falls[19]; (8) periodic reduction of hyperkeratotic lesions and dystrophic nails, which cause pain and difficulty with braces and shoes; and (9) reinforcement of recommendations regarding reducing activity level, particularly in individuals with PPS. Simple office procedures such as dispensing over-the-counter pads or protectors known as "orthodigita" (Fig. 7), construction of custom silicone appliances for management of severe digital deformities, appropriate shoe recommendations, sclerosing injections of neuromas, and corticosteroid injections of inflammatory processes can usually lead to spontaneous resolution of pain complaints.

ORTHOTIC MANAGEMENT

Examples of bracing options include a posterior leaf spring AFO for flaccid dorsiflexor weakness and a solid AFO for those with both plantar and dorsiflexor weakness. Patients with equinovarus can be treated with a solid AFO or a short leg brace with a lateral T strap.[31] Plastic molded AFOs made of polyethylene or polypropylene permit custom design of lightweight flexible to rigid orthoses, depending on the ratio of flexible monomer.[25] A double metal upright brace should be used when there is significant loss of sensation or foot ulcers, fluctuating edema, or simply if the individual

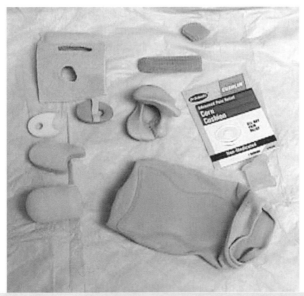

Figure 7. Orthodigita.

prefers this type of brace option. The foot interface can range from soft, accomodative orthoses primarily functioning for soft tissue supplementation to rigid orthoses with extrinsic posts for correction of flexible foot deformities of the forefoot and hindfoot (Figs. 8 and 9). Sometimes the simplest modifications such as metatarsal bars and rocker-bottom soles can drastically reduce focal pressures under the metatarsal heads. Medial and lateral oversoles can improve the amount of control that bracing provides. Recently, knee-ankle-foot orthoses (KAFOs) are offering many more options, particularly with "smart" knee joints that allow patients who traditionally would have to walk with a locked knee to bend their knees during swing phase and early stance phase. When prescribing braces, attention should be given to preconditioning of joints and muscles through home exercises, physical therapy, and gradual incorporation of the appliance into daily life. This break-in period can drastically decrease the transient "adjustment" discomfort and overall patient frustration and noncompliance.

TREATMENT OF COLD FEET

Complaints of cold feet are prevalent in a number of studies, yet although patients are likely to note this condition on subjective surveys, they rarely complain of the symptoms in the clinic because of more pressing issues. When evaluated, patients should be questioned at the first visit about cold sensations of the feet, purplish discoloration, sensitivity to pain when cold, loss of strength when cold, or fainting when rising quickly or when getting out of a warm bath. Cutaneous temperatures are quantified through use of infrared dermal thermometry. If abnormal cold sensitivity is suspected, instructions are given to the patient to minimize symptoms. Patients are instructed to dress as if they are "one season colder" and to use Thinsulate-lined socks during cold months. A number of commercially available gadgets can warm the socks and feet. Often these can be found through suppliers in outdoor, mountaineering, or skiing equipment.[22]

SURGICAL INTERVENTIONS

Occasionally, surgical intervention is indicated in polio survivors with the following objectives: (1) arthrodesis or replacement of arthritic joints; (2) removal of loose or broken hardware; (3) tendon lengthening and transfers for equinus and dropfoot; (4) treatment of unresolved deformities through arthroplasty, osteotomy, and arthrodesis; (5) revisional surgery of overcorrected deformities; and; (6) correction of severe limb length disorders. The overall goal is to relieve pain and, in some cases, create a plantigrade and braceable foot. Faraj successfully treated postpolio patients, including correction of claw foot deformity using a modified Jones procedure[9] and used a talonavicular joint arthrodesis for forefoot instability.[10] Graves et al. have used the triple arthrodesis to fuse painful arthritic joints and to provide a plantigrade foot for ambulation.[15] Any contemplated surgical procedure, however, must be weighed against the increased morbidity associated with the poliomyelitis survivor and stresses that will be induced on more proximal joints. Surgeons must also be aware of psy-

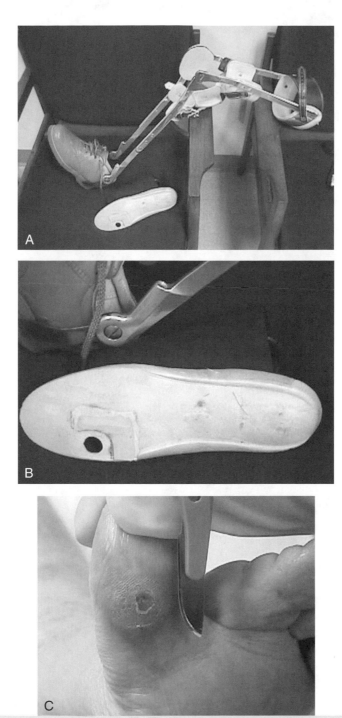

Figure 8. Modified knee-ankle-foot orthosis (KAFO). *A*, KAFO with insert. *B*, Close-up of insert with modifications to treat keratosis under 1st metatarsal head. *C*, Sharp debridement of keratosis.

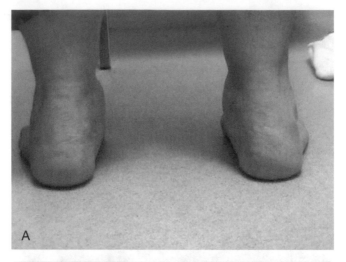

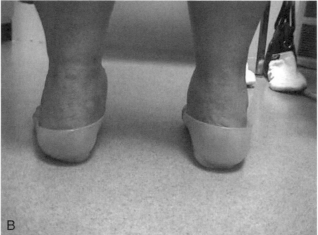

Figure 9.   Posterior tendon dysfunction. *A*, Associated heal eversion. *B*, Control of deformity with deep heel cup and extrinsic post on orthotic.

chological factors given that many polio survivors endured both physical and emotional trauma by undergoing numerous surgeries as children[11] and should spend additional time to review risks and benefits as well as the postoperative protocols with the patient.

PERIOPERATIVE CONSIDERATIONS

The orthopedic or podiatric surgeon follows a strict perioperative protocol. The physiatrist is involved with overall treatment and rehabilitation issues. Ideally, patients should also be evaluated preoperatively by a physical therapist, with specific attention to developing a plan for postoperative offweighting if necessary. Preoperative physical therapy assists in training in the use of temporary assistive devices for safe postoperative ambulation and transfers and also evaluating the home setting, so that the patient can manage optimally in his or her home environment after surgery. Also, specialized phase conversion training of muscles is performed if out-of-phase tendon transfers (e.g., a posterior tibial tendon transfer) are planned. In some facilities, a computerized gait analysis examination is also performed preoperatively.

OPERATIVE CONSIDERATIONS

Some anecdotal reports have shown polio survivors to be abnormally sensitive to anesthesia, which is theorized to possibly be caused by damage to the reticular activating system in the brain.[5] Anesthesia may also be complicated by pulmonary muscle weakness, either from the intial polio or from PPS. Other than very limited forefoot procedures that are performed as an outpatient under local anesthesia, surgeons and anesthesiologists should consider the possible risks associated with various types of anesthesia, and pulmonary function studies should be contemplated. Operating room temperatures are ideally adjusted to warm the room moderately, and an inflatable body warming device can be applied to the upper body and torso to avoid the thermoregulatory problems typical in polio survivors.

POSTOPERATIVE TREATMENT

Gentle physical therapy is instituted in bed to decrease the common occurrence of muscle spasms. Pneumatic sequential compression boots are routinely used on the nonsurgical extremity to prevent deep vein thrombosis, while the Robert Jones dressing provides gentle compression to the veins on the surgical limb. Pain is controlled through aggressive elevation of the extremity to prevent swelling. Opioids are typically safe for polio survivors, but respiratory complications should be monitored. Special attention to adequate availability of bedside commodes, grab bars, and overhead frames for transfers and other assistive devices for mobility and activities of daily living is important.

SPECIFIC SURGICAL PRINCIPLES

When possible, complex reconstructive procedures involving the foot, ankle, and lower leg that historically would necessitate strict non–weight bearing for 2 months or more are often now performed with a multi-ring external fixation system. Many surgeons have found that external fixation is superior in poliomyelitis patients for the following reasons: (1) multiple pins allow better fixation of osteoporotic bone than standard internal screw fixation; (2) multi-ring fixation allows the postoperative variability and versatility necessary for dynamic revision of complex deformities; (3) it avoids the shortening that is typical with standard osteotomies and internal fixation in an already shortened foot or leg through the concept of bone and soft tissue distraction; and (4) the supreme stability of the frame allows early weight bearing on the limb, which helps avoid worsening of the deconditioning in the already weakened polio patient (Figs. 10–12). Also, surgeons often order a dynamic, spring-loaded ankle

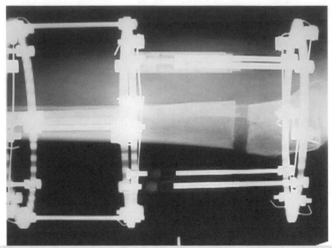

Figure 10. Long leg multi-ring external fixator for concomitant triple arthrodesis and tibial corticotomy and lengthening.

foot orthosis to be attached to the frame in the operating room (Fig. 13). This device can be adjusted to variable tensions to allow dynamic dorsiflexion of the forefoot and avoids the common complication after triple arthrodesis (Fig. 14) and subsequent non–weight bearing of flexion contracture of the forefoot.[17] Modern surgeons also make use of cannulated screws and soft tissue anchor systems, both of which decrease the amount of dissection and increase the predictability of fixation compared with systems that were available when patients with acute polio were treated decades ago.

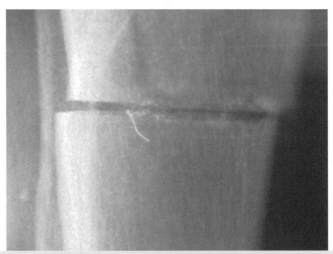

Figure 11. Close-up of tibial corticotomy site.

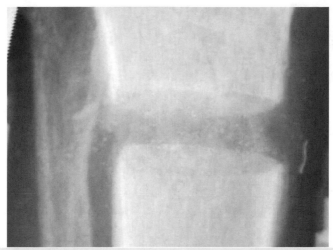

Figure 12. Tibial corticotomy after distraction; early mineralization of soft bone callous.

Bone growth stimulators are standard in arthrodesis procedures in polio survivors because of the historically slow healing of bone in these patients. If appropriate, ankle arthroscopy is used rather than arthrotomy to access intraarticular and periarticular ankle pathology, thereby limiting pain and recuperation time. All attempts are made to decrease the size of incisions, pain, and the overall morbidity of any particular procedure that could be catastrophic to the weakened extremities of polio patients. In patients with standard internal fixation, postoperative offweighting is performed with

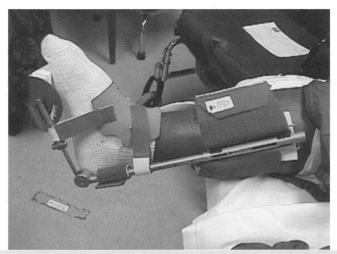

Figure 13. Dynamic stretching with low load after tibialis anterior tendon transfer.

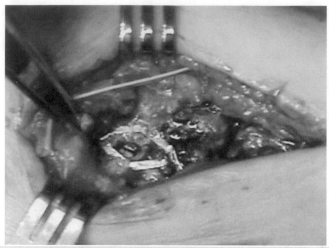

Figure 14. Calcaneocuboid joint resection during triple arthrodesis.

either total contact casting in the Carville method or a removable patellar tendon bearing brace.[25] These modalities adequately unload the hindfoot while keeping the patient mobile. They also decrease the need for crutch trauma on the upper extremities while also adding to a sense of warmth of the extremity, thereby decreasing postoperative pain in the polio survivor.

Additional attention is made in polio survivors being surgically treated for equinus (Fig. 15). A full examination is necessary to preoperatively assess for gastrocnemius versus gastrosoleal equinus. Additionally, the strength of the quadriceps and any genu recurvatum of the knee is assessed. Many times, the equinus deformity is a necessary compensation for a weak quadriceps, and aggressive lengthening of the Achilles may make ambulation impossible.[17] The muscles of the calf are very important in stabilizing the knee during the single-limb stance portion of the gait cycle.[33] Also, pseudo-equinus secondary to anterior ankle joint bone spurs must be ruled out to avoid inadequate correction through soft tissue release alone. A preoperative charger-type radiograph of the ankle is standard to rule out this condition. The manual squeeze test of the calf helps differentiate between tightness of the gastrocnemius versus the gastrocsoleus conjoined tendon. Additionally, the surgeon considers that long-standing equinus in polio patients may lead to widening of the anterior dome of the talus, which may limit correction somewhat despite full release of the Achilles and ankle/subtalar joint contractures. If this is expected, application of an Ilizarov frame is considered with two half pins in the calcaneus and gradual correction of the deformity.[21] Immediate correction using this method is avoided because of a high occurrence of pin site necrosis. Surgery is warranted if the contracture directly leads to an unstable gait. The surgeon must be able to make an expert decision as to the need for isolated gastrocnemius recession, Achilles tendon lengthening, full posterior capsular

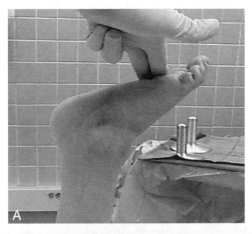

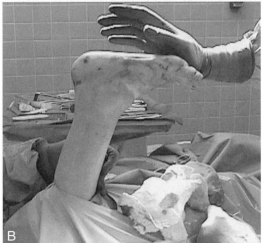

Figure 15. Treatment of equinus. *A*, preprocedure deformity. *B*, Post-Achilles and ankle joint lengthening.

release, or arthroscopically assisted osteophyte excision so that full correction will occur with minimal dissection and disruption of compensatory mechanisms.

CONCLUSION

The literature demonstrates that foot deformities and foot pain are common in polio survivors. The review of data from clinical studies reveals that many polio survivors have foot disorders, including degenerative joint disease, pes cavus, equinus, drop foot, limb length discrepancy, and toe deformities as well as old fusions such as a triple arthrodesis. In many cases, the foot can be the limiting or aggravating factor in the patients' overall ability to function and can exacerbate symptoms of PPS. It is therefore important to inquire about foot problems at each visit and to evaluate the feet, limb length, shoes, and orthotic devices during the physical examination. Of note is the fact that male polio survivors may be less likely to seek help for foot problems than female patients, despite the fact that foot pain is equal among genders. Ancillary studies, including plain radiographs, computer-assisted scanagrams, and computerized gait analysis can be helpful in diagnosis and planning. Most polio foot disorders can be managed nonsurgically through the use of shoes, orthotics, assistive devices, and other appliances. This can be achieved through a referral to an orthotist, pedorthist, or podiatrist. Only occasionally is surgical treatment indicated, but it can provide relief in severe cases. Special perioperative precautions are warranted to prevent complications in this special population. Any surgeon attempting reconstruction of the lower extremity in a polio patient must have expertise in the anatomy and biomechanics of the polio foot. Last but not least, the surgeon should have basic knowledge of PPS itself so as not to fall into the trap of chastising patients to "work harder in therapy," only leading to frustration, increased weakness, and pain for the patient. As Federico Stelo-Ortiz, stated in *Disorders of the Foot and Ankle:*

> The eradication of poliomyelitis in highly developed countries resulted in neglect of facilities once available for acute, subacute and residual cases. Physiotherapy and rehabilitation departments and diagnostic and therapeutic facilities disappeared or were converted for other uses, as no more cases were seen—when a sporadic case of poliomyelitis presents, residual paralysis is incorrectly managed, jeopardizing the life of the patient by improper surgery or fitting of the wrong brace.[17]

References

1. Armstrong DG, Boulton JM: Activity monitors: Should we begin dosing activity as we dose a drug? J Am Podiatr Med Assoc 91:152–153, 2001.
2. Barrett GR, Meyer LC, Bray EW: Pantalar arthrodesis: A long-term follow-up. Foot Ankle 1(5):280–283, 1981.
3. Berman A, Gartland JJ: Metatarsal osteotomy for the correction of adduction of the fore part of the foot in children. J Bone Joint Surg 53A:498–506, 1971.
4. Boughton B: Time is not on their side. Biomechanics (Mar):87–92, 2001.
5. Bruno RL: The knife is not so rough if.... Post-Polio Netw Newslett 31:3–13.
6. Currarino G: Premature closure of epiphyses in the metatarsals and knees: A sequela of poliomyelitis. Radiology 87:424–428, 1966.
7. Dekel S, Weissman SL: Osteotomy of the calcaneus and concomitant plantar stripping in children with talipes cavo-varus. J Bone Joint Surg 55B:802–808, 1973.
8. Dwyer FC: The present status of the problem of pes cavus. Clin Orthop Rel Res 106:254–275, 1975.
9. Faraj AA: Modified Jones procedure for post-polio claw hallux deformity. J Foot Ankle Surg 36(5):356–359, 1997.
10. Faraj AA: Talonavicular joint arthrodesis for paralytic post poliomyelitis forefoot instability. J Foot Ankle Surg 35:166–168, 1996.
11. Frick NM: Proceedings of the Ontario March of Dimes Conference on Post-Polio Sequelae. Toronto, Ontario, March of Dimes, 1995.
12. Gawne AC, Bernstein BH: Foot problems in polio survivors. Arch Phys Med Rehabil 82(9), 2001.

13. Gawne AC, Halstead LC: Pathophysiology and clinical management of post-polio syndrome. CRC Crit Rev Rehabil 7:147–188, 1995.
14. Gawne AC, Richards RS, Petrosky G: Post-polio muscle pain in polio survivors. Arch Phys Med Rehabil 81(10):770–776, 2000.
15. Graves SC, Mann RA, Graves KO: Triple arthrodesis in older adults. J Bone Joint Surg 75A:355–362, 1993.
16. Irwin CE: The calcaneous foot. South Med J 44:191–197, 1951.
17. Jahss MH: Disorders of the hallux and first ray. In Disorders of the Foot and Ankle, 2nd ed. Philadelphia, W.B. Saunders, 1991, pp 943–1174.
18. Jahss MH: Tarsometatarsal truncated-wedge arthrodesis for pes cavus and equinovarus deformity of the fore part of the foot. J Bone Joint Surg 62A:713–722, 1980.
19. Janisse DJ: Footwear for polio survivors. Polio Netw News 17(1):6–9, 2000.
20. Kling C, Persson A, Gardulf A: The health-related quality of life of patients suffering from the late effects of polio. J Adv Nurs 32:164–173, 2000.
21. Kocaoglu M, Eralp L, Atalar AC: Correction of complex foot deformities using the Ilizarov external fixator. J Foot Ankle Surg 41:30–39, 2002.
22. Kozak P: Circulatory changes of the paretic extremities after acute anterior poliomyelitis. Arch Phys Med Rehabil 49:77–81, 1968.
23. Langenskiold A, Ritsila V: Supination deformity of the forefoot. Acta Orthop Scand 48:325–333, 1977.
24. M'Bamali EI: Results of modified Robert Jones operation for clawed hallux. Br J Surg 62:647–650, 1975.
25. Meyer PR: Lower limb orthotics. Clin Orthop Rel Res 102:58–72, 1974.
26. National Center for Health Statistics Research Data Center website: http://www.cdc.gov/nchs/.
27. Parsons PE: National Center for Health Studies [personal communication]. 1987.
28. Perry J, Fontaine JD, Mulroy S: Finding in post-poliomyelitis syndrome: Weakness of muscles of the calf as a source of late pain and fatigue of muscles of the thigh after poliomyelitis. J Bone Joint Surg 77A:1148–1153, 1995.
29. Perry J, Keenan MA: Post-polio corrective surgery: Then and now. Polio Netw News 11(3), 1995. Available at http://www.post-polio.org/ipn/pnn11-3.html.
30. Sharma JC, Gupta SP, Sankala SS, Metha N: Residual poliomyelitis of lower limb: Patterns and deformities. Ind J Pediatr 58:233–238, 1991.
31. Sobel E, Giogini RJ: Podiatric management of the neuromuscular patient. Podiatry Today.com (Jan):1–10, 2001.
32. Tachdjian MO: Pediatric Orthopedics. Vol. 2. Philadelphia, W.B. Saunders, Philadelphia, 1972, p 967.
33. Tachdjian MO: Pediatric Orthopedics, Vol. 2. Philadelphia, W.B. Saunders, 1972, p 972.
34. Tachdjian MO: Pediatric Orthopedics, Vol 2. Philadelphia, W.B. Saunders, 1972, p 977.
35. Tillet SG, Mozena JD: The reappearance of polio, postpolio syndrome. J Am Podiatr Med Assoc 89(4):183–187, 1999.
36. Wahl M: Cutting the cord. Quest 5:18–23, 2001.
37. Weil LS, Roukis TS: The calcaneal scarf osteotomy: Operative technique. J Foot Ankle Surg 40(3):178–182, 2000.
38. Wider M, Ahlstrom G: Experiences and consequences of pain in persons with post-polio syndrome. J Advance Nurs 28(3):606–613, 1998.
39. Wilson H, Kidd D, Howard RS: Calf hypertrophy following paralytic poliomyelitis. Postgrad Med J 76:179–181, 2000.

Gait, Orthoses, Footwear, and Assistive Devices

Dorothy D. Aiello, PT, MS

Gait has been studied and categorized based on norms. According to Perry, "the natural mix of joint mobility, muscle strength, neural control and energy leads to a customary walking speed, stride length and step rate. These time and distance factors, in combination with the swing and stance times, constitute the person's stride characteristics." The gait cycle is equal to a stride. A stride is a basic unit of walking, occurring from initial contact of one limb to initial contact of the same limb. Stride is divided into stance and swing period. Generally, at a comfortable walking speed, stance comprises 60% of the gait cycle and swing 40% of the cycle.[2–4] The gait cycle is further subdivided into eight phases (Fig. 1).[2]

Figure 1 also diagrams ground reaction forces (GRFs). GRFs are the upward forces exerted by the ground at the body's point of contact. Physics principles such as GRF are important to consider for gait because of their influence on stability. For example, if the GRF passes anterior to the knee joint, it produces an extension moment at the knee that increases knee stability. Conversely, if the GRF passes posterior to the knee joint, it produces a flexion moment at the knee that decreases knee stability.

During the normal walking cycle, displacement of the center of mass is approximately 2 inches.[5] Minimizing the displacement of the center of mass is considered important for minimizing energy expenditure.[1] Increases in the displacement of the center of mass increase the energy expenditure required for walking.[2] This is an important concept to remember when assessing pathological gait, as is the concept that normal walking is most energy efficient at moderate speeds.[1,2]

GAIT IN PATIENTS WITH A HISTORY OF POLIO

The assessment of gait is an essential component of the physical evaluation in patients with a history of polio. Such patients often experience difficulty with their functional mobility or increased weakness, in the case of those with postpolio syndrome (PPS) caused by a combination of factors, including fatigue, weakness, decreased flexibility, and impaired balance.[6,7] In Nollet et al.'s study of subjects with a history of polio, 46% reported that walking outdoors is a major problem.[8] In a survey done by Halstead and Rossi, 82% of PPS subjects reported progressive loss of the ability to ambulate.[9]

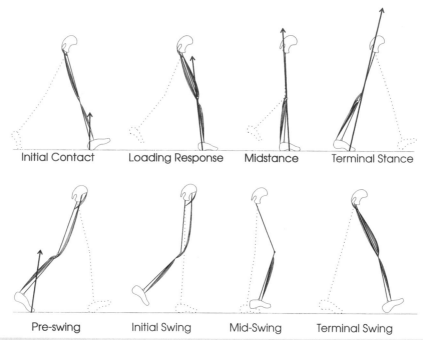

| Initial Contact | Loading Response | Midstance | Terminal Stance |

| Pre-swing | Initial Swing | Mid-Swing | Terminal Swing |

Figure 1. The eight phases of the gait cycle are initial contact, loading response, midstance, terminal stance, preswing, initial swing, midswing, and terminal swing. The ground reaction force vector is represented by a solid line with an arrow. The active muscles are shown during each phase of the gait cycle. The uninvolved limb is shown as a dotted line. (From Kerrigan DC, Schaufele M, Wen MN: Gait analysis. In DeLisa JA, Gans BM (eds): Rehabilitation Medicine: Principles and Practice, 3rd ed. Philadelphia, Lippincott Williams & Wilkins, 1998, pp 167–187, with permission.)

Polio survivors who lack movement or strength use compensatory techniques.[10] They may use joint structure and ligaments to enhance stability in stance and momentum and stronger muscle groups to assist movement in swing phase. Polio survivors may have a functional leg length discrepancy attributable to polio's effects during growth; scoliosis; or knee recurvatum, varus, or valgus. Some polio survivors had surgeries such as ankle fusions and tendon transfers that also influence gait.

Because polio affects people differently in regard to severity and muscles affected, there is a wide spectrum of possible gait deviations. In a study by Perry et al. gait was evaluated in a sample of polio survivors with a grade 0 to 3 of the calf and grade 4 to 5 of the vastus lateralis. In this sample, most patients used more then one substitution method; substitutions included quadriceps overuse, hip extensor overuse, plantar flexion contracture, and avoidance of loading the limb during knee flexion.[10] Hurmuzlu et al. assessed gait deviations in a sample of 17 postpolio patients for sagittal plane gait deviations. As compared to controls, the postpolio patients presented with excessive hip flexion in swing, and knee hyperextension and excessive plantar flexion in stance.[11] In many postpolio patients, the knee remained extended during the load response phase of gait instead of moving into flexion for shock absorption as expected.[11] Hurmuzla et al. used a mapping gait analysis procedure to assess dynamic stability in postpolio patients compared with a non–polio-affected control group with no gait pathology.[11] They concluded that during stance, postpolio patients were significantly less stable than the control group and the weaker postpolio subjects were even less stable.[11] In patients with a weak gluteus medius (hip abductors), a gait deviation known as *Trendelenburg gait* or a *gluteus medius gait* is characterized by dropping of the pelvis or hip to the opposite side during stance. In some patients who compensate for this, a lateral lean of the trunk to the weak side during stance is seen (compensated Trendelenburg gait).[2,12]

Perry et al. examined stride and muscle strength in a sample of 24 polio survivors with no lower extremity joint contractures or pain.[13] Patients with weak hip abductor muscles presented with both a contralateral pelvic drop and a lateral trunk lean to the weak side. The muscle torque that was the best predictor for gait velocity was plantar flexion. This study also showed that in polio survivors, both plantar flexion and hip abduction torques affect stride length. In this sample, the patients compensated best for quadriceps weakness.[13]

Normally, during the mid-stance phase of gait, tibial progression and ankle dorsiflexion occur.[1,2] If the patient is unable to dorsiflex the ankle, there are a few possible compensatory movements. Perry et al. noted that the patient may compensate by knee hyperextension, forward flexion at the hips, or increased arm support with an assistive device.[14] In another study, they used dynamic electromyography (EMG) to assess muscle use during gait in polio survivors. The biceps femoris was most frequently overused (82%), followed by the quadriceps (53%).[15]

Practitioners should be aware of the significance of individual polio survivors' compensatory strategies and consider if the compensatory strategies should be altered. The most important questions to answer in regard to this are:

1. Is the patient's gait pattern safe?
2. Is the patient's gait pattern functional?

If the patient's gait is both safe and functional, it is not as crucial to intervene to alter his or her gait pattern. However, there are several other important considerations, including the patient wanting to change his or her walking pattern, pain, fatigue, energy conservation, and a progressively limited functional ability, that should also be considered.

A "safe" gait pattern can be defined as no recent history of falls (within the past year) and no significant increased falls risk while walking (e.g., tripping). Silver and Aiello surveyed polio survivors and noted a high incidence of falls.[16] Of the 233 subjects surveyed, 64% reported falling at least once within the past year. This same study also related falls in polio survivors with a high incidence of fractures; 82 of 233 surveyed (35%) reported that they had a history of at least one fracture caused by a fall.[16] Comparatively, in community-dwelling elderly individuals (age > 65 years), approximately 30% fall each year; of those falls, fewer than 1 in 10 results in a fracture.[17] This is a significant difference, especially because the average age of the survey population was 56 years.

Because of osteoporosis in paralyzed limbs, polio survivors may be more susceptible to injuries.[18,19] A recent study indicated that bone mineral density percentage significantly affected fractures in severely disabled people.[20] Generally, osteoporotic fractures that are related to falls are associated with high health care costs and with increased morbidity and mortality.[21–25] Few studies have been done that address falls in polio survivors. Aiello studied 31 polio survivors with a history of falling. In this sample, both intrinsic and extrinsic (environmental) factors were identified as reasons for their falls.[26] Lord et al. examined predictive factors for falling and found an association between lower extremity weakness and falling.[27] Silver and Aiello studied 233 polio survivors and noted tripping to be predictive of falling. They also found a statistically significant correlation between trips and falling and the fear of falling and falling.[16,28] Because tripping is a risk factor for falling, practitioners should address interventions such as patient education, exercise, pacing, gait training, orthotic training, and home safety to minimize tripping risk.

Functionally, minimizing compensatory movement and ambulating at a moderate, comfortable rate are energy efficient for gait.[1,2] This also helps with complaints of fatigue by conserving energy. Treatment recommendations for this are addressed in the orthotic and assistive device sections that follow.

Pain during gait can be debilitating. One of the gait deviations commonly noted in polio survivors is genu recurvatum, or "back knee." Repetitive long-term genu recurvatum can injure the posterior aspect of the knee. "Injury to these tissues may cause pain, ligamentous laxity, and eventually bony deformity."[2] Treatment recommendations for this are also addressed in the orthotic and assistive device sections that follow.

ASSESSING GAIT AND FUNCTIONAL MOBILITY

Observational gait analysis is the most commonly used method for assessing gait. It is used to qualify movement. It is not as reliable and valid as gait laboratory analysis, but it is an appropriate starting point. Observational gait analysis is considered best for more notable gait deviations, and it might not detect subtle gait deviations. Gait laboratory analysis evaluates kinematics and kinetics and provides more specific information regarding gait.[1,2] It may include oxygen consumption monitoring, "optoelectronic motion analysis systems to measure kinematics, force plates to help measure external kinetics and a multichannel dynamic EMG apparatus to measure muscle activity."[2] It measures stride length and gait speed. Gait laboratory analysis is very time consuming and expensive, but for some complex cases, it may be warranted.

Observational gait analysis should be done under different conditions for a more comprehensive clinical picture. In polio survivors, it is recommended that gait be assessed while the patient is barefoot, if possible. Some subtle foot gait deviations might include toe clawing in the stance phase or excessive great toe extension in the swing phase. If the patient normally uses orthoses, he or she should also be assessed with his or her usual orthoses, footwear, and assistive device. Videotaping can be helpful to assist thorough analysis, especially if pain or markedly decreased endurance are issues.[2]

Because fatigue is often an issue for polio survivors, gait assessment should include some walking while the patient is fatigued (i.e., 10–20 feet). Grimby et al. have done extensive research in regard to the pathophysiology of polio.[29] Their enzyme-histochemical examination of muscle biopsy suggests a loss of aerobic enzyme activity and greater reliance on anaerobic metabolic capacity, which is a highly fatigable energy source.[29] This may help to explain why in muscles that have been affected by polio repeated use can result in decreased muscle performance. For example, a patient with a history of polio affecting the anterior tibialis may have normal dorsiflexion range and a manual muscle test of 4-/5, but after walking 200 feet, this same patient may begin to have difficulty with toe clearance. Differences in performance with fatigue are important for treatment consideration.

The Sickness Impact Profile (SIP) and Short-Form 36 (SF-36) are both health-related quality of life surveys that include a physical functioning section. The SF-36 has been shown to be useful in evaluating physical functioning in polio survivors.[30,26] A recent study to validate the use of the SIP and the SF-36 in community-dwelling polio survivors noted that because of a ceiling effect, the SIP was less sensitive to discriminating levels of physical function than the SF-36.[30] Therefore, the SF-36 is recommended for ambulatory community-dwelling polio survivors and the SIP for other samples of polio survivors. Both the 2-minute walk test and the 6-minute walk test have been correlated to the SF-36 physical functioning section.[31-33] These walk tests are functional measures that evaluate distance walked. Depending on the patient's functional level, these walking tests may be appropriate as part of evaluation. In a more impaired patient, the timed get-up-and-go test (TUG) may be a better measure for assessing functional mobility. The TUG is a timed test in which the patient is asked to rise from a chair, walk 3 meters, and then turn walk back and sit. The TUG has been shown to be reliable and valid in quantifying functional mobility.[26,34,35]

ORTHOSES

Often polio survivors' complaints of lower extremity pain, muscular fatigue, and new weakness can be related to gait deviations that promote biomechanical imbalances and muscular overuse of the legs.[36,37] Studies have shown that gait deviations increase energy expenditure.[38-40] Waring et al. showed that appropriate orthotic prescription markedly improved ambulation ability in polio survivors.[36] Therefore, improving mobility and efficiency of ambulation helps to enhance functional mobility for people who have had polio.

The goal of an orthotic device is to achieve a balance between stability and mobility. Bracing is used to enhance stability, but it is very important not to overbrace, thereby limiting mobility. Using light-weight materials and physics principles for alignment can help to achieve this. The weight of the orthosis is a critical consideration in prescribing a brace for individuals with distal lower extremity weakness because it has been shown that ankle weighting significantly increases energy expenditure.[41] Thus, in a patient with marginal strength, the weight of the orthosis may significantly impact his or her ability to ambulate.

In patients with a history of polio, it is important to use caution in altering long-standing gait patterns and not to inhibit compensatory movements that are helpful.[42] As you analyze the appropriate orthotic for a patient, consider the following:

1. Range of motion (ROM)
2. Strength
3. Balance
4. Pain
5. Fatigue
6. Current functional ability
7. Gait pattern, including compensatory strategies
8. Prior orthotic intervention
9. History of trips or falls
10. Tone
11. Sensation
12. Edema
13. Cognition
14. Current assistive devices or orthoses
15. Dexterity
16. Compliance
17. Family support

Each of these should be considered; collectively, they represent impairments, functional mobility, and social status. Individual patients have different factors that are crucial. These are discussed in detail in the orthotic subsections that follow.

In patients with a history of polio, knowledge of prior orthotic intervention can be very helpful. Ideally, directly examine the orthoses. Seeing the orthoses and hearing the patient's feedback give the orthotist a baseline for what was and was not appropriate for the individual in regard to materials used, alignment, and degree of control and stability. This relates to compliance because if the patient found something to be uncomfortable or lack function, there will not be carryover. Cognition, dexterity, and family support also influence compliance.

Patients with a history of polio have low tone and normal sensation unless there is a comorbidity such as diabetes or upper motor neuron pathology present.[42] Because decreased sensation and edema are precautions for bracing presence of edema should also be assessed. Fluctuating edema and pitting edema pose the greatest concerns for bracing because of girth changes, decreased skin integrity, and risk of skin breakdown. First, the edema should be medically assessed and managed. Next, when considering bracing seek to minimize contact with the skin and pad areas that are in contact with the skin. Then orthotic trial fitting and use should be closely monitored and progressed gradually.

KNEE-ANKLE-FOOT ORTHOSES

For patients who have both weak dorsiflexors and markedly weak quadriceps, a locked-knee knee-ankle-foot orthosis (KAFO) has been the only option available to truly control knee buckling. Initially, patients with a history of polio with markedly weak quadriceps were fitted with metal KAFOs with a locked knee joint.[43,44] Advances in the types of material used in orthotics have reduced the weight of these braces, and now a KAFO can be made of plastic or carbon fiber (Fig. 2). The manufacturer Townsend (Bakersfield, CA) even makes a brace that they call a "polio

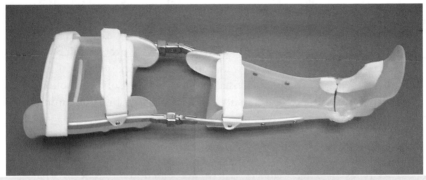

Figure 2.   Knee-ankle-foot orthosis.

brace," which has laminated graphite shells. One other possible hinge option is an off-set hinge. But because of the risk of knee buckling, this type of hinge can be dangerous for those with weak quadriceps to use on a decline or on uneven terrain.

Until recently, there was not a safe alternative to locking the knee joint. A locked knee joint increases energy expenditure and reduces walking speed.[1] Because the knee acts as a shock absorber during gait, restricted knee flexion has been shown to increase mechanical stress on the ankle and hip.[45] Interestingly, this increased mechanical stress was present bilaterally in unilateral orthotic users.[45] This increased stress may increase the risk of arthritis and back and hip pain for locked-knee KAFO users.

To address knee control with quadriceps weaker than a 3/5 manual muscle testing (MMT) while allowing for knee flexion and extension, a new knee joint has been designed by Horton Technology, Inc. (Little Rock, AR). It is called a "stance control orthotic knee joint."[46] It has three modes: locked in full extension, free motion, and "stance control" mode. The stance control mode operates on the same basic principle as a prosthetic weight-activated friction knee. The stance control mode is set to lock with minimal pressure and will lock in the bent position to allow safe stair use in this mode. As the patient weight shifts to his or her non-orthotic side, the orthotic knee releases, allowing flexion in swing.[46] This knee joint took 7 years to develop, and clinical trials were done in August of 2001 by Horton Technology. The initial clinical trials included two patients with a history of polio.[46] The initial trials indicate this brace may be promising for use in polio survivors. Since this brace has been out on the market, competitors have sought to develop their own versions. This should further enhance development of this design and help to control costs.

In a patient who has never been braced or has not been braced for a long time, it is advisable to try a short leg brace first before a long leg brace (KAFO), even in the presence of notable quadriceps weakness. The increased bulk and weight of a KAFO and the significant changes in gait make it less desirable if a short leg brace will suffice. An anterior shell may be added to the short leg brace proximally to provide additional tactile feedback to aid in quadriceps control. The ankle may also be set in a few degrees of plantar flexion to assist in optimizing knee control. The short leg brace should be constructed such that metal uprights could be added to it if, in trial fitting, the patient response indicates that a long leg brace is needed to control knee buckling.

The exception to trying a short leg brace first is a patient with a weak ankle and extreme knee pain. Repetitive long-term knee recurvatum or excessive knee varus or valgus forces can cause marked knee pain in polio survivors caused by tissue injury and ligament laxity.[11,36] In this case, the unstable knee joint must be controlled orthoticly with metal uprights; this external stability can decrease irritability and minimize pain, thus improving function.

KNEE ORTHOSES

The two types of knee orthoses (KOs) are patellofemoral joint orthoses and tibiofemoral joint orthoses.[47] Patellofemoral orthoses are prescribed for patellofemoral joint dysfunction and are primarily designed to assist proper patella tracking during knee movement and to minimize patellar compression.[47,48]

The indications for tibiofemoral KO use in polio survivors are ligament laxity and pain (arthritic or muscular). Muscular pain or chondromalacia may be alleviated by the use of a neoprene wrap or sleeve for neutral warm and pressure. Arthritic pain may be alleviated by a hinged KO or a joint-unloading KO. Joint-unloading KOs are designed to unload the arthritic joint compartment. Because there is a varus moment at the knee during most of the stance phase, knee osteoarthritis is more common in the medial compartment than the lateral compartment[2] (Fig. 3). Functional knee braces are used to provide external stability for a knee with ligament laxity.[47,49] Because many knee orthoses are available over the counter, it is often possible to trial the patient with one. This gives the orthotist the opportunity to evaluate the impact on pain as well as functional mobility. Although these are relatively light weight braces, they can pose a mobility problem for polio survivors because of the increased weight. The risk-to-benefit ratio should be carefully evaluated in patients with a history of polio.

ANKLE-FOOT ORTHOSES

There are a variety of choices for types of ankle-foot orthoses (AFOs). Typically, because of the increased weight of a metal brace (aluminum or steel), they are only used when edema or marked skin integrity issues are present. There are four general types of ankle joints for metal braces: solid, simple hinge, Klenzak, and double action.[50] Whereas the Klenzak joint stops or assists movement in one direction, the double action joint can either stop or block or assist movement in both directions.[50] These ankle joints are also available for plastic AFOs.

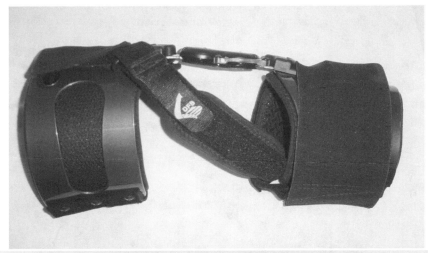

Figure 3. Medial unloading knee orthosis.

Possible materials include aluminum, steel, titanium, plastic, laminated plastic, carbon fiber, Kevlar, and other lightweight composites. Possible designs for plastic AFOs include solid ankle, semisolid ankle, posterior leaf spring AFO, hinged AFO (including additional joint type options that are not available for metal AFOs), and floor reaction orthoses.

For patients with a foot drop (weak anterior tibialis), an AFO is often set in dorsiflexion or adjusted with a dorsiflexion assist to allow foot clearance in swing.[50] However, if a patient has weak quadriceps muscles, dorsiflexion will produce a flexion moment at the knee during stance that could cause knee buckling. Because a weak tibialis anterior and quadriceps are often both present in polio survivors, other design considerations should be made. In polio survivors, Perry et al. have reported good functional results with use of a plastic hinged AFO with a dorsiflexion stop (approximately 5–10°) and a plantar-flexion stop (approximately 15–20°).[10] These authors noted that because plantar flexion was allowed with the knee extended, there was a notably decreased demand on the quadriceps.[10]

Compliance with orthotic use can be an issue for patients with a history of polio.[36,51] Patients may cite appearance or bulk of a brace as reasons for noncompliance. Minimizing the weight and optimizing the appearance of an orthosis can aid in compliance. For example, color choices are available for plastic orthoses (e.g., white, beige, and black), and lightweight orthotic options are also available. Educating patients as to the functional need can also enhance compliance. If possible, having demonstration models for patients to see and try can be very helpful.

For patients who have both weak dorsiflexors and quadriceps muscles, using a floor re-action orthosis (FRO) can be advantageous. This design aids foot clearance during swing, and the anterior shell assists knee stability during stance. The anterior floor reaction AFO design has been used successfully in individuals who have paralysis,[52] and it has recently become available in lighter weight materials such as carbon fiber.[53] This orthosis may also be set in slight plantar flexion to assist stability during stance; plantar flexion of the ankle in stance helps to create an extension moment at the knee, which minimizes the risk of knee buckling. Figure 4 shows an AFO set in plantar flexion.

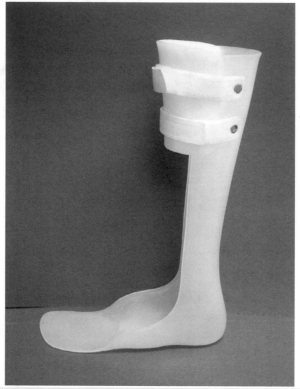

Figure 4. Ankle-foot orthosis set in plantar flexion.

Polio survivors with a history of an ankle fusion during the initial onset of polio may present with loosening of the fusion site that is usually painful. When bracing for this problem, ideally use a solid-ankle design for stability. Also consider a semisolid design if the patient is not willing to use a solid AFO because of the trim lines. The foot and ankle should be set in its functional neutral position.

In some cases, polio survivors may not be ready or willing to accept the most appropri-ate orthotic prescription because of aesthetics or reluctance to change. Polio survivors who have used leather and metal braces for a long time may want to continue to use the same type of brace. In this case, it is important to educate them in regard to weight and energy expenditure and to work with them to determine the most appropriate orthotic device for them. Also, if an AFO is prescribed for a polio survivor, he or she may not be willing to use one but may be open to using an ankle orthosis (AO). Use of an AO first can be considered an intermediary step. If a patient has difficulty with medial-lateral ankle stability in stance, it may be a helpful first step.

SUPRAMALLEOLAR ORTHOSES, ANKLE ORTHOSES, AND UNIVERSITY OF CALIFORNIA AT BERKELEY LABORATORY ORTHOSES (UCBLs)

"The design of a supramalleolar orthosis (SMO) mimics the effect of a high-top sneaker or shoe but provides more intimate control of the ankle-foot complex because of its custom-molded fabrication"[54] (Figs. 5 and 6). An SMO is indicated to assist in controlling ankle medial-lateral stability during stance but because of the shortened lever arm, it is not considered to be very effective in controlling sagittal plane motion.[54] An SMO can also control for rearfoot position and pronation and supination of the foot. If the only goal is to provide medial-lateral control of the ankle, an AO will usually suffice (Fig. 7). AO options include lightweight sports plastic and Velcro models, lacing AOs, neoprene sleeves, and ankle wraps. A University of California at Berkeley Laboratory orthosis (UCBL) is indicated to control rearfoot position as well as midtarsal joint position during stance.

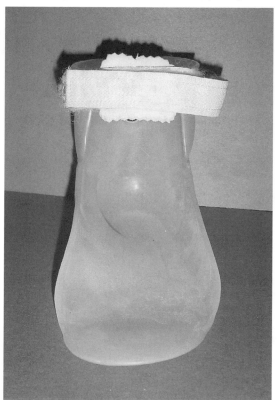

Figure 5. Supramalleolar orthosis—front view.

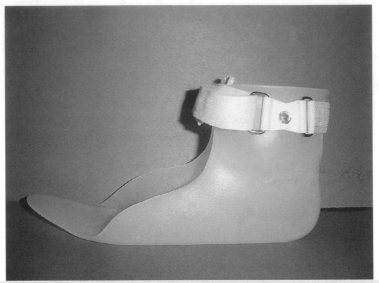

Figure 6. Supramalleolar orthosis—lateral view.

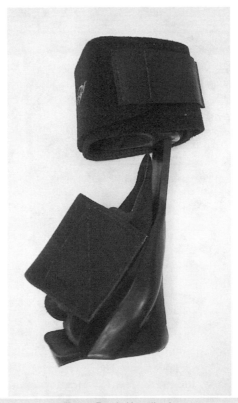

Figure 7. Ankle orthosis.

FOOT ORTHOTICS

The biomechanical function of the foot is an important part of gait. Normally during gait, the foot pronates from initial contact to midstance to assist with shock absorption and supinates from midstance to preswing to act as a rigid pushoff lever.[55] Orthotic intervention for the foot is a very complex subject. This section provides a brief overview of foot orthotics.

Generally, the goal of foot orthotics is to decrease pain and improve function. More specifically, these orthotics may accommodate or correct deformities and provide shock absorption for the foot.[56]

Some soft over-the-counter orthotics that assist in shock absorption. Some of these also provide some arch support. These soft orthotics are generally inexpensive and may be appropriate for patients with minimal biomechanical faults. However, for significant biomechanical issues, a custom orthotic is necessary. A custom orthotic may be soft, semirigid, or rigid. A soft orthotic may not provide enough control, but a rigid orthotic may be too controlling. A semirigid orthotic is generally a good functional choice to provide adequate support and shock absorption.

Ideally, for polio survivors, to address both biomechanics and shock absorption, prescribe a custom semirigid orthosis with a soft, shock-absorbing cover.

FOOTWEAR

Footwear is the foundation for walking. It should aid stability but without being heavy. The weight of the shoe is significant because ankle weighting significantly increases energy expenditure.[41] Thus, in a patient with leg weakness, lightweight shoes should be selected because heavy shoes may adversely impact functional ambulation. For a patient with a metal orthosis that needs to be attached to the shoe, it is important that the sole is proper to support the brace.

The fit of the shoe is also important. Shoes are constructed over a form called a *last* that determines the contour of the base of the shoe.[55] Lasts are made for different foot types, and a certified pedorthist is qualified to select the proper last for different foot types.[55] Shoe size should be determined by "arch" length rather than foot length. "The proper shoe size is the one that accommodates the first metatarsal joint in the widest part of the shoe."[57]

Some general considerations to optimize footwear for all foot types include the following:

- A firm heel counter for good rearfoot support
- Lacing or Velcro closure to assist in proper foot position
- A soft insert with an arch support to assist in positioning and absorbing shock

Adapting a shoe can enhance stability and function. Adaptations to consider include a lift, medial wedge, lateral wedge, rocker bottom, and leather toe tips. A lift is indicated to correct for a leg length discrepancy; typically, 3/8 inch or less is accommodated for within a shoe, and greater than 3/8 inch modification is attached to the outside of the shoe. Medial and lateral wedging are used to correct rearfoot position.

A medial wedge is used to help correct for calcaneal valgus, and a lateral wedge is used to help correct for calcaneal varus.[57] A rocker bottom is designed to decrease midfoot motion and metatarsal stress while still allowing a smooth rollover.[55] Indications for a rocker bottom include foot pain caused by arthritis, deformities, or neuromas.[57]

Leather toe tips are indicated for a patient with difficulty in the swing phase of gait. For example, a polio survivor with proximal weakness may have difficulty clearing his or her limb in swing, especially with increased fatigue. If the patient has some type of rubber or grip sole and the toe of the shoe catches, he or she is more likely to trip or stumble than if the tip of the shoe has decreased friction and can slide more easily.

SPINAL ORTHOSES

Spinal orthoses in polio survivors may be indicated for any of the comorbidities that are seen in the general population. They may be used for pain management, improved posture, or increased function. This section gives a brief overview of some of the more commonly used orthoses for polio survivors.

In patients with low back pain, a lumbosacral orthosis may be used.[58] It is important for the patient to not always wear it, because doing so will contribute to increased trunk weakness. Usually, for a polio survivor, it is recommended that this type of orthosis be used during a taxing activity or at the end of the day because of fatigue. The possible types of orthoses include a lumbosacral Warm-n-form, corset, or wrap support. Use of these may improve a patient's functional tolerance.

Patients with a fixed scoliosis may choose to use a brace for aesthetics, pain management, or increased function. A range of possible orthoses exist, from the soft to the rigid and restrictive. Because the intent is not true spinal correction, as it is with growing children, a very rigid and restrictive brace is not necessary. Usually a soft body jacket or a thoracolumbar sacral orthosis (TLSO) with metal stays is most appropriate. Sometimes a patient's standing scoliosis is partially correctable if it is caused by progressive weakness. If weakness is a problem, the patient should be referred to physical therapy for nonfatiguing strengthening exercises.

UPPER EXTREMITY ORTHOSES

In polio survivors, upper extremity orthoses may include shoulder supports to correct subluxation or nerve protection orthoses. In a patient with an atrophied upper extremity, shoulder subluxation may be present. If the shoulder subluxation is painful, a shoulder subluxation support is recommended. There are Velcro and plastic supports that can be fitted to the patient. Typically, these are appropriate. In some cases, a custom version is required for a greater level of stability. Usually a custom version is needed more if a patient has distal upper extremity strength on the same side as the subluxed shoulder and is, therefore, using the arm more functionally.

The typical nerve protection orthoses are for the median and ulnar nerves. In cases of median and ulnar neuropathy, they are recommended. A soft wrist splint in neutral is tried first for median neuropathy or carpal tunnel syndrome (CTS).[59] If the soft splint is not sufficient, a custom-molded plastic version is fabricated. For ulnar neuropathy at the elbow, elbow pads are recommended for protection during the day, and a resting night splint may be recommended for use when sleeping. Balanced forearm orthoses or mobile arm supports may also be useful in assisting the patient with elevation of the arm.

ASSISTIVE DEVICES AND ENERGY EXPENDITURE

Several possible assistive devices are available for walking, including canes (straight, offset handle, ergonomic, lightweight, small base quad cane, large base quad cane), axillary crutches, Everett crutches, Loftstrand crutches, standard walker, and rolling walkers (without hand brakes; tripod with hand brakes; four-wheeled rolling walker with handbrakes, with and without a seat). Ideally, trialing multiple assistive devices with a patient helps to determine which is most appropriate. Walking aids may improve stability, minimize muscle stress and overuse, and decrease pain. In polio survivors, assistive devices are also believed to improve function because of the decreased muscle overuse.[60]

The wider base of support that an assistive device provides increases stability and should help to minimize fall risk. Because walking aids decrease the load and pressure on joints, they are effective for pain reduction of painful joints.[61] Contralateral cane use has been shown to decrease joint stress more than ipsilateral cane use.[62] In determining appropriate unilateral assistive device use in polio survivors, there may be confounding factors such as a nonfunctional upper extremity or significant CTS. Dean and Ross studied 144 elderly community cane users and noted no increased fall frequency or decrease in function associated with ipsilateral cane use.[63] Therefore, in polio survivors with upper extremity impairment, it is reasonable to try ipsilateral assistive device use. In patients with CTS or hand arthritis, an ergonomic grip such as Ortho-Ease or a "pistol grip" should be considered.

Compared with unilateral device use, bilateral assistive devices provide more stability and decreased joint stress. Foley et al. studied older adults with an average age of 60 years and assessed ambulation without a device, with a standard walker, and with a rolling walker.[64] They calculated that "ambulation with the use of a standard walker was shown to require 212% more oxygen per meter than unassisted ambulation and 104% more oxygen per meter than ambulation with a wheeled walker."[64] These are important statistics because polio survivors are often concerned with fatigue and must practice energy conservation. A rolling walker is more appropriate for conserving energy than a standard walker. Wheel types for the rolling walker should also be considered. Pivoting wheels of increased size (approximately 5-inch diameter) are more easily maneuverable than the standard 3-inch nonpivoting wheels. Some models are available with a seat to help with energy conservation; the only models that are considered to be safe are those that allow the patient to lock the handbrakes before sitting. The handbrakes are a good safety feature, especially for declines, and a walker basket is a useful to assist function.

Gonzales et al. evaluated the energy cost of ambulation and determined "the normal values at a comfortable walking speed of 80 m/min = 0.063 kcal/m/kg."[65] In patients with arthritis, assistive device use has been assessed, and walker use produced the highest energy expenditure; no assistive device use produced the least energy expenditure.[1] Figure 8 shows the energy expenditure associated with assistive devices.[1] Increased weight adversely affects energy expenditure. In a study by Foster et al., obese people with significant weight loss markedly improved energy expenditure during gait.[66]

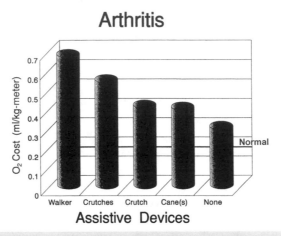

Figure 8.   Oxygen cost in arthritis patients requiring different types of upper extremity assistive devices. (From Perry J: Gait Analysis. Thorofare, NJ, Slack, 1998, with permission.)

"There is a general consensus that the energy cost of ambulation is directly proportional to the severity of neurologic deficit or the degree of loss of limb or its function."[67] Luna-Reyes et al. assessed ambulation in a group of children who had lower extremity deficits from polio compared with a control group of children with no significant medical history.[67] They found that the most efficient mobility was the control group's normal gait. Interestingly, ambulating with a unilateral orthosis in the group with polio produced less energy expenditure per minute than ambulating for the control group. However, in order to achieve this decreased energy expenditure, the children with a history of polio markedly reduced gait speed, thereby reducing the efficiency of gait. This was the second most efficient form of mobility, followed by wheelchair propulsion. Wheelchair propulsion expended 16% more energy than normal gait. Walking with bilateral crutches required 41% more energy than normal walking. In children who normally wore a brace, ambulating without the brace resulted in a 109% increase in energy expenditure compared with control group walking.[67] The increase in energy expenditure noted when not ambulating with a prescribed orthotic is significant. This indicates that noncompliance with orthotic use can significantly increase energy expenditure, which would adversely affect fatigue. This hypothesis is supported by a study by Waring et al.[36] In follow-up with patients who were prescribed orthotics, those who complied with orthotic use daily experienced less fatigue than those who did not comply with decive use or were inconsistent with using the device. The compliant group also had a significant improvement in walking ability, weakness, and knee pain.

Differences in terrain are associated with changes in energy expenditure. Gonzales and Edelstein noted that "the energy cost of walking on a 10–12% grade is approximately twice the energy expenditure of walking on level ground. On a 20–25% upgrade, the cost is tripled. On downgrades the energy expenditure is lowest at a 10% grade and rises again on steeper down slopes."[65] "Stairs require 29% more energy than a 5% ramp and 45% more time."[65] These statistics explain why considering a scooter or a stairlift can be important for energy conservation in polio survivors. Energy conservation can assist in preserving mobility.

CONCLUSION

Optimizing gait in patients with a history of polio involves achieving a balance between stability and mobility. The biomechanics of gait should be carefully assessed to assist in determining safety, function, and energy expenditure. Minimizing energy expenditure can help to manage fatigue, thereby improving function. Proper orthotic intervention has been shown to enhance function in polio survivors.

References

1. Perry J: Gait Analysis: Normal and Pathological Function. New York, McGraw-Hill, 1992.
2. Kerrigan DC, Edelstein JE: Gait. In Gonzalez EG, Myers SJ, Edelstein JE, et al (eds): Downey & Darling's Physiological Basis of Rehabilitation Medicine. Boston, Butterworth Heinemann, 2001, pp 397–416.
3. Ayyappa E, Mohamed O: Clinical assessment of pathological gait. In Lusardi MM, Nielsen CC (eds): Orthotics and Prosthetics in Rehabilitation. Boston, Butterworth Heinemann, 2000, pp 33–52.
4. Ounpuu S: Clinical gait analysis. In Spivack BS (ed): Evaluation and Management of Gait Disorders. New York, Marcel Dekker, 1995, pp 1–35.
5. Kerrigan DC, Viramontes BE, Corcoran PJ, LaRaia PJ: Measured versus predicted vertical displacement of the sacrum during gait as a tool to measure biomechanical gait performance. Am J Phys Med Rehabil 74:3–8, 1995.
6. Halstead LS (ed): Managing Post-Polio: A Guide to Living Well with Post-Polio Syndrome. Washington, DC, NRH Press, 1998.
7. Grimby G, Thoren Jonsson AL: Disability in poliomyelitis sequelase. Phys Ther 74:415–424, 1994.
8. Nollet F, Beelen A, Prins MH, et al: Disability and functional assessment in former polio patients with and without post-polio syndrome. Arch Phys Med Rehabil 80:136–143, 1999.
9. Halstead LS, Rossi CD: New Problems in old polio patients: Result of survey of 539 polio survivors. Orthopedics 8:845–850, 1985.
10. Perry J, Fontaine JD, Mulroy S: Findings in post-poliomyelitis syndrome. Weakness of muscles of the calf as a source of late pain and fatigue of muscles of the thigh after poliomyelitis. J Bone Joint Surg 77A:1148–1153, 1995.
11. Hurmuzlu Y, Basdogan C, Stoianovici D: Kinematics and dynamic stability of post-polio patients. J Biomechan Eng 118:405–411, 1996.

12. Shumway-Cook A, Woollacott MH: Motor Control: Theory and Practical Applications, 2nd ed. Philadelphia, Lippincott Williams & Wilkins, 2001.

13. Perry J, Mulroy SJ, Renwick SE: The relationship of lower extremity strength and gait parameters in patients with post-polio syndrome. Arch Phys Med Rehabil 74:165–169, 1993.

14. Perry J: The mechanics of walking: A clinical interpretation. Phys Ther 47:778–801, 1967.

15. Perry J, Barnes G, Gronley JK: The post-polio syndrome: An overuse phenomenon. Clin Orthop 233:145–162, 1988.

16. Silver JK, Aiello DD: Polio survivors: Falls and subsequent injuries. Am J Phys Med Rehabil 81:567–570, 2002.

17. Gillespie LD, Gillespie WJ, Robertson MC, et al: Interventions for preventing falls in elderly people. Cochrane Database Syst Rev 3:CD000340, 2001.

18. Silver JK: Aging, comorbidities, and secondary disabilities in polio survivors. In Halstead LS (ed): Managing Post-Polio: A Guide to Living Well with Post-Polio Syndrome. Washington, DC, NRH Press, 1998.

19. Silver JK, Aiello DD: Bone density and fracture risk in male polio survivors. Arch Phys Med Rehabil 81:1329, 2001.

20. Kawada T: Factors influencing bone fractures in severely disabled persons. Am J Phys Med Rehabil 81:424–428, 2002.

21. Kannus P, et al: Genetic factors and osteoporotic fractures in elderly people: Prospective 25 year follow-up of a nationwide cohort of elderly Finnish twins. Br Med J 319:1334–1337, 1999.

22. Melton LJ 3d: Hip fractures: A worldwide problem today and tomorrow. Bone 14:51–58, 1993.

23. Cooper C, et al: Population-based study of survival after osteoporotic fractures. Am J Epidemiol 137:1001–1005, 1993.

24. Kannus P, Parkkari J, Niemi S: Age-adjusted incidence of hip fractures. Lancet 346:50–51, 1995.

25. Birge SJ: Can falls and hip fracture be prevented in frail older adults? J Am Geriatr Soc 47:1265–1266, 1999.

26. Aiello DD: Polio Survivors: A Comparison of Fallers versus Non-fallers on a Functional Task and a Disability Measure. Ann Arbor, MI, UMI Dissertation Services, Bell & Howell Company, 2001.

27. Lord SR, Allen GM, Williams P, Gandevia SC: Risk of falling: Predictors based on reduced strength in persons previously affected by polio. Arch Phys Med Rehabil 83:757–763, 2002.

28. Silver JK, Aiello DD: Risk of falls in survivors of poliomyelitis [abstract]. Arch Phys Med Rehabil 81:1272, 2000.

29. Grimby G, Tolback A, Muller U, Larsson L: Fatigue of chronically overused motor units in prior polio patients. Muscle Nerve 19:728–737, 1996.

30. Noonan VK, Dallimore M: The relationship between self-reports and objective measures of disability in patients with late sequelae of poliomyelitis: A validation study. Arch Phys Med Rehabil 81:1422–1427, 2000.

31. Rossier P, Wade DT: Validity and reliability of 4 mobility measures in patients presenting with neurological impairment. Arch Phys Med Rehabil 82:9–13, 2001.

32. Brooks D, Parsons J, Hunter JP, et al: The 2-minute walk test as a measure of functional improvement in persons with lower limb amputation. Arch Phys Med Rehabil 82:1478–1483, 2001.

33. Miller WC, Deathe AB, Speechley M: Lower extremity prosthetic mobility: A comparison of 3 self-report scales. Arch Phys Med Rehabil 82:1432–1440, 2001.
34. Mathias S, Nayak USL, Isaacs B: Balance in elderly patients: The "get-up and go'" test. Arch Phys Med Rehabil 67:387–389, 1986.
35. Podsialdo D, Richardson S: The timed "up and go": A test of basic functional mobility for frail elderly persons. J Am Geriatr Soc 39:142–148, 1991.
36. Waring WP, Maynard F, Grady W, et al: Influence of appropriate lower extremity orthotic management on ambulation, pain, and fatique in a postpolio population. Arch Phys Med Rehabil 70:371–375, 1989.
37. Silver JK, Aiello DD: What internists need to know about post-polio syndrome. Cleve Clinic J Med 69:704–712, 2002.
38. Gussoni M, Margonato V, Ventura R, Veicsteinas A: Energy cost of walking with hip joint impairment. Phys Ther 70:295–301, 1990.
39. Walters RL, Perry J, Conaty P, et al: The energy cost of walking with artritis of the hip and knee. Clin Orthop Rel Res 214:278–284, 1987.
40. Waters RL, Yakura JS: The energy expenditure of normal and pathological gait. Crit Rev Phys Rehabil Med 1:187–209, 1989.
41. Barrack RL, Skinner HB: Ankle weighting effect on gait in able-bodied adults. Arch Phys Med Rehabil 71:112–115, 1990.
42. Silver JK, Aiello DD: Post-polio syndrome. In Frontera WR, Silver JK (eds): Essentials of Physical Medicine and Rehabilitation. Philadelphia, Hanley & Belfus, 2001, pp 678–686.
43. Natarajan K, Joshi JB, Yadav BP: Muscle recovery in the lower limbs in poliomyelitis. Indian J Pediatr 35:173–179, 1968.
44. Stewart E, Rooney M: Cosmetic caliper for use with flail leg. Med J Aust 1:969–970, 1976.
45. Cook TM, Farrell KP, Carey IA, et al: Effects of restricted knee flexion and walking speed on the vertical ground reaction force during gait. J Orthop Sports Phys Ther 25:236–244, 1997.
46. Horton Technology, Inc. Web site: www.stancecontrol.com.
47. Nawoczenski DA, Epler ME: Orthotics in Functional Rehabilitation of the Lower Limb. Philadelphia, W.B. Saunders, 1997.
48. Eisele SA: A precise approach to anterior knee pain. Phys Sports Med 19:126–139, 1991.
49. Knecht JF: Knee orthoses. In Lusardi MM, Nielson CC (ed): Orthotics and Prosthetics in Rehabilitation. Boston, Butterworth Heinemann, 2000, pp 177–190.
50. McGuire JB: Orthoses used in the management of neurologic and muscular disorders. Clin Podiatr Med Surg 16:153–174, 1999.
51. Silver JK: Post-polio Syndrome: A Guide for Polio Survivors and Their Families. London, Yale University Press, 2001.
52. Lin RS: Thermoforming plastic improves floor reaction orthoses. Biomechanics 9:69–75, 1998.
53. Silver JK, Aiello DD, Drillio RC: Lightweight carbon fiber and Kevlar floor reaction AFO in two polio survivors with new weakness. Arch Phys Med Rehabil 80:1180, 1999.
54. Lin RS: Ankle-foot orthoses. In Lusardi MM, Nielson CC (eds): Orthotics and Prosthetics in Rehabilitation. Boston, Butterworth Heinemann, 2000, pp 159–175.
55. Bordelon RL: Orthotics, shoes and braces. Orthop Clin North Am 20:751–757, 1989.
56. Nole R, Garbalosa JC: Functional foot orthoses. In Lusardi MM, Nielson CC (eds): Orthotics and Prosthetics in Rehabilitation. Boston, Butterworth Heinemann, 2000, pp 129–158.

57. Bottomley JM: Footwear: Foundation for lower extremity orthotics. In Lusardi MM, Nielson CC (eds): Orthotics and Prosthetics in Rehabilitation. Boston, Butterworth Heinemann, 2000, pp 159–175.

58. Flanagan P, Gavin TM, Gavin DQ, Patwardhan AG: Spinal orthoses. In Lusardi MM, Nielson CC (eds): Orthotics and Prosthetics in Rehabilitation. Boston, Butterworth Heinemann, 2000, pp 231–251.

59. Vender MI, Ruder JR, Pomerance J, Truppa KL: Upper extremity compressive neuropathies. In Kasdan ML (ed): Occupational Hand and Upper Extremity Injuries and Diseases, 2nd ed. Philadelphia, Hanley & Belfus, 1998, pp 83–96.

60. Halbritter T: Management of a patient with post-polio syndrome. J Am Acad Nurse Prac 13:555–559, 2001.

61. Joyce BM, Kirby RL: Canes, crutches and walkers. Am Fam Physician 43:535–542, 1991.

62. Edwards BG: Contralateral and ipsilateral cane usage by patients with total knee or hip replacement. Arch Phys Med Rehabil 67:734–740, 1986.

63. Dean E, Ross J: Relationships among cane fitting, function, and falls. Phys Ther 73:494–500, 1993.

64. Foley MP, Prax B, Crowell R, Boone T: Effects of assistive devices on cardiorespiratory demands in older adults. Phys Ther 76:1313–1319, 1996.

65. Gonzalez EG, Edelstein JE: Energy expenditure during ambulation. In Gonzalez EG, Myers SJ, Edelstein JE, et al (eds): Downey & Darling's Physiological Basis of Rehabilitation Medicine. Boston, Butterworth Heinemann, 2001, pp 397–416.

66. Foster GD, et al: The energy cost of walking before and after significant weight loss. Med Sci Sports Exerc 27:888–894, 1995.

67. Luna-Reyes OB, Reyes TM, So FY, et al: Energy cost of ambulation in healthy and disabled Filipino children. Arch Phys Med Rehabil 69:946–949, 1988.

Powered Mobility for Polio Survivors

Pima S. McConnell, PT, ATP

The wheelchair is widely viewed as a symbol of illness and loss. Becoming a wheelchair user is thought of as a failure, to be avoided at all costs, even when conditions cry out for an alternative method of mobility. Those with no disability (a temporary condition, it is said, for most people), recoil in horror at the thought of being "wheelchair-bound." In their minds, it is a mark of tragedy, of lost dreams, of pity, grueling effort, and regret. These beliefs are simply not true. The wheelchair is a tool that enhances quality of life. The right wheels facilitate their (wheelchair users') ability to be out in the world, continuing their life, partaking of the many realms of human experience.[1]

Although health care professionals may see clearly that the "right wheels" for polio survivors would be powered mobility, this is a monumental decision not easily reached. Hugh G. Gallagher speaks eloquently for polio survivors:

[W]e feel a real sense of failure: we have fought the good fight—and lost it. In my own case, for many years I refused to admit that I needed an electric (power) wheelchair. When I was forced to transfer to an electric wheelchair, I was surprised by how greatly the quality and independence of my life improved. Better equipment makes for better living.[2]

Many polio survivors are now experiencing debilitating fatigue, new muscle weakness, joint and muscle pain, cold intolerance, difficulty sleeping, dysphagia, and respiratory complications. Although both muscle and joint pain are associated with reduced quality of life,[3] fatigue is cited as the most common and most disabling problem. Lifestyle changes are necessary to cope with these issues. "Wishful thinking that the problem is temporary is detrimental," according to Halstead and Wiechers.[4]

In a 1985 survey, more than 90% of polio survivors reported that fatigue was triggered by physical overexertion. For polio survivors, this is caused by compensating for more severely affected muscle groups by substituting stronger, but not necessarily unaffected, muscles groups. This ultimately leads to chronic overuse of the substituted muscles. This is true for crutch ambulators as well as manual wheelchair users.[5]

Polio survivors who have used manual wheelchairs for many years are now reporting increasing difficulty in maintaining their independence in mobility. The years of demand on their upper extremities for wheelchair propulsion and activities of daily living (ADLs) have taken a toll. They are now experiencing the results of the chronic musculoskeletal overuse as fatigue, joint and muscle pain, and new muscle weakness. Research shows that their upper extremity muscle group strength is deteriorating at a rate higher than that associated with normal aging.[6] Intervention that is directed at reducing these stresses must include powered mobility. Powered mobility should be considered for both crutch ambulators and manual wheelchair users.

But why powered mobility? Why not a manual wheelchair for a current crutch ambulator? This is a question asked by polio survivors as well as physicians, therapists, and funding sources. Some have even suggested that a manual wheelchair is a better choice because it serves as a means of exercise. This is erroneous logic. A wheelchair is *not* an exercise prescription; it is a means of independent mobility. If upper extremity exercises are appropriate, they should be done separate from mobility. For polio survivors, the most crucial contraindication for continuing or initiating manual wheelchair use is the continued stress to the overused muscles of the upper extremities.

Powered mobility is an appropriate component of the interventions required to alleviate the chronic musculoskeletal overuse so prevalent in this population. It significantly reduces the energy expenditure needed for mobility. It can also be considered a means to conserve energy to allow for short distance ambulation and transfers. A power wheelchair can significantly improve quality of life for polio survivors who are becoming limited because of mobility issues.[2,7] By no longer depending on upper extremity effort for mobility, power wheelchair users can once again be active participants in life. Powered mobility allows users to independently go whatever distance necessary, safely and comfortably. Steep inclines and ramps are no longer a challenge. Rough terrain can be negotiated safely. Just getting to a destination is no longer exhausting and thereby a limiting factor in life choices. Energy is still available for work or pleasure activities.[2,7–9]

Despite convincing arguments by health care professionals for powered mobility, polio survivors are often reluctant to comply. This is a population that viewed discarding braces and wheelchairs as a "victory" over polio. To return to the use of assistive devices (e.g., a wheelchair) represents a "failure." Many polio survivors may initially reject powered mobility. It is essential for health care professionals who are involved in recommending and providing powered mobility to be aware of the significance of this choice to polio survivors. "Compassion, patience, and understanding are essential," state Fletcher et al.[10]

EVALUATION

The ideal setting for a polio survivor to be evaluated for powered mobility is a seating clinic staffed with practitioners knowledgeable about the history and current issues of polio survivors. The team should include the polio survivor, the referring physician, a physical or occupational therapist, and a rehabilitation technology supplier. The family or caregiver for the polio survivor should also be included whenever possible. The team approach is most effective when the polio survivor is viewed as an integral part of the team. As Gallagher explains:

> Only *I* know what it takes for me to remain functional in my daily living. I do not mean that I know more about medicine than does my physician. Not at all. I know more about *me*. When I consult my doctors, they bring to the conference their knowledge of medicine, and I bring my knowledge of my paralyzed body. Together, we analyze what is wrong, what treatment is advisable, and what impact that treatment is likely to have on the problem and on my ability to function independently.[2]

With this perspective in mind, the initial evaluation by the therapist includes the medical history and a physical examination to assess current functional status. Functional activities such as style of transfers, toileting techniques, and methods of accomplishing other ADLs are observed or discussed. Many survivors have developed unorthodox methods that, although effective, may be dangerous. Strategies may need to be introduced to decrease the risk of falls.[11]

The next consideration is the polio survivor's previous and current mobility equipment. It is critical to discover the features or components important to the user. Some polio survivors require a specific armrest type and height to perform independent transfers. Many have custom wheelchair modifications that are essential for independent function. An example is zippered-back upholstery that is used for transferring backwards onto a toilet. These must be duplicated for continued independence. Equally important is discovering what has failed in the past.[11,12]

Next, the home and work environments are considered. A polio survivor may have made extensive home or worksite modifications to accommodate his or her current manual wheelchair. It is often crucial to duplicate the current wheelchair's seat to floor height, seat depth, and overall width to allow continued independence. This is a particular challenge when transitioning from a manual to a power wheelchair or from a standard (dedicated) power wheelchair to a modular power base wheelchair with a power recline or power tilt system. Manual wheelchair users who have gotten by with being bumped up a step or two at home will now be forced to have a ramp built. Powered mobility devices are much too heavy for this technique to be effective.[11]

Finally, the type of transportation used by the polio survivor must be considered. A folding-frame manual wheelchair can easily be stowed in the backseat or trunk of a car. Transportation of powered mobility device is not as convenient. Although some types of powered mobility devices can be disassembled for transport, the component parts are heavy and often cumbersome. This is rarely the best option for polio survivors. An accessible vehicle with a power lift or ramp/lift system that does not require upper extremity strength to load the powered mobility device is ideal. An outside platform lift systems mounted at the trunk is frequently used with automobiles. Trunk lifts can be used in vans, station wagons, trucks, sports utility vehicles, and motor homes. Power lift or ramp/lift systems are typically used in modified vans. A tie-down system mounted in the vehicle is a necessity to secure the powered mobility device for safe transport. Some tie-down systems are contact or electronically activated. This allows the polio survivor to be independent in securing the powered mobility device and in transportation.[1]

Specific recommendations are made upon completion of a thorough evaluation and consideration of all of the above factors. Ideally, equipment is available in the seating clinic to allow the polio survivor to experience the recommended mobility device and seating system. A trial use in the clinic is an opportunity to experience different options. It can highlight areas that should be reconsidered. Modifications can be made to accommodate the specific needs of the patient.

POWERED MOBILITY EQUIPMENT

Powered mobility can take many forms. It includes standard power wheelchairs, modular power bases, scooters (power operated vehicles), and other powered vehicles used as a means of independent mobility. Hybrid power add-on units for manual wheelchairs can also be included. All of these devices run on rechargeable battery power.[13]

Power add-on units for lightweight, manual wheelchairs are usually some form of wheelchair hub power assist, a friction drive system with a joystick, or a fifth wheel with either a joystick or scooter-type tiller. Although power add-on units do reduce the energy expenditure and stress on the upper extremities, they can be cumbersome and heavy to attach and detach from the manual wheelchair for transport. They also add a significant amount of weight to an otherwise lightweight, manual wheelchair. And unfortunately, they often accelerate wear and tear on the manual frame by subjecting it to excess stress. These are usually considered an "unauthorized attachment" and may void the manufacturer's warranty on the manual wheelchair frame. Although they are considered by some to be a "best of both worlds" solution, this is rarely true for polio survivors.[8,14]

Power operated vehicles (POVs) or scooters are often the preference of those wanting only occasional powered mobility. A POV is considered by some to be more "socially acceptable" than a wheelchair. A POV has either three or four wheels. The three-wheel POV is less stable and may tip over when taking a corner too fast or turning onto a surface with a sideways slope. The four-wheel drive POV is more stable but does have a larger turning radius. A POV may have either a front wheel or rear wheel drive system. A front wheel drive POV is often smaller, is generally more maneuverable, and does better on level terrain. A front wheel drive POV may use a belt and chain or a two-belt system. These systems require more maintenance because of the belts and chains. A rear wheel drive POV has better traction, more power, and is generally better equipped to handle inclines and uneven terrain. A rear wheel drive POV typically has a direct drive system that is more durable and requires little maintenance.

A POV is a fairly generic device with limited options compared with power wheelchairs that can be significantly customized. A POV typically has a basket attached to the front of the tiller for transporting materials. A crutch or cane holder or oxygen tank holder can be added to the back of some models. A POV is generally steered with a tiller in front, which requires significantly more upper extremity effort and range of motion than a joystick. Because the tiller is in front of the user, it is an obstacle to accessing tables and desks. The user must pull alongside and rotate the seat (which is mounted on a stem and held in place by a lock-and-release mechanism) to face the table or desk. This leaves the user's feet unsupported. Because of these aspects of the POV, it is not ideal for everyday use in the home or office unless the user is able to easily transfer to another chair. Very few seating options or modifications exist for a POV. The user is usually limited to the fishing boat type seat or van type seat that is standard with each model. A powered lift seat system is available on some POV models. A POV may disassemble for transportation in the trunk of a car. However, the component parts are often too heavy for polio survivors to lift.[8,14]

All-terrain vehicles or golf carts are an alternative for outside use only. They are often used by the general public as well as polio survivors in planned communities with cart paths to many destinations. However, transfers in and out of these vehicles may be difficult. Some polio survivors use these to work in the yard or manage rural properties. However, they are not options for everyday mobility within the home or work environments.

Standard power wheelchairs are similar in design to manual wheelchairs in which the seat is an integral part of the wheelchair. They may have either a folding or a rigid (nonfolding) frame. The folding frame style can be disassembled for transport. The motors and wheels do not detach from the frame. This results in a heavy and awkward item to lift into a vehicle.

Standard power wheelchairs generally come in a limited range of seat sizes. They are usually less expensive than modular base power wheelchairs, although they have many of the same options available. They are typically driven with a proportional joystick. The electronics may be integrated or remote. The standard power wheelchair electronics typically have less programmability than the modular base power wheelchairs. The standard power wheelchair usually has a smaller overall visual impact, which is often an attractive feature to a new powered mobility user. They cannot typically be modified to allow for a power recline system, power tilt system, or power lift seat system. However, because these options may not be needed or desired by many polio survivors, a standard power wheelchair can be an excellent choice.[14]

Modular base power wheelchairs are the most versatile of all forms of powered mobility, and an infinite variety of options are available to meet polio survivors' needs. They are designed specifically to maximize power with motors attaching directly to the wheels (direct drive). A modular power base wheelchair can have a standard seat in a wide range of seat sizes, or it can be modified with a power recline system or power tilt system for pressure relief. Power lift seat systems or power standing systems are also options on some power bases. The typical means of driver control is with a proportional, remote joystick positioned on the user's right or left distal to the front of the armrest. An advantage of the remote joystick is that it can be mounted in various positions as needed for ease of access. The most common alternatives to a proportional, remote joystick drive system are head drive, chin drive, and pneumatic (sip-and-puff) systems.[1]

Modular base power wheelchairs are available in three different drive wheel configurations. Each offers advantages and disadvantages to polio survivors. The rear wheel drive (RWD) configuration is the most common. RWD mimics the manual wheelchair design with the drive wheel in the rear. This design enhances control and stability over rough terrain. However, RWD is less maneuverable than front wheel drive (FWD) or mid-wheel drive (MWD) systems.

The FWD configuration, with the drive wheel in the front, allows for going over a small curb or threshold because the larger wheels make contact first. The turning radius with a FWD is smaller than with a RWD. However, the FWD may be more difficult to control. The MWD configuration is the most recent alternative. The MWD design uses six wheels: two casters in the front, two drive wheels in the middle, and two casters in the rear. The MWD is often standard with a van type seat rather than a standard wheelchair seat. The MWD with the van type seat typically has a flipdown footplate platform rather than swing-away footrests. The van type seat is available in limited sizes, can seldom be custom modified, and typically cannot be modified with a power recline or power tilt system. The main advantage of a MWD is its tight turning radius. This maneuverability is a significant functional benefit in small home or work environments. The MWD design also helps to improve traction because the user's body weight is over the drive wheels. One disadvantage of the MWD is the typically higher seat-to-floor height inherent in the design. Some people also object to the motor shroud that makes the wheelchair appear larger and bulkier.[1,8]

OPTIONS

Many options available on a modular power base wheelchair should be considered for polio survivors initially or for the future. Many polio survivors with impaired upper extremity function are no longer able to adequately shift their weight for pressure relief. This can result in significant discomfort as well as place them at risk for skin breakdown. Although a pressure-relief cushion is indicated, an independent means of weight shift is required to prevent skin breakdown. A power tilt system or power recline system to periodically redistribute pressure can be added to a modular power base initially or can be retrofitted when needed. These systems can be activated by the user by a toggle switch, through the joystick, or by an alternative switch.

Power lift seat systems are available on some modular power base wheelchairs, usually MWDs. These systems are usually activated through the joystick or by a toggle switch. The vertical excursion of the seat is often adequate to improve functional reach for continued independence in ADLs such as cooking. The elevated seat height can also assist in transfers. One disadvantage is the relative instability of the seat in the elevated position.

Power standing systems are available on only a few FWD modular power base wheelchairs. Power standing systems are also usually activated through the joystick or by a toggle switch. The power standing system allows the users the freedom to access many areas of their home or work environments that would otherwise be inaccessible in a seated position. Physiologic benefits of standing include pressure relief to prevent skin breakdown, improved bowel and bladder function, improved circulation, osteoporosis prevention through weight bearing, and contracture prevention. Contraindications include knee and hip flexion contractures, orthostatic disorders, cardiac disorders, and bone brittleness. Disadvantages of power standing systems include the limited seating options typically available and the bulky appearance.

WHEELCHAIR ACCESSORIES

Beyond the standard equipment provided, some special options are available that enhance polio survivors' function in a power wheelchair. It is difficult to access tables and desks from a power wheelchair because of the position of the remote joystick at the distal end of the armrest pad. This can be corrected by the use of a swing-away joystick mount. This allows the user to swing the remote joystick back in line with the armrest pad when approaching a table or desk. The user is then able to drive up under the edge of the table or desk for a more functional position for activities. This is an option that should be offered to all power wheelchair users with a remote joystick drive system.

Many other accessories are available to power wheelchair users. Polio survivors who use braces and crutches for transfers need a means to transport the crutches. A crutch or cane holder can be added to the back of the power wheelchair. Caddy arms can be mounted to the footrest hangers to transport a briefcase. An oxygen tank holder or vent tray can be mounted to the back of the wheelchair. Many other specialty accessories are available such as cup holders, cell phone holders, and even umbrellas.

SEATING FOR POWERED MOBILITY

Seating must be considered for power wheelchair users. Because poliomyelitis is an anterior horn cell disease, sensation is normally intact. However, polio survivors are not exempt from pressure problems. Comorbidities may have resulted in diminished sensation, or impaired upper extremity function may have impaired the ability to independently weight shift for pressure relief. A pressure-mapping system evaluation is helpful in documenting this for polio survivors. Conversely, many polio survivors are hypersensitive and find seating solutions uncomfortable. If the only seating used in the past has been standard sling seat upholstery (i.e., cloth or vinyl), a solid cushion may be difficult to accept.[11]

Many options are available in wheelchair seating products. The component materials range from simple single-density foam (such as polyurethane or viscoelastic) in various thicknesses to multidensity foam, air bladder, air bladder–foam combinations, fluid–foam combinations, gel, gel–foam combinations, and thermoplastic urethane honeycomb biomaterials. The component materials have variable qualities of postural support and pressure distribution, which must be considered. Some cushions are simply flat surfaces (planar), but others are pre-contoured with a pelvic well, leg troughs, and a pommel. Many polio survivors need custom contouring to accommodate fixed deformities such as a pelvic obliquity or leg length discrepancy, to correct flexible deformities, or to accommodate thigh bands on long leg braces. A solid seat (wood or molded plastic) may be used under the cushion if the wheelchair does not have a solid seat pan to provide a level sitting surface. The cushion cover must also be considered because the fabric may be an obstacle to the patient's style of transfer.

Wheelchair seating is not limited to the wheelchair seat cushion. Wheelchair back cushions (in materials similar to wheelchair seat cushions) are available to replace sling-back upholstery. A supportive wheelchair back that provides postural support can significantly increase comfort and function for the wheelchair user. Planar or linear style backs, similar to the posture panel inserts many polio survivors used in the past, are available. Precontoured or custom-contoured backs provide other options and are often angle adjustable. Some styles can be modified to accommodate fixed deformities or correct flexible deformities such as scoliosis or kyphosis. Wheelchair backs are a convenient surface for attachment of trunk laterals or headrests as needed. A successful seating solution (cushion and back) requires providing options to the polio survivor for trial use in the seating clinic.

CONCLUSION

Polio survivors present a unique challenge to the seating clinic team. Knowledge of the history of poliomyelitis and the current issues of the polio survivor are necessary to achieve successful seating and powered mobility solutions. A willingness to view the polio survivor as an integral part of the process of finding the "right wheels" is a necessity for success.

References

1. Karp G: Life on Wheels: For the Active Wheelchair User. Sebastopol, CA, O'Reilly & Associates, Inc., 1999.
2. Halstead LS, Grimby G (eds): Post-Polio Syndrome. Philadelphia, Hanley & Belfus, 1995.
3. Vasiliadis HM, Collet JP, Shapiro S, et al: Predictive factors and correlates for pain in postpoliomyelitis syndrome patients. Arch Phys Med Rehabil 83:1109–1115, 2002.
4. Halstead LS, Wiechers DO (eds): Late Effects of Poliomyelitis. Miami, Symposia Foundation, 1985.
5. Bruno RL: The Polio Paradox. New York, Warner Books, 2002.
6. Klein MG, Whyte J, Keenan MA, et al: Changes in strength over time among polio survivors. Arch Phys Med Rehabil 81(8):1059–1064, 2000.
7. Silver JK: Post-Polio Syndrome: A Guide for Polio Survivors and Their Families. New Haven, CT, Yale University Press, 2001.
8. Karp G: Choosing a Wheelchair: A Guide for Optimal Independence. Sebastopol, CA, O'Reilly & Associates, Inc., 1998.
9. Miles-Tapping C, MacDonald LJ: Lifestyle implications of power mobility. Phys Occupat Ther Geriatr 12:31–49, 1994.
10. Fletcher GF, Banja JD, Jann BB, Wolf SL (eds): Rehabilitation Medicine: Contemporary Clinical Perspectives. Malvern, PA, Lea & Febiger, 1992.
11. Leonard RB: Seating and mobility issues for polio survivors. Rehabil Manage 10:44–46, 1997.
12. Batavia M: The Wheelchair Evaluation: A Practical Guide. Woburn, MA, Butterworth-Heinemann, 1998.
13. Field D: Powered mobility: A literature review illustrating the importance of a multifaceted approach. Assist Technol 11:20–33, 1999.
14. Cook AM, Hussey SM: Assistive Technologies: Principles and Practice. St. Louis, Mosby, 1995.

The Role of Occupational Therapy in the Management of Polio Survivors

Beth Kowall, MS, OTR

O ccupational therapy enables people to do the day-to-day activities that are important to them despite impairment, disability, or handicap.[22] A person with postpolio syndrome (PPS) has new symptoms that may include fatigue, muscle weakness, muscle atrophy, and muscle or joint pain. Some of these symptoms may also be seen in those who have a residual deficit from their bout with paralytic poliomyelitis but do not meet the criteria for PPS.[7] Occupational therapists work with both polio survivors who are experiencing new symptoms as well as those who are not but may be at risk of developing the symptoms in the future. The role of the occupational therapist is to assist clients in: (1) establishing lifestyle modifications; (2) adopting a healthy balance of work, rest, and leisure; (3) using appropriate assistive and orthotic devices; (4) making environmental or home modifications; and (5) developing new adaptive and coping responses for optimal functioning within their communities and engagement in meaningful daily activities.

OCCUPATION

Occupational therapists are concerned with how clients engage in purposeful occupations in the performance of (1) activities of daily living (ADLs; e.g., personal care, hygiene, mobility), (2) work and productive activities (e.g., meal preparation, household cleaning, work), and (3) leisure activities (e.g., recreation, leisure pursuits).[4] The occupational therapist examines the individual and his or her family; the daily tasks the person does and how they are done; and the home, social, and work environments. People with chronic impairments, such as polio survivors, are assisted in engaging in occupations in a healthy way by developing and using specific skills to achieve their goals.[26]

APPROACH

CLIENT CENTERED

Mary Law stated that occupational therapy, at its best, is client centered, with a collaborative partnership between the therapist, the client, and the family.[17] She noted that client-centered therapy promotes participation, exchange of information, client decision making, and respect for choice. Individuals with polio can benefit from this approach when their expertise about their bodies is valued, their needs are respected, and they can gain a sense of control within their environment to make healthy choices for management of postpolio symptoms. The occupational therapist values the strengths, competencies, and life stories that the person with polio brings to the therapeutic environment.

CARING AND EMPATHY

Occupational therapists investigate the impact of PPS on the physical, psychological, social, cultural, and spiritual aspects of clients' lives. Halstead contended that sometimes caregivers listen without responding, knowing that just talking can be therapeutic, and just listening is a way of affirming that what a patient is feeling is understandable, normal, natural.[12] When an occupational therapist uses good communication and interpersonal skills, the therapeutic relationship can be strengthened. A genuine caring and empathetic approach can have a positive impact on the well-being and health of the client.

UNDERSTANDING PREVIOUS COPING STYLES

People who had polio and endured the initial onset and rehabilitation often adopted the attitudes and values of that time to help them survive a life-threatening event. Some of the coping styles included working very hard through rigorous exercises, pushing themselves, minimizing limitations, and ignoring pain. Halstead[10] notes that these former coping patterns are no longer the appropriate response to the challenges of postpolio problems and symptoms. Occupational therapists guide and assist clients in developing new coping responses and stress management techniques that are more suitable in managing PPS.

UNDERSTANDING VIEW OF SELF

If polio survivors fought so hard during their initial rehabilitation to avoid feeling or looking "disabled," how are new physical limitations affecting their self-concept? Do they feel "disabled" now, or do they believe others perceive them as a person with a disability? Thoren-Jonsson and Moller[36] found that whereas some people perceived their disability as a restriction or a negative, others perceived their disability as mostly a practical obstacle to be overcome and compensated for in different ways. They implied that negative attitudes toward a disability might be an additional hindrance to future changes (e.g., in using new mobility aids). It is imperative for the occupational therapist to understand how the polio survivor is now perceiving him- or herself with these limitations.

Thus, using these four approaches can positively impact the therapeutic relationship and the choices the polio survivor makes for lifestyle change. The polio survivor is supported and empowered to be responsible for making changes in his or her life to help manage new symptoms. Also, it is important that the occupational therapist be aware of the research literature on PPS because this can be a method for choosing the best and most effective assessments and interventions for the client.[38]

OCCUPATIONAL THERAPY PROCESS

The occupational therapy process involves interactions and activities between the therapist, client, and family. This includes referral, evaluation, intervention plan, intervention, and discharge and follow up.[21] The time to adequately follow through and complete the stages of this process may depend on many factors, including time constraints of the client, the number of therapy visits allowed through insurance coverage, or the client's readiness to participate in therapy and follow through with recommendations. Occupational therapists need to be flexible throughout the therapy process and provide quality and cost-effective services to satisfy the client, his or her family, and other payers of service.

EVALUATION

Evaluation methods include interviews, observation of the client performing a task, and standardized measures such as questionnaires or checklists that note the client's strengths, limitations, and individual needs. For polio survivors who believe they are not currently experiencing new symptoms, it is important to identify those clients who are at risk of developing PPS or who have early signs of PPS.[9] It is vital that these polio survivors be aware of PPS symptoms and know where to seek medical advice in the future, if necessary. The occupational therapist assesses the client's current status, takes a polio history, obtains a baseline evaluation, and then makes recommendations for lifestyle changes for optimal health and wellness.

Polio History

For polio survivors exhibiting new symptoms, the therapist seeks a thorough polio history from the client and family members to assess the age of onset of the original polio and the extent of the polio (e.g., limbs involved, surgical history, history of respiratory involvement). Other medical issues are noted, and overall general health is discussed. Maynard and Headley found that comorbidities (i.e., other medical conditions), in addition to previous paralytic poliomyelitis, may contribute to and compound a person's health problems and cause a decrease in daily activities.[20] They noted that comorbidities may be related to previous paralytic polio such as scoliosis or osteoarthritis or unrelated disorders such as cancer or diabetes.

Current Functioning

Current functioning is evaluated to see if changes in activity and performance level have occurred for the polio survivor within the past several years. Areas to be explored include functioning before initial polio, changes in function since their period of stability, and present functional status. This can be assessed by determining if the patient reports having more difficulty performing daily tasks at home or work or in the community, if his or her current braces remain effective or there is difficulty with mobility, or if the patient is able to pursue previous leisure interests. Kling et al.[14] found patients mainly report that their physical abilities are affected by PPS. The occupational therapist determines how decline in physical functioning affects the patient's overall lifestyle and activity level on a daily basis.

Postpolio Syndrome Symptoms

Although there are other symptoms of PPS, the most frequently reported problems— fatigue, pain, and new weakness—should be evaluated as to how they impact daily activities. Concerning fatigue, Schanke and Stanghelle[30] found that polio survivors are affected mainly by physical fatigue, primarily because of their physical health with both polio-related problems and comorbidity. Halstead[11] described that for some, fatigue is muscular and for others, fatigue refers to a generalized sensation felt throughout the body that is described as an overwhelming exhaustion that tends to get worse as the day progresses. Thus, the polio survivor should report the type of fatigue they are experiencing such as extreme tiredness or lack of energy, when it occurs during the day, and how it interferes with daily activities.

The second symptom is muscle and joint pain. Many of the problems that appear to be related to overuse of weak muscles and abnormal joint movements may simply represent the inevitable consequences of chronic disability.[11] Widar and Ahlstrom[44] found that the most commonly reported pain was in the joints of the extremities and that pain was a part of everyday life. Willen and Grimby[45] studied polio survivors and found that the experience of pain is related to level of physical activity and that pain influences energy level, mobility, sleep, and emotional reactions. Thus, the occupational therapist evaluates the type, intensity, and duration of pain and how it influences the patient's participation in daily activities.

The third symptom, new weakness, is often most prominent in the muscles that were severely involved in the initial illness and then underwent good recovery.[11] New weakness is found not only in those muscles originally involved but also in the "good" limb that was believed to be spared; however, it had been overworking for years to compensate for the more involved limb.[11] Evaluating new weakness includes understanding when it started, if it has progressed, when it is worse, and how it interferes with daily tasks.

Performance Areas

The three main performance areas the occupational therapist evaluates are ADLs, work and productive activities, and leisure. The therapist documents how changes in activity level impact upon the patient's independence and quality of life. Some of the tasks under each performance area are described here, but a complete list is found in the American Occupational Therapy Association's "Outline of Uniform Terminology for Occupational Therapy."[4]

Activities of Daily Living. Dressing, personal hygiene, bathing, grooming, and mobility are some of the tasks in this performance area that the therapist assesses in the clinic or at a home visit. For each task, it is important to explore if the activity is done independently, if assistance from family is needed to perform the task, if the task can not be performed at all, and if the client is willing to use assistive devices or modifications to perform an activity. It is also noted how long it takes to accomplish a task now compared with several years ago. If the client has difficulty performing an activity, the therapist determines if it is caused by fatigue, pain, or weakness.

In exploring how these symptoms affect ADLs, the occupational therapist asks the client 1) what his or her daily routine is like on an hourly basis; 2) which ADLs are most important for him or her to continue; 3) how fatigue influences mobility or ability to do personal hygiene tasks; 4) when fatigue is worse during the day; 5) if he or she tends to fall when fatigue increases; 6) if pain limits activities; or 7) if weakness causes difficulty in personal hygiene, climbing stairs, or getting up from a sitting position.

Work and Productive Activities. Inquiry into this performance area focuses on home management and job activities. The therapist obtains information about the clients' environment, which may include an onsite visit to the client's home or job site. The practitioner asks polio survivors (1) how fatigue affects their ability to maintain and clean the home; (2) what activities are most important to them and their family in this performance area; (3) if they are able to prepare a meal and clean up afterwards; (4) if they do their own shopping or need assistance; (5) if they are working, and if so, how many hours a day they work, if their job requires lifting, sitting, standing, or climbing stairs, or if they are able to take rest breaks during the day; (6) if they find that they are exhausted by the end of the work week and spend the weekend resting up to begin the next work week; and (7) if they encounter environmental barriers in the community or at their worksite.

Leisure. Thoren-Jonsson et al.[35] found that pain and lack of energy prevent leisure activity. Although a polio survivor may value his or her leisure activities, they often become a lower priority because all available energy is used for personal care, work, or family obligations. When evaluating leisure activities, the therapist asks: if the client's participation in leisure has decreased, if he or she is choosing more sedentary activities, if he or she can participate in the same recreational activities with the family compared with several years ago, or which leisure activities are important for him or her to continue.

Thus, the occupational therapist chooses the appropriate evaluation methods and gathers data about how postpolio symptoms affect the tasks and roles in these three performance areas. The input of the client and the family is essential in gaining an accurate account of the health status of the polio survivor. The results of the evaluations assist the therapist in understanding the scope of postpolio involvement and the priorities that the client has in these performance areas.

Performance Components
Range of Motion. Performance components encompass many areas, but the specific components to be addressed here are range of motion (ROM), muscle strength, and psychosocial skills.[4] ROM measurements are taken to determine if limitations affect function, additional range is needed for function, or orthotic or assistive devices are needed.[23,40] Pain and weakness may limit ROM, so the therapist documents if there is an increase or decrease in these symptoms during interventions.

Muscle Strength. Muscle strength is measured to establish a baseline, determine if weakness is limiting performance, and determine if orthotic or assistive devices are needed.[15] For many years, polio survivors compensated for weak muscles by using other compensatory muscle patterns to maintain function. When muscle testing, it is essential that the practitioner is aware of these adaptive patterns.

Grimby and Stalberg reported that, in the 1960s, Beasley found that manual muscle testing does not give reliable information in muscles with strength levels of fair (3/5) or above.[8] Muscles that had appeared normal or good on clinical examination may have significant weakness because these polio involved muscles have had to work harder than a truly normal muscle.[25] A careful history of how the patient's muscles function on a daily basis and how he or she performs routine activities that require repetitive muscle contractions, such as walking or climbing stairs, can provide a semiquantitative picture of declining strength.[11] Thus, the therapist can use both the manual muscle test and a functional assessment to get a better indication of muscle strength in the polio survivor.

Other upper extremity conditions such as arthritis, tendinitis, carpal tunnel syndrome, and shoulder overuse are evaluated as to how they impact function and muscle strength. In polio survivors, carpal tunnel syndrome and overuse of the shoulder occur because of long-term use of crutches, canes, or a manual wheelchair.[32] Klein et al.[13] indicated that people with lower extremity weakness are at risk to develop shoulder overuse problems because they tend to increase reliance on their upper extremities for mobility and ADLs. By evaluating how the polio survivor ambulates and uses assistive devices, the occupational therapist can determine if there is a risk for shoulder overuse or if it already exists.

The occupational therapist also evaluates functional endurance and how it relates to the performance of ADLs. A polio survivor may now have difficulty working full time, completing household cleaning tasks, participating in community activities, or walking through a shopping mall. Methods of evaluation include timing how long clients can participate in activities (e.g., meal preparation, house cleaning) before requiring a rest or monitoring clients' perception of how hard they are working or how tired they are after a given amount of time at a specific workload.[15]

Psychosocial Skills. The therapist evaluates psychosocial skills and responses by examining issues such as how polio survivors feel about their new physical limitations, how their new symptoms affect their self-concept and body image, if these new changes are losses to them, or if they have changed how they view themselves. Wenneberg and Ahlstrom[42] found that polio survivors were not looking forward to again being dependent on others for daily care, instead wanting to be independent as long as possible. Being unable to perform or participate in activities that were achievable several years ago can have a detrimental effect on the emotional well-being of the polio survivor. It is critical for the therapist to understand how the psychosocial responses to changing health status may affect participation in interventions and clients' outlook for the future.

INTERVENTION PLAN

After examining the evaluation results, the therapist along with the polio survivor and his or her family, as well as other members of the team, if appropriate, develop a therapy plan that includes intervention methods and goals.[21] The therapist also addresses performance components such as ROM, muscle strength, or coping skills because they are linked to occupational performance.[1] The length of time to accomplish these goals and to use appropriate interventions varies with each individual. A polio survivor may need additional time and support to adjust to new assistive devices or other modifications.

In formulating goals, the importance of culture and spirituality in the client's life should be acknowledged because it may affect the choice and methods of interventions. Cultural environment, values, and beliefs are considered as well as understanding the occupations that are meaningful to the client. Planning for interventions includes addressing how occupations are performed, the roles and relationships within the cultural group, and the occupational performance according to the group's standards and expectations.[33] The importance of spirituality in the client's life is established to determine if it can assist him or her in dealing with the effects of PPS. Spirituality may help the client attain contentment and focus on different or more pleasurable aspects of life.[39] A sense of spirituality can also assist the client in following through with interventions and in gaining health and well-being in daily life.

Occupational therapy services can achieve beneficial outcomes, including an increased independence level, symptom status improvement, improvement in quality of life, and improved emotional well-being.[21] Watson stated that outcomes are the end results of care and describe what happened to the client after he or she received care.[41] In collaboration with the occupational therapist, the polio survivor and the family establish positive outcomes that are significant to them for wellness and a sense of meaning in their lives.

INTERVENTION

Interventions are tasks or activities that promote health and improve occupational performance.[21] Polio survivors can participate individually or in a group educational setting, such as that proposed by Young.[47] Interventions can be most effective when initiated and accomplished on a gradual basis to provide time for these new adjustments to lifestyle. Halstead[11] stated that changes that enable polio survivors to retain a sense of control may enhance compliance. He added that some of the interventions to manage the effects of PPS include (1) the use of orthoses and assistive technology devices, (2) environmental modifications at home and work, (3) the use of community support groups, (4) new coping and adaptive strategies, (5) lifestyle modifications and energy conservation, and (6) an individualized exercise program.

Orthoses for the Upper Extremity

Upper extremity splints are prescribed to avoid overuse, support and assist weak muscles, provide rest to decrease inflammation, and reduce pain in the management of postpolio symptoms. Daily repetitive activities such as use of canes, crutches, computers, or certain leisure activities can result in overuse syndrome and an increased workload of the upper extremities. Besides splinting, occupational therapists also teach interventions such as use of prescribed exercise, use of rest and work periods, joint protection, correct posture and use of ergonomic keyboards, and energy conservation. To protect and preserve the shoulder and conserve energy, the therapist can recommend a scooter or electric wheelchair for use during daily activities.

Upper extremity conditions include peripheral mononeuropathies (e.g., carpal tunnel syndrome), de Quervain's syndrome, and tendinitis and osteoarthritis in the hand or wrist. Besides splinting, patient education is an important intervention to help the polio survivor learn about the condition, how to decrease symptoms, how to avoid overuse, and how to balance work and rest. The therapist can also use a variety of modalities (e.g., iontophoresis, ultrasound, cryotherapy) to reduce acute symptoms of pain and inflammation.

The balanced forearm orthosis or mobile arm support is used for polio survivors with increased proximal weakness in the upper extremity. It is attached to a chair or wheelchair and consists of a ball-bearing hinge joint at the elbow with a forearm trough.[29] This intervention improves independence in ADLs such as feeding and hygiene by helping lift the arm to the face.

Polio survivors may have difficulty complying with orthotic devices because it makes them "feel disabled." To improve chances for compliance, it is vital for the practitioner to understand what the device means to the client, what support the client has from family and friends, and what expectations the polio survivor has for the device. The polio survivor needs time and support to use these devices in order to show how these aids can improve functioning in their daily activities.

Assistive Technology

Assistive technology devices are defined as any item, piece of equipment, or product system, whether acquired commercially (off the shelf), modified or customized, that is used to increase, maintain, or improve functional capabilities of individuals with disabilities.[19] These wide range of items can be used by polio survivors to help manage postpolio symptoms because these devices assist in conserving energy, decreasing pain and fatigue, improving independence, and increasing functional ability to perform daily tasks. Compliance with these devices is dependent on factors such as effectiveness in performance, comfort, motivation of the client, and the importance of the task being performed. Riemer-Reiss and Wacker found that involving the client in the decision-making process influences the likelihood that the client will continue using the device.[28] The therapist, client, and family collaborate to identify the most appropriate device for the client's specific needs and environment. Adapting to new methods of functioning takes self-acceptance.[6] Thus, there are physical and psychological components to using these devices, and the polio survivor needs education, support, and time to be compliant.

Many interventions exist to improve occupational performance and roles, as found in resources such as Krantz et al.[16] and Mann and Lane.[19] Interventions for the home include a phone ear- or headset; a reacher; built-up pens and pencils; arm rests for chairs; long-handled cleaning devices; a lifting chair; adjustable work heights; a mouthstick; a page turner; environmental control devices to operate lights, phone, or appliances; and adaptations to the mouse and keyboard of a home computer (e.g., voice-activated software).

For mobility, interventions include modifying a car or van to accommodate a lift for a scooter or power wheelchair, hand controls, or adaptations to the joystick for a wheelchair.

Interventions for the kitchen include built-up utensils, an electric knife, adapted cutting boards, one-handed jar opener, a hand mixer, or use of a food guard for a plate.

Concerning the bathroom, Thoren-Jonsson and Grimby[34] reported that frequent types of renovations include removing a tub and installing a shower, removing high thresholds, and use of handrails and grab bars. Raised toilet seats with a safety frame, a shower chair, long-lever handles on faucets, a roll in shower, or a hand-held shower are other bathroom devices.

For dressing, interventions include a long-handled shoe horn, slip-on shoes, Velcro fasteners, or a dressing stick.

In a work situation, interventions include modifications to a work station such as modified handles on tools, an ergonomic keyboard, wrist support or an arm rest for computer use, or use of voice recognition for computer access or environmental control systems.

Interventions for leisure include use of a book holder, adapted recreational equipment, and careful selection of modified or new activities. Assistive technology devices are chosen, modified, or created according to the client's needs; occupational performance; functional level; and home, work, or community environment.

Modifications at Home and Work

Modifying and adapting environments enhances performance and safety in daily life roles.[5] When choosing the most appropriate modification, the cost factor to the client and his or her family can be a major part of the decision-making process. Environmental modifications are prescribed to avoid overuse, decrease pain and fatigue level, increase safety measures to prevent falls, and have greater accessibility to the home and work setting.

In the home, modifications include eliminating scatter rugs to prevent falls, proper seating and use of cushions, rearranging work areas for easier reach, delegating chores and asking for help, obtaining a home cleaning service, and moving the laundry facilities to the main living area to avoid use of stairs.

Kitchen modifications include use of a wheeled utility cart, use of a chair to sit on while preparing meals, use of lower countertops or work surfaces, appliances with dials toward the front, a cut-out area under the sink, use of nonskid surfaces, and rearranging shelves so that the heavier or more frequently used items are on lower shelves or kept on the countertop.

In the bathroom, modifications include use of nonskid surfaces in the tub or shower, a tub or shower bench, a bath transfer bench, or a long-handled bath mitt or sponge.

For mobility in the community or at work, use of a scooter, power wheelchair, or use of a community van service for people with disabilities can be recommended. Major renovations to the home such as ramps, adapting an existing bathroom for a roll in shower, or kitchen renovations involve building professionals with knowledge of requirements of the Americans with Disabilities Act (ADA) and accessibility. The team approach in which the client, therapist, and builder work together to maximize the client's functioning within the home environment allows each participant to contribute knowledge and skills for the renovation process.[27]

In the work environment, many modifications can be recommended, including lowering or raising work surfaces; rearranging work areas for optimal efficiency and energy conservation; correct posture and positioning; using a proper chair with appropriate cushions and arm rests; using rest breaks; proper body mechanics for sitting, standing, and bending; ergonomic keyboard for computer and use of ergonomic principles; and use of an elevator instead of the stairs. Other minor or major renovations should be done in conjunction with the employer and in agreement with ADA requirements. Printed materials can be given to the polio survivor and the family to reinforce these techniques and modifications. Modifications are individualized for the specific needs and work environment of the polio survivor.

Support Groups

Community support groups are used as an intervention because they can provide emotional support, educational information, information on community resources, and a network of people in similar situations. These groups focus on wellness, sharing ideas and feelings, and problem solving. They provide a supportive environment where persons with polio feel they are "not alone" in dealing with postpolio symptoms. People who lack nurturing relationships become more socially isolated and more susceptible to depression.[31] To help survivors enrich their coping resources, it is important to have a social support system in which the emotional and physical reality of ongoing adaptation is acknowledged and strategies found helpful by survivors are known and shared.[43]

Postpolio support groups are also an important resource for family and friends of polio survivors because they are also dealing with the impact of PPS on a daily basis. Caregivers and family members need ongoing support and education to help them maintain their health and well-being. Thus, it is important that occupational therapists know about these valuable community resources and share information about local groups with polio survivors and their families so they can use them now or in the future.

Coping and Adaptation

The onset of new postpolio symptoms may create feelings of stress, sadness, loss, or fear. Polio survivors learn and use new coping strategies as interventions to cope with the impact of PPS in a healthy way. Thoren-Jonsson et al. identified strategies that people with PPS use to manage their daily occupations, such as setting priorities, restoring activity and role balance, problem solving, and compensating.[37] Other effective coping interventions also used with other disability groups include optimism, information seeking, positive reinterpretation, expressing feelings, and seeking social support.[18] The therapist and client recognize that using these new strategies can be a long-term and ongoing process. As polio survivors gradually gain success with these new skills, their competence, self-esteem, and independence level can improve. Polio survivors need to acknowledge rather than deny their limitations before changes can occur. With family support and the support of therapists, clients recognize that new coping interventions can have positive influences on their health and quality of life.

Lifestyle Modifications
Pacing, energy conservation, and lifestyle modifications are significant interventions to manage postpolio symptoms. Pacing, the balance of activity and rest, can decrease pain and fatigue, prevent falls, avoid overuse, and preserve energy for activities that are more important to the polio survivor. Agre and Rodriquez demonstrated that pacing of physical activities with work–rest programs decreases local muscle fatigue, increases work capacity, and results in recovery of strength in symptomatic postpolio patients.[2] By planning, prioritizing, and pacing, polio survivors are instructed in how to use their energy in an efficient and careful way. Small changes made throughout the day in what clients accomplish and how they perform tasks can produce an impressive change in energy level and sense of well-being.[11] Lifestyle modifications include use of a scooter, sitting instead of standing, getting help with household tasks, decreasing hours at work, and scheduling rest breaks during the day. Although occupational therapists may find these interventions practical and achievable, psychologically, they may be the most difficult for clients.

Exercise Program
The use of exercise as an intervention is an individualized and closely supervised program that is customized to each person's needs, residual strength, and symptom patterns.[11] Exercises are beneficial physically and psychologically, and they range from gentle stretching to aerobic training. Polio survivors are instructed to "listen to their bodies' signals" and avoid muscle overuse, exhaustion, and pain, which are indications of overwork. Conversely, inactivity and lack of any exercise can lead to disuse and deconditioning; therefore, the therapist and client collaborate to design a healthy, balanced exercise program to fit the client's lifestyle.

Muscle stretching and ROM exercises help improve function in daily activities and decrease pain when there is muscle weakness.[20] Conditioning or aerobic exercises to improve endurance, such as a program of non-swimming exercises in a heated pool, have been found to have a positive impact on polio survivors.[46] The warm water minimizes the stress on joints and muscles and can impact pain level, but even with these underwater nonresistive exercises, overuse and fatigue should be avoided. In weak muscles, the general guideline is to perform nonfatiguing exercises.[31] Muscle fatigue is avoided by interspersing bouts of activity with rest breaks; it has been found that this technique also improves strength recovery after activity.[2] People with PPS who are able to exercise at a level that avoided overuse experience positive results.[3] Individualized exercise regimes should start off slowly, and changes can be made at any stage of the program. The type of exercise, how often it is performed, the amount of exercise or activity, and the level of intensity is individualized for each polio survivor. Persons with postpolio symptoms are closely monitored for any adverse effects from the exercises such as an increase in pain or fatigue. Perry[24] proposed that an exercise program should not begin until polio survivors have redesigned their lifestyles in order to avoid muscle strain, fatigue, and weakening. Thus, the daily activities, motivation, current functional and health status, and muscle strength of the polio survivor are important factors to consider when developing and recommending an exercise program.

DISCHARGE AND FOLLOW-UP

Clients are discharged from occupational therapy services when goals have been met, insurance coverage has ended, or the client requests to be discharged because he or she is not psychologically ready for participation and use of interventions. The polio survivor may, at a later date, return for follow-up visits if functional status changes; if there is a change in living situation; assistive devices need modifications; or the client is now ready to learn and use interventions at home, work, or in the community.[21] Because dealing with a chronic illness is an ongoing and long-term process, periodic rechecks with the therapist can assist the polio survivor with problem-solving skills, coping strategies, and updating assistive devices and modifications to manage the effects of postpolio symptoms.

CONCLUSION

By using modified, energy-efficient strategies to perform daily skills, having a supportive environment, and being willing to adopt new lifestyle changes and interventions, polio survivors are empowered to manage the effects of PPS to achieve optimal functioning and quality of life. Occupational therapists support the health and wellness of polio survivors at risk for developing postpolio symptoms as well as polio survivors who have been diagnosed with PPS. Interventions in the areas of ADLs, work and productive activities, and leisure help polio survivors accomplish their goals and regain a sense of purpose and meaning through engaging in daily activities that are important to them. Therapists help polio survivors integrate lifestyle changes; a balance of activity and rest; new assistive devices and modifications; and new coping responses into their daily life at home, work, and in the community to improve the level of competence and independence. Ideally, health care professionals can blend the humanistic (i.e., caring and empathy) and scientific components in medicine to provide a framework for rehabilitation healing and care of people with polio and PPS.[12] With the support of family, friends, caring professionals, and other polio survivors, polio survivors can make healthy choices and changes in their daily lives that will have a positive impact on their health, well-being, and participation in society.

References
1. Acquaviva JD: Effective Documentation for Occupational Therapy, 2nd ed. Bethesda, MD, American Occupational Therapy Association, 1998.
2. Agre JC, Rodriquez AA: Intermittent isometric activity: Its effect on muscle fatigue in postpolio subjects. Arch Phys Med Rehabil 72:971–977, 1991.
3. Agre JC, Rodriquez AA: Muscular function in late polio and the role of exercise in post-polio patients. Neurorehabilitation 8:107–118, 1997.
4. American Occupational Therapy Association: Uniform terminology for occupational therapy, 3rd ed. Am J Occup Ther 48:1047–1054, 1994.
5. American Occupational Therapy Association: Definition of OT practice for the AOTA model practice act. Am J Occup Ther 53:608, 1999.
6. Bieniek LL: Emotional bridges to wellness. Polio Netw News 17:1–4, 2001.
7. Gawne AC, Halstead LS: Post-polio syndrome: Pathophysiology and clinical management. Crit Rev Phys Rehabil Med 7:147–188, 1995.
8. Grimby G, Stalberg E: Muscle function, muscle structure, and electrophysiology in a dynamic perspective in late polio. In Halstead LS, Grimby G (eds): Post-polio Syndrome. Philadelphia, Hanley & Belfus, 1995, pp 15–24.
9. Habel M, Strong P: The late effects of poliomyelitis: Nursing interventions for a unique patient population. Medsurg Nurs 5:77–84, 1996.
10. Halstead LS: The residual of polio in aged. Topics Geriatr Rehabil 3:9–26, 1988.
11. Halstead LS: New health problems in persons with polio. In Halstead LS (ed): Managing Post-polio: A Guide to Living Well with Post-Polio Syndrome. Washington, DC, NRH Press, 1998, pp 20–53.
12. Halstead LS: The power of compassion and caring in rehabilitation healing. Arch Phys Med Rehabil 82:149–154, 2001.
13. Klein MG, Whyte J, Keenan MA, et al: The relation between lower extremity strength and shoulder overuse symptoms: A model based on polio survivors. Arch Phys Med Rehabil 81:789–795, 2000.
14. Kling C, Persson A, Gardulf A: The health-related quality of life of patients suffering from the late effects of polio (post-polio). J Adv Nurs 32:164–173, 2000.
15. Kohlmeyer K: Evaluation of performance components. In Neistadt ME, Crepeau EB (eds): Willard and Spackman's Occupational Therapy. Philadelphia, Lippincott-Raven, 1998, pp 223–290.
16. Krantz GC, Christenson MA, Lindquist A: Assistive Products—An Illustrated Guide to Terminology. Bethesda, MD, American Occupational Therapy Association, 1998.
17. Law M (ed): Client-centered Occupational Therapy. Thorofare, NJ, Slack Inc., 1998.
18. Livneh H: Psychosocial adaptation to cancer: The role of coping strategies. J Rehabil 66:40–49, 2000.
19. Mann WC, Lane JP: Assitive Technology for Persons with Disabilities, 2nd ed. Bethesda, MD, American Occupational Therapy Association, 1995.
20. Maynard F, Headley J (ed): Handbook on the Late Effects of Poliomyelitis for Physicians and Survivors. St. Louis, Gazette International Networking Institute, 1999.
21. Moyers P: The guide to occupational therapy practice. Am J Occ Ther 53:251–289, 1999.
22. Neistadt ME, Crepeau EB: Introduction to occupational therapy. In Neistadt ME, Crepeau EB (eds): Willard and Spackman's Occupational Therapy. Philadelphia, Lippincott-Raven, 1998, pp 5–12.
23. Pedretti LW: Evaluation of joint range of motion. In Pedretti LW (ed): Occupational Therapy—Practice Skills for Physical Dysfunction, 4th ed. St. Louis, Mosby, 1996, pp 79–107.
24. Perry J: Why are "old polios" who were stable for years now losing function? What should they do about it? Polio Network News. Gazette International Networking Institute 16:1–2, 2000.

25. Perry J, Fleming C: Polio: Long-term problems. Orthopedics 8:877–881, 1985.
26. Porn I: Health and adaptedness. Theoret Med 14:295–303, 1993.
27. Pynoos J, Sanford J, Rosenfelt T: A team approach for home modifications. OT Pract 8:15–19, 2002.
28. Riemer-Reiss ML, Wacker RR: Factors associated with assistive technology discontinuance among individuals with disabilities. J Rehabil 66:44–50, 2000.
29. Rodstein B, Kim D: Orthoses and adaptive equipment in neuromuscular disorders. In Younger DS (ed): Motor Disorders. Philadelphia, Lippincott Williams & Wilkins, 1999, pp 453–467.
30. Schanke AK, Stanghelle JK: Fatigue in polio survivors. Spinal Cord 39:243–251, 2001.
31. Silver JK: Post-polio—A Guide for Polio Survivors and Their Families. New Haven, Yale University Press, 2001.
32. Smith LK: Lifestyle changes: Taking charge. In Halstead LS (ed): Managing Post-polio: A Guide to Living Well with Post-polio Syndrome. Washington, DC, NRH Press, 1998, pp 84–106.
33. Spencer J, Krefting L, Mattingly C: Incorporation of ethnographic methods in occupational therapy assessment. Am J Occup Ther 47:303–309, 1993.
34. Thoren-Jonsson AL, Grimby G: Ability and perceived difficulty in daily activities in people with poliomyelitis sequelae. J Rehabil Med 33:4–11, 2001.
35. Thoren-Jonsson AL, Hedberg M, Grimby G: Distress in everyday life in people with poliomyelitis sequelae. J Rehabil Med 33:119–127, 2001.
36. Thoren-Jonsson AL, Moller A: How the conception of occupational self influences everyday life strategies of people with poliomyelitis sequelae. Scand J Occ Ther 6:71–83, 1999.
37. Thoren-Jonsson AL, Moller A, Grimby G: Managing occupations in everyday life to achieve adaptation. Amer J Occup Ther 53:353–362, 1999.
38. Tickle-Degnen L: What is the best evidence to use in practice? Am J Occup Ther 54:218–221, 2000.
39. Trieschmann RB: Spirituality and energy medicine. J Rehabil 67: 26–32, 2001.
40. Trombly CA: Evaluation of biomechanical and physiological aspects of motor performance. In Trombly CA (ed): Occupational Therapy for Physical Dysfunction, 4th ed. Baltimore, Williams & Williams, 1995, pp 73–156.
41. Watson DE: Evaluating Cost and Outcomes: Demonstrating the Value of Rehabilitation Services. Bethesda, MD, American Occupational Therapy Associaton, 2000.
42. Wenneberg S, Ahlstrom G: Illness narratives of persons with post-polio syndrome. J Adv Nurs 31:354–361, 2000.
43. Westbrook M, McIlwain D: Living with the late effects of disability: A five-year follow-up survey of coping among post-polio survivors. Aust Occup Ther J 43:60–71, 1996.
44. Widar M, Ahlstrom G: Pain in persons with post-polio. Scand J Caring Sci 13:33–40, 1999.
45. Willen C, Grimby G: Pain, physical activity, and disability in individuals with late effects of polio. Arch Phys Med Rehabil 79:915–919, 1998.
46. Willen C, Stibrant Sunnerhagen K, Grimby G: Dynamic water exercise in individuals with late poliomyelitis. Arch Phys Med Rehabil 82:66–72, 2001.
47. Young GR: Treating post-polio syndrome. OT Practice 19:10–14, 2001.

Energy Conservation and Pacing

Maria H. Cole, OTR, and Laura A. Ryan, OTR

How we perceive and use our energy determines our ability to function in everyday life. New weakness and fatigue can impact one's ability to perform functional tasks. In the case of polio survivors with already weakened muscles, a change in energy level and increased fatigue can be devastating. Between 50% and 85% of polio survivors are now experiencing new symptoms of increased weakness, fatigue, pain and muscle atrophy.[1] The incidence of developing postpolio syndrome (PPS) varies from 22% to 85%.[2] Although the statistics vary, it is known that many people who had acute poliomyelitis will eventually develop symptoms of PPS.[2,3] The most likely theory for the new onset of progressive muscle weakness is years of overusing muscles left functioning after the acute attack.[4] Studies suggest that avoiding overuse of muscles, decreasing fatigue and pain, and addressing physical activity are paramount in the treatment of patients with PPS.[2,5,6] Embracing energy-conservation and work simplification techniques can help relieve the symptoms of PPS, prevent further decline in function, and allow polio survivors to carry on with their lives, albeit in adapted ways.

DEFINING ENERGY CONSERVATION AND WORK SIMPLIFICATION

Neidstadt and Crepeau simply and accurately define *work simplification* as the "performance of a task in an organized, planned and orderly way, such that body motions, work load and fatigue are reduced to a minimum."[7] Webster's Dictionary defines *energy conservation* as "preservation."[8] The goal of energy conservation and work simplification is to maximize energy levels to then be used for other more meaningful tasks and to prevent fatigue. Hugh Gregory Gallagher, a noted author and polio survivor, likens endurance and muscle power to coins in a purse. He writes, "I only have so many and they will only buy so much, I must live within my means and to do this I have to economize: what do I want to buy and how can I buy it for the least possible cost?"[4] This is a wonderfully concrete way to illustrate how something as intangible as energy can be quantified. Each activity, no matter how simple, costs a coin. Tasks that

Table 1. BASIC ENERGY CONSERVATION AND PACING TECHNIQUES: FOUR EASY STEPS TO CONSERVE ENERGY
1. Pacing 2. Prioritizing 3. Planning 4. Posture

are more physically or mentally taxing cost more. When those "coins" are gone, you are essentially out of energy. Similar to any budget, it is not advisable to borrow from the next day's worth. When polio survivors use energy-conservation techniques, they are buying an activity for the least amount of coins possible (Table 1).

THE IMPORTANCE OF ENERGY CONSERVATION

Polio survivors often use more energy than their able-bodied counterparts in order to complete everyday tasks. Moreover, studies have shown that polio muscles that may test normal or good on a manual muscle test actually must work 2.5 times harder as a truly normal muscle to do the same job.[9] Additionally, muscles that polio survivors thought were not affected by the polio virus because of their "normal" strength actually may have been affected. Luna-Reyes et al. reported that the energy consumption by postpolio children with leg weakness was three times greater when a leg brace was not used.[10] Agre notes that postpolio subjects do not perform daily activities at the same relative level of effort as do other individuals.[5] Muscles affected by polio may have to work at much closer to maximal strength in order to perform activities that nonpolio subjects can easily perform at a much lower relative level of effort. Consequently, polio survivors expend an enormous amount of energy performing everyday tasks and are often unaware of this. Agre and Jubelt note that those with PPS who exert their already weakened muscles to the point of exhaustion may require 2–3 days to recover from the muscle fatigue.[11] Thus, it is imperative to address the energy output by polio survivors in order to provide relief to their overworked muscles.

Polio survivors complain of muscular weakness, leading to difficulty with the physical aspects of life and overwhelming weariness preventing them from initiating an activity or concentrating on a task for a length of time. Polio survivors often also report sudden and encompassing tiredness and the need to abruptly cease all activity. This is frequently referred to as "hitting the wall."[3–6] Halstead and Rossi reported that 43% of polio survivors experience this phenomenon.[6] This type of fatigue is most commonly experienced in the mid- to late afternoon. The authors also noted that increasing rest time and reducing overall activity could avoid this phenomenon.

Fatigue is not unique to patients with PPS; it is also known to be associated with other diseases such as multiple sclerosis, arthritis, and cardiopulmonary disorders such as chronic obstructive pulmonary disease. Energy conservation techniques are used widely in the treatment of patients with these diseases with good effect. Mathiowetz et al.[12] studied the efficacy of energy conservation education for those with multiple sclerosis and found that teaching energy-conservation and work simplification principles in a small group setting had a positive and lasting effect on patients' reported level of fatigue.[12] The study participants reported less fatigue and a greater satisfaction with their lives after incorporating energy-conservation techniques into their daily routines. Furst et al. studied rheumatoid arthritis and energy conservation and determined that the use of energy conservation techniques was quite successful with occupational therapy treatment sessions.[13]

TEACHING ENERGY CONSERVATION

Occupational therapists (OTs) use a variety of tools to evaluate the physical demands polio survivors face each day. Understanding the type of activities engaged by polio survivors allows therapists to provide specific feedback on prioritization, planning, and pacing. Therapists use their knowledge of adaptive devices, home modifications, and assistive technology to help polio survivors reduce energy expenditure and improve performance in everyday activities. Although handouts provide a wealth of information, a program that is individually tailored to the particular polio survivor is more successful. Grace Young, OT and polio survivor, developed an energy-conservation program that includes education on the neurophysiological basis of polio, the causes of excessive fatigue, and techniques to implement energy conservation for polio survivors.[14] Young notes that the key to successful lifestyle modification is patient education: "If the polio survivor does not understand his or her disorder, it is very difficult to implement necessary interventions and strategies."[14] Occupational therapists can provide this much-needed education and offer practical and helpful solutions to problems with fatigue and weakness.[15]

IMPLEMENTING AN ENERGY CONSERVATION PROGRAM

A successful energy conservation program should ideally be completed over several visits with the OT. Asking the polio survivor to make changes is often opposite to what he or she was brought up to believe. When seeking treatment, the polio survivor's goal is usually the development of an appropriate exercise program, and using energy conservation techniques is not a priority. A program that includes education on the physiologic components of polio and how the motor neurons have been affected is crucial to the basis of a successful energy conservation program. The program should include a review of a 3-day log, activity analysis of the daily tasks of the polio survivor, education on the principles of energy conservation and specific recommendations on assistive devices, home modifications, and the modification of activities to ensure they are done safely and efficiently.

Although specific recommendations on how to conserve energy are critical, providing education on the general principles of energy conservation gives polio survivors a solid foundation on which to incorporate these principles within their daily routines. Because every detail of polio survivors' energy demands cannot be explored, this information enables polio survivors to come up with their own solutions to each individual scenario (Table 2). The general principles used in our clinic were adapted from

Table 2. HELPFUL SUGGESTIONS FOR CONSERVING ENERGY

Home Modifications
- Use a raised toilet seat and shower chair.
- Keep all frequently used items within easy reach.
- Use a rolling cart to transport items.
- Install a stair glide if stairs are difficult to climb.
- Use a home cleaning service.

Car and Driving Adaptations
- Change gas pedal to left side if right leg is weak.
- Consider hand controls.
- Use cruise control in the car.
- Install an automatic car starter.
- Obtain a handicapped plate or placard.

Assistive Technology
- Install automatic door openers.
- Install automatic lights.
- Use voice-activated software.
- Consider a motorized scooter or wheelchair.

Workstation
- Use forearm supports.
- Use a headset or speakerphone.
- Use a reduced tension keyboard.
- Use a track ball instead of a mouse.

Work Simplification Tips
- Establish a work triangle with the primary project in front and all necessary supplies to the sides.
- Keep the main work area at your midline and extending no more than 12 inches from your body.
- Keep all work surfaces at a uniform height.
- Sit in a chair with a back whenever possible with feet supported.
- When standing, the height of the work surface should be at the level of your stomach.

Linda Dempster Ogden's book *OT and Cardiac Rehabilitation* (Table 3).[7] There are ten basic principals.

ORGANIZE AND PLAN YOUR DAY AHEAD OF TIME

This principle involves forward thinking and anticipating. The polio survivor must look ahead at the days coming and judge when the best time would be to complete heavy-duty tasks. Having a month-at-a-glance calendar is very useful in keeping track of obligations and days that are busier than desired. If the current day appears light and the individual has jobs that are time or labor intensive, this may be a good time to complete them. One must also keep in mind the preceding and following days. Within the current day, one must also plan accordingly. One larger task for the morning and one for the afternoon with plenty of time in between to eat and rest is the ideal schedule. Performing all the daily chores or errands in the morning may not

Table 3. TEN STEPS TO ENERGY CONSERVATION
1. Organize and plan your day ahead of time.
2. Prioritize.
3. Take frequent rest periods.
4. Pace yourself throughout the day.
5. Breathe easy.
6. Use good body mechanics.
7. Perform actives in comfortable temperatures.
8. Avoid straining and vigorous arm movements.
9. Relax.
10. Use adaptive equipment or assistive aids.

be the best solution. If the day is anticipated to be a busy one, skipping tasks that are unnecessary will conserve energy for the more important jobs lying ahead. Keeping frequently used items close at hand and using an organized, well-thought-out work-space is ideal and saves unnecessary steps.

PRIORITIZE

Prioritization is crucial to energy conservation. The emphasis should be on selecting activities that are most important to the polio survivor. Many people fear that by acknowledging their limits, they will be forced to give up the activities they love. One polio survivor reported that he no longer drove long distances or went hiking and avoided spending time with his family. He was employed full time and essentially spent all his energy completing his work duties. By mapping out his weekly routines, this patient was able to clearly see where his energy "coins" were being spent and make changes to his life in order to regain the energy to engage in his hobbies and so-cialize with his family and friends. This individual decided to begin carpooling in or-der to minimize the energy spent driving to work and began a strict work schedule en-suring he rarely worked more than an 8-hour day. By intentionally eliminating tasks that were not essential, enjoyable, or simply too "energy greedy," polio survivors are able to direct their energy to the more meaningful aspects of their lives. Determining which tasks should stay versus which should go requires close inspection of one's daily routine as to which tasks, even if they are part of a well-organized schedule, can be banished. Prioritizing encourages polio survivors to take control of their lives in a proactive and positive way.

TAKE FREQUENT REST PERIODS

The prevailing recommendation here is to alternate rest with activity. If a task is, by nature, long and arduous, it is best to separate it into smaller steps with resting in be-tween. Always schedule rest periods. One should avoid the thought that rests can be taken when the task is over because doing so is a definite avenue to overuse and fa-tigue. Rather than planning on resting after a particular task has been done, the polio survivor should strive to rest at preplanned intervals (e.g., every 30 minutes). Using an egg timer set to a predetermined time will help cue the individual to stop all activity and rest. Keep in mind that resting does not mean that one must sleep. Having a comfortable chair close by and sitting to listen to soft music also may help prevent fatigue. When at work, planning consistent lunch breaks and scheduling meetings mid-morning and mid-afternoon allows for some down time during the day. These techniques all ensure proper pacing and lead to the next principle.

PACE YOURSELF THROUGHOUT THE DAY

This is often difficult for polio survivors. There is a tendency to overdo on a good day with the result being the individual is incapacitated for several days afterward. This can turn into a vicious cycle of overuse, fatigue, and "bottoming out." Often polio survivors feel so good after a period of rest that they are anxious to use the time and race around trying to complete as much as they can. Many polio survivors do not realize they are playing catch-up on the weekends or after a busy day. Asking thought-provoking questions on how polio survivors spend their time is an opportunity to teach the art of pacing and offer them insight into habits that are less than ideal. It is optimal to avoid hitting the wall and have several more days of energy and vigor if they can adapt to a paced routine.

BREATHE EASY

Deep breathing is relaxing and improves ventilation. Respiratory problems are common in polio survivors. Often patients will complain of shortness of breath with activity.[16] It is also worthwhile to note that the arm muscles (which many polio survivors use extensively for mobility) are small and have less oxygen storage capacity; therefore, they require more frequent work from the heart and lungs to keep working. A good breathing routine in which the individual takes in a maximum and constant oxygen supply ensures that the muscles stay healthy and strong.

USE GOOD BODY MECHANICS

Assessing the posture of polio survivors is important and is often overlooked. Slumping and poor spinal alignment may cause the neck, back, and arm muscles to be overworked. Promoting good posture and alignment allows those muscles to do the job they are meant to do and not overuse other accessory muscles. If a person has a hard time sitting up, providing lumbar and lateral supports improves head and neck alignment and allows the person to have improved eye contact. Keeping arms supported when doing a task that involves upper back and arm use, such as crafts, handwork, or reading, greatly decreases the amount of energy expended. A workstation analysis is also important. Photographs of the office or work areas at home can be very helpful to both the therapist and patient. The therapist can problem solve with the polio survivor and recommend appropriate equipment that maximizes good postural alignment. Recommending ergonomic equipment such as arm supports, a telephone headset or earset, and wrist supports can reduce the amount of effort a polio survivor uses when at work, thus allowing muscles to be used for other tasks. For the most part, sitting to perform activities is recommended. Improper height of a workstation can cause neck, back, and upper extremity strain. Distributing work over several sets of muscles or alternating from the left to the right hand is also helpful.

PERFORM ACTIVITIES IN COMFORTABLE TEMPERATURES

It is well documented that one of the symptoms of PPS is cold intolerance.[3,4,6] Polio survivors often complain that air conditioners can cause them to be uncomfortable. Advising patients on proper attire for both indoors and outdoors is helpful. Some of the new materials available, such as Polartech, Gore-Tex, and microfibers, are lightweight and help with heat retention. Even flannel or fleece-lined pants and shirts are helpful in keeping one warm without adding too much weight or bulk. Dressing in layers allows the option of tailoring outfits to any type of weather. If possible, polio survivors should try to avoid heavy clothing because the added weight can sap energy. When purchasing a car, patients should install an automatic car starter and upgrade to heated seats. The body uses up more energy trying to regulate its temperature if it is too hot or cold.

AVOID STRAINING AND VIGOROUS ARM MOVEMENTS

Arm work can be more demanding on the heart than legwork. As stated previously, the heart and lungs have to work harder when patients are using their arms rather than their legs. Many times, polio survivors are unaware that the initial polio virus affected their arms. Because polio muscles need to work harder and at greater capacity to perform the same activity as muscles not affected by polio,[5,9,11] recommendations should include an appropriate nonfatiguing exercise program along with avoiding repetitive and strenuous arm movements. Dr. Julie Silver notes, "Your arms are your key to independence."[3] Minimizing the use one's arms when doing daily tasks is advisable. When using a computer, patients should consider using voice-activated software program and place their arms in forearm supports. They should take advantage of electricity. When cooking, they should use an electric mixer, can opener, food processor, and electric knife. For self-care, they should use an electric toothbrush and install a mount for the hair dryer. They should use a self-propelled vacuum cleaner to eliminate pushing a heavy object over a carpet. Pushing a manual wheelchair is a good example of strenuous arm movements, and a power wheelchair or scooter should be prescribed instead. Stairs can be strenuous on both the arms and the legs. A stair glide provides much needed relief to both the arms and the legs.

RELAX

It may be easy to tell polio survivors to relax, but it may be difficult for them to do so. Polio survivors have often told stories of how they kept up with their able-bodied counterparts and sometimes surpassed them in physical activities. Relaxation often goes against their basic beliefs; however, relaxation techniques have been proven to relieve stress and anxiety and should be included in a good rest cycle.[17] If the polio survivor has trouble with the more passive forms of relaxation such as guided imagery or relaxation tapes, more active forms of relaxation such as progressive muscle relaxation and yoga maybe good choices. Progressive muscle relaxation involves systematically contracting and relaxing the muscles of the body from head to toe, ensuring that each muscle group is relaxed. This is also an especially good form of relaxation because it teaches polio survivors to become more in tune with how their bodies are feeling. Yoga is another form of relaxation that focuses on posture, breathing, and meditation.

USE ADAPTIVE EQUIPMENT OR ASSISTIVE AIDS

The use of adaptive aids can greatly reduce energy output. One must be very careful how this subject is introduced. Frequently, polio survivors state that they are "giving in" or state that they are "not ready." Therapists must introduce this subject with empathy and tact. Some simple suggestions to make in this area include using a chair in the bathtub to allow the polio survivor to sit while bathing, a rolling cart in the kitchen to help transport food items and using adaptive equipment such as longer shoehorns and elastic shoelaces to minimize exertion with lower body dressing. Even the popular stair basket, found in many homes, is a good example of using an item to reduce energy expenditure when tidying up the home.

THE 3-DAY LOG

When teaching the principles of energy conservation, occupational therapists must encourage patients to evaluate their daily routines. This can be done very effectively through the completion of a 3-Day Activity Log in which patients record their activities and how they are feeling in 1-hour increments for 3 consecutive days (Table 4). The therapist and patient then analyze the log, and the therapist provides specific recommendations. This exercise is beneficial in many ways. First, it is a concrete and valid testament as to how busy the polio survivor is. It is also an excellent way to illustrate one of the prevailing concepts of energy conservation, which is to alternate rest with activity. Often when analyzing the log, one of the first things noted is how busy the earlier hours of the day are, followed by a distinct drop in activity in mid-afternoon. Correlating with the decrease in activity are comments of fatigue or pain. It

Table 4. ORGANIZING A 3-DAY ACTIVITY LOG
1. Ask the patient to use a notebook and write down what he or she is doing each hour of the day for 3 days.
2. Have the patient note next to the activity whether he or she is experiencing pain or fatigue and how severe it is (you can use a numeric scale for this).
3. Review the log with the patient, and using three different highlighters, mark the activities in the categories of low, moderate, and high energy.
4. Analyze the log together. Are there too many high-energy activities? Do they correlate with increased pain or fatigue?

is not uncommon to find notations of naps or rest mid-afternoon and into the early evening hours. Another benefit of the 3-day log is the ability to better analyze the activities being performed. The steps that must be taken before an actual task can be done are just as taxing as doing the task itself. Frequently, polio survivors do not take into account the work they have performed in preparation. Finally, the log allows patients to learn the importance of prioritization. Seeing the energy spent on areas less desirable to them is one of the first steps that needs to be taken to modify their lifestyles.

ACTIVITY ANALYSIS

Polio survivors may readily complain of feeling tired and at the same time resist any change in routine. A continual and careful analysis of the vocational and avocational activities polio survivors engage in on a day-to-day basis allows therapists to determine where energy is spent. Polio survivors may comment that their jobs or exercise regimens are not difficult or too taxing. However, when one accounts for how much energy is consumed completing self-care, commuting, parking, and ambulating to the office, the physical aspects of working can be more taxing than the person may have thought.

> *Case example:* Joe is a 9th grade math and science teacher who reports he is tired but doesn't feel that he works his muscles too hard. Initially, Joe stated that he sits down while he is teaching. When going through the steps of his day more thoroughly, Joe reported that he has three different computers located throughout the classroom that he uses regularly to illustrate different points but that he always sits when he gets there. With further questioning, Joe estimated that he probably gets up four to five time during a class period to move to another computer. Joe did not feel that this was a lot of work. When reminded that he teaches five classes a day for 50 minutes each, he suddenly realized how much effort he was expending. He stated, "Oh my, I did not realize how much I had been moving!"

Activity analysis breaks down each specific task into individual steps. After an activity has been closely analyzed, it is much easier to eliminate the unnecessary steps within the entire task, thereby ensuring no energy is spent frivolously.

ROADBLOCKS TO EMBRACING ENERGY CONSERVATION

Although between 62% and 89% of polio survivors complain of a new onset of fatigue and 52–85% report new difficulties with walking, many survivors are slow to make changes or adapt to their new levels of functioning.[2] From early in their lives, polio survivors were taught to keep exercising, get rid of any assistive devices, and move on with life.[3,4] Many polio survivors have overcome great odds to perform the most basic of tasks after their initial polio experience. To tell such an individual after "winning the war" that he or she must again adapt their ways can be profoundly disheartening. Historically, these individuals were faced with significant disability and trauma, often at a very young age. Those with polio were encouraged to disregard their disabilities and carry on with their life's work, be it schooling, a career, or parenting, without another regard to polio. Most notably, President Franklin Delano Roosevelt hid his disability by ensuring he had an aide on either side of him to assist with ambulation, thereby eliminating the need for a cane or crutch.[18] As a result of this frame of mind, many polio survivors developed very high standards for themselves and a strong desire to overcome their limitations and participate fully in their roles and responsibilities. Rhoda Olkin, a polio survivor and psychologist writes:

> We weathered its acute onset and then we proceeded to carry on to the best of our abilities. The prevailing motto was "use it or lose it." Use it we did. We were taught to push ourselves, not to impose or accept limits . . . Then suddenly, after a lifetime of messages that we could be anything, do anything we set our mind to, that there are no limits— after all that—we learned we had a new diagnosis: post polio syndrome. Now the motto became "conserve it to preserve it."[4]

This succinctly puts into perspective how many polio survivors present. They are often perfectionists, time and results driven, and accept few boundaries. Creange and Bruno[19] looked at the effect of type A behavior and its correlation to compliance with PPS treatment. They found that polio survivors with type A behaviors were significantly less likely to comply with a treatment program that included resting during the day, decreasing one's pace, eliminating strenuous activities, and using assistive devices. After exploring why this was true, they concluded that type A behavior is a manifestation of low self-esteem, a heightened sensitivity to criticism, and a deep-rooted belief that one should not appear disabled. Young[14] notes that the current physical problems affecting polio survivor necessitate new coping styles that are totally in conflict with those learned during the initial illness.

Another potential roadblock to the success of a treatment program incorporating energy conservation and work simplification techniques is the fact that we all lead very busy, complex lives. Multitasking is expected in this day and age. We have developed technology that allows us to virtually work at all times. With the advent of cell phones and laptops, it is common to work longer hours—even at 30,000 feet in the air. The height of the polio epidemics in the United States (and other developed countries) occurred in the early 1950s, with more than 60,000 cases reported in 1952.[3] Therefore, many polio survivors are now in their 40s, 50s, and 60s—essentially in the prime of their lives and at the pinnacles of their careers.[19] Younger survivors are frequently facing greater financial strain because their children are likely entering college. The older survivors may be facing a limited amount of years left to save for retirement and can be facing greater pressure to perform in the workplace as the workforce grows younger and more dynamic. It can be difficult to accommodate such expectations with the need to rest frequently.

For polio survivors to embrace general principles of energy conservation, it is important to understand their life roles. We all have different roles we play in our everyday world. For example, women are mothers, daughters, friends, wives, employees, and employers. Understanding polio survivors' life roles and support systems provides specialists with information on how to approach energy conservation. Creange and Bruno have shown that the compliance of polio survivors often depends on their support systems.[19] They found that a significant number of polio survivors did not request assistance from their family members even if the intervention was sure to assist in their well-being. Although studies have noted that polio survivors are married more so than other disabled populations,[14,20] their support systems may not be good. The well spouse may see the polio survivor struggling and encourage him or her to slow down or offer to complete the task, but the individual may see this as giving in or the inability to be a productive member of the family. Conversely, the spouse may say he or she understands the polio survivor's level of fatigue but may then want to shop at three or four stores during the afternoon or may become annoyed because the lawn is not mowed or the laundry is not done. Encouraging the polio survivor's spouse, partner, or other family members to come to the sessions is helpful and provides an open forum for discussion, which may lead to a better understanding between the patient and people in his or her support system. These are issues specialists must explore when interviewing polio survivors. From a treatment perspective, it is apparent that having unconditional family support offered to polio survivors is ideal but not always available.

OTHER FACTORS THAT IMPACT ENERGY LEVELS

It is well documented that fatigue is the number one complaint of polio survivors. Studies show that between 62% and 89% report fatigue as their greatest problem.[2] This fatigue can prevent polio survivors from carrying out activities that they were once able to do with little or no effort. Burger and Marincek performed a study to determine the prevalence of fatigue in those with PPS.[21] When comparing a group with PPS, 68% complained of fatigue during daily activities versus 22% in the control group. Although the polio survivors had less difficulty with bathing and dressing, they did report greater amounts of difficulty with home management and community activities such as shopping and working.[21] Willen and Grimby studied pain and disability and noted polio survivors who reported more exhaustion scored higher in the dimensions of increased pain and decreased physical mobility.[22]

Fatigue and low endurance can have many causes. With the onset of progressive weakness, polio survivors may be faced with increasingly sedentary lives. Weight gain occurs frequently.[3] Additional weight can place an undue burden on already weakened muscles. Addressing weight loss should be considered in conjunction with recommended lifestyle changes.

When polio survivors complain of fatigue, the quality of their sleep should be investigated. Reasons for poor sleep quality include mechanical obstructions; medical problems such as anemia, cancer, or heart disease; poor sleep habits; sleep apnea; and excessive stress. Normal aging can also contribute to poor sleep, with close to half of all persons older than age 65 years demonstrating apnea during their sleep cycles.[3] Those with a history of polio may have weakened respiratory muscles related to the initial polio attack.[24] Complaints of fatigue in the morning, not feeling "refreshed" after a night's sleep, and reports of snoring or restlessness are signs of sleep disorders and can cause excessive fatigue. If poor sleep patterns are caused by physiologic problems, energy conservation techniques may not be helpful, and a referral to a sleep specialist is indicated.

Another factor to consider is the polio survivor's psychological status. In her book *Post-Polio Syndrome: A Guide for Polio Survivors and their Families,* Silver writes, "The fatigue caused by depression may be confused with the fatigue caused by PPS."[3] Kemp et al. studied depression and life satisfaction and note that those diagnosed with PPS were more depressed than the control group and polio survivors without symptoms.[23] Depression often leads to low energy and fatigue. It is important that depression is addressed because it may impact the success of an energy conservation program.

CONCLUSION

The human spirit is difficult to squelch. Each polio survivor has his or her unique tale of life to tell. Over the years, polio survivors have learned to adapt to their limitations and, as a result, have usually led fulfilling lives. It is this quest for independence and autonomy that should be tapped into when educating a patient about the importance of pacing and prioritizing. Isaac Asimov said, "knowledge is indivisible."[25] By understanding the physical aspects of each activity, polio survivors can then make sound choices and have greater control over their lives. Adapting one's lifestyle is not a process that happens quickly. Similar to breaking an undesirable habit, setting priorities and incorporating energy conservation techniques is most successful when it is done gradually and ultimately at the polio survivor's discretion. Empowering people to change through the offering of knowledge is a powerful tool in the quest for continued independence.

References
1. Thoren-Jonsson A, Hedberg G, Grimby G: Distress in everyday life in people with poliomyelitis. J Rehabil Med 33:119–127, 2001.
2. Thorsteinsson G: Management of post polio syndrome. Mayo Clinic Proc 72:627–638, 1997.
3. Silver JK: Post Polio Syndrome: A Guide for Polio Survivors and Their Families. New Haven, CT, Yale University Press, 2001.
4. Halstead LS: Managing Post-Polio: A Guide to Living Well with Post-Polio Syndrome. Washington, DC, NRH Press, 1998.
5. Agre J: Local muscle and total body fatigue. In Halstead LS, Grimby G (eds): Post-polio Syndrome. Philadelphia, Hanley & Belfus, 1995, pp 35–67.
6. Halstead LS, Rossi CD: New problems in old polio patients: Results of a survey of 539 polio survivors. Orthopedics 8:845–850, 1985.
7. Neidstadt M, Crepeau E: Willard and Spackman's Occupational Therapy, 9th ed. Philadelphia, Lippincott-Raven, 1998.
8. Webster's II New Riverside Dictionary. Boston, Houghton Mifflin, 1985.
9. Perry J, Fleming C: Polio: Long-term problems. Orthopedics 8:877–881, 1985.
10. Luna-Reyes OB, Reyes TM, So FY, et al: Energy cost of ambulation in healthy and disabled Filipino children. Arch Phys Med Rehabil 69:946–949, 1998.
11. Jubelt B, Agre JC: Characteristic and management of post polio syndrome. JAMA 284:412–414, 2000.

12. Mathiowetz V, Matuska K, Murphy M: Efficacy of an energy conservation program for persons with multiple sclerosis. Arch Phys Med Rehabil 82:449–456, 2001.

13. Furst GP, Gerber LH, Smith CC, et al: A program for improving energy conservation behaviors in adults with rheumatoid arthritis. Am J Occup Ther 41:102–111, 1987.

14. Young GR: Energy conservation, occupational therapy and the treatment of post polio sequelae. Orthopedics 14:1233–1239, 1991.

15. Young GR: Occupational therapy and post polio syndrome. Am J Occup Ther 43:97–103, 1988.

16. Silver JK, Aiello DD: Postpolio syndrome. In Frontera WR, Silver JK (eds): Essentials of Physical Medicine and Rehabilitation. Philadelphia, Hanley & Belfus, 2001, pp 678–686.

17. Thayer RE, Newman R, McClain TM: Self-regulation of mood: Strategies for changing a bad mood, raising energy and reducing tension. J Personality Soc Psychol 67:910–925, 1994.

18. Gallagher HG: FDR's Splendid Deception: The Moving Story of Roosevelt's Massive Disability and the Intense Efforts to Conceal It from the Public, 3rd ed. Arlington, VA, Vandemere Press, 1999.

19. Creange SJ, Bruno RL: Compliance with treatment for post polio sequelae. Am J Phys Med Rehabil 76:378–382, 1997.

20. Halstead LS: Post post polio sequelae: Assessment and differential diagnosis for post-polio syndrome. Orthopedics 14:1209–1217, 1991.

21. Burger H, Marincek C: The influence of post-polio syndrome on independence and life satisfaction. Disabil Rehabil 22:318–322, 2000.

22. Willen C, Grimby G: Pain, physical activity and disability in individuals with late effects of polio. Arch Phys Med Rehabil 79:915–919, 1998.

23. Kemp BJ, Adams BM, Campbell ML: Depression and life satisfaction in aging polio survivors versus age-matched controls: Relation to postpolio syndrome, family functioning and attitude toward disability. Arch Phys Med Rehabil 78:187–192, 1997.

24. Shanke AK, Stanghelle JK: Fatigue in polio survivors. Spinal Cord 39:243–251, 2001.

25. Asimov I: The Roving Mind. New York, Prometheus Books, 1983.

17

Aging with Polio

Dorothy D. Aiello, PT, MS, and Julie K. Silver, MD

Aging is a complex process, and skeletal muscle changes can interfere with optimal muscle function. The pathophysiology of aging skeletal muscle with a history of polio complicates normal aging issues. It makes getting older with a history of polio more difficult. Hubert et al.[1] noted that a history of polio is a risk factor for greater disability with aging. Polio survivors lose strength at a quicker rate than their age-matched peers.[2]

Comorbidities are also an issue for polio survivors. For example, they are at risk for cardiac disease, respiratory disease, aspiration, sleep dysfunction, osteoporosis, falls, fractures, and depression. Evidence supports that polio survivors are at increased risk compared with their age-matched peers for aspiration, sleep dysfunction, osteoporosis, falls, and fractures.[3–12]

Because of residual respiratory muscle weakness, restrictive respiratory disease is a known complication of polio.[3,4] This restriction is worse in obese patients because of the excess weight over the rib cage and abdominal cavity. Respiratory problems are more significant for patients with a history of bulbar polio.[3,4] Alba et al. found decreased vital capacity in a convenience sample of polio survivors ($n = 35$).[13] Thirty-three of these patients were complaining of new symptoms. In their sample, vital capacity was especially decreased for subjects with a history of smoking or a history of respiratory involvement when they initially had polio.[13]

Cardiac disease has not been specifically documented to be more of an issue for polio survivors than their age-matched peers, but research indicates that being sedentary increases the risk of cardiac disease. Therefore, sedentary polio survivors are at increased risk for heart problems. This is significant because polio survivors have more difficulty with mobility than their age-matched peers.[14,15] Alba et al.[13] ($n = 35$) and Owens and Jones[16] ($n = 22$) noted deconditioning in their convenience samples of polio survivors. Alba et al. noted more severe deconditioning in their non-ambulatory subjects.[13] Safe, appropriate exercise is recommended for polio survivors to decrease the negative effects of deconditioning.[13,16–18]

Another important aspect of cardiac fitness is lipid and lipoprotein levels. Agre et al. found hyperlipidemia in a convenience sample of polio survivors ($n = 64$) at a rate of 16 of 24 (66%) men and 10 of 40 (25%) women.[19] Based on their results, Agre et al. recommended screening polio survivors for lipid and lipoprotein disorders.[19]

Interventions to minimize the adverse affects of aging with polio are crucial to optimize function. These interventions should address both intrinsic and extrinsic factors. This chapter discusses the unique aspects of aging with polio and interventions to improve patients' health.

SKELETAL MUSCLE

Normal aging skeletal muscle loses force production ability. Starting in our thirties, arm, leg, and back strength decrease at an overall rate of 8% per decade.[20] This rate of strength decrease is not linear over the life span.[20] It is characterized by an accelerated rate of decline later in life.[20] Research indicates that this is primarily caused by decreased muscle cross-sectional area and a smaller percentage of contractile tissue in muscle.[21] Aging skeletal muscle is more likely to be injured during eccentric exercise,[22] but it has been shown that endurance and strength training of appropriate intensity can help to minimize the adverse effects of aging.[20-22]

SKELETAL MUSCLE AFFECTED BY POLIO

Klein et al. reported strength loss in polio survivors at a rate greater than expected with normal aging; they noted lower extremity flexor and extensor weakness as well as upper extremity weakness.[2] Grimby et al. examined knee flexion and extension strength in polio survivors with a history of lower extremity involvement; they noted a 20% reduction in strength over a 4–5-year period.[23]

During the acute phase of polio, motor neurons are lost and collateral sprouting of existing motor neurons occurs. Sprouts reinnervate denervated muscle fibers, resulting in larger-than-normal motor units.[24] The burden on each of these remaining motor neurons is higher than under normal conditions because fewer motor units are present. As part of the aging process, gradual loss of some motor neurons occurs.[24,25] Polio survivors are more aware of this loss because they have fewer to begin with. They have a compromised ability to compensate with collateral reinnervation compared with their peers who did not have polio.[25]

A threshold level of muscle strength is needed for achieving functional tasks. After muscles' capabilities drop below that threshold, patients become unable to perform certain tasks.[6] Polio survivors may be functioning at or close to threshold levels for some time, but it is usually only when they are below task threshold levels that they notice new weakness because they are longer be able to perform functional tasks.[24,26]

Some studies have shown that muscles in subjects who had polio are composed of a greater percentage of type I fibers than in nonpolio subjects.[27,28] Grimb et al.'s enzyme-histochemical examination of muscle biopsy samples in polio survivors with chronic muscle overuse supports this.[28] He chose to examine the resistance to fatigue in overused muscles. Because this can be measured by metabolic capacity, Grimby et al. examined the metabolic capacity in polio survivors by measuring succinate dehydrogenase (SDH), a marker for mitochondrial enzyme activity and calcium-stimulated myofibrillar ATPase, a marker for adenosine triphosphate (ATP) utilization.[28] In type I muscle fibers, the SDH activity was lower and the calcium-stimulated ATPase activity was higher in postpolio patients versus controls subjects. The ratio of SDH to ATPase activity may be a predictor of muscle fatigue resistance because it suggests a loss of aerobic enzyme activity and greater reliance on anaerobic metabolic capacity, which is a highly fatiguable energy source.[28]

According to this study, "in prior polio patients, residual muscle was used on an all-or-nothing basis and there was no room for a fiber differentiation."[28] Although the muscle fibers were primarily classified as type I, their characteristics were more consistent with type II fibers.[28] Polio survivors' muscle fibers were noted to have good force output ability but very limited endurance.[28,29]

In polio survivors, muscle fatigue has also been attributed to chemical instability resulting in impaired neuromuscular transmission.[30,31] Tam et al. recently conducted a study that supported this theory.[32] The study showed "a link between this progressive muscle weakness and the increased jitter [on electromyography] indicative of synaptic instability and impaired neuromuscular transmission."[32]

ASPIRATION

According to videofluoroscopic studies, most patients with postpolio syndrome (PPS) have swallowing difficulty.[6] This is true of those with and without bulbar involvement.[33] It is of note that about 50% of them are asymptomatic.[7]

Because the risk of aspiration pneumonia and choking is life threatening, these patients should be referred to speech therapy for proper exercise and dietary guidelines. For safety, they and their loved ones should be trained in the Heimlich maneuver.

SLEEP DYSFUNCTION

Sleep dysfunction has been linked to an increased risk of cardiopulmonary disease.[8] The most common types of sleep dysfunction are sleep apnea (obstructive, central, mixed), central hypoventilation, and restless leg syndrome. Nocturnal respiration can be a problem, even for patients with normal daytime respiration.[9] This is partially because rapid eye movement (REM) sleep comprises about 20% of the sleep cycle and intercostal muscles and accessory respiratory muscles are not active during REM sleep.[9]

In normal subjects, there is a specific sequence of events that occurs before REM sleep. This sequence was studied in polio patients with and without a history of bulbar involvement. In those with past bulbar involvement, the latency between events was significantly longer than those without bulbar involvement.[34] This may be because of damage of the pontine tegmentum that has resulted in prolonged neuron recruitment time.[34] Central sleep apnea is more likely to be present in patients who have had bulbar polio because of possible damage to the medullary area of the brain stem where there are neurons responsible for respiration.[35]

The statistics in regard to frequency of sleep dysfunction vary. In the general population, there is a wide range of values based on how the sample was selected (e.g., medical history, age, weight, gender). In normal subjects, increased age is associated with increased risk of sleep dysfunction.[8] The lowest value reported in normal individuals is 4% for middle-aged adults.[36] It is suspected that there may be a greater incidence of sleep-disordered breathing in postpolio individuals compared with their age-matched peers because of intrinsic muscle weakness of the larynx and damage to the respiratory control centers from the acute polio viral infection.[8] Labanowski et al. ($n = 60$) studied subjects with neuromuscular disease and found that 42% had sleep-disordered breathing.[9] Cosgrove et al. reported that sleep disturbance affected 31% of their postpolio patient sample.[37] Van Kralingen et al. ($n = 43$) reported that approximately 50% of their postpolio patients had sleep complaints, including "tiredness on waking up and during the day, headache on waking up, daytime sleepiness and restless legs. These complaints were significantly higher compared with the control group."[38]

Dean et al. studied 10 patients with PPS who all tested positive for sleep apnea.[10] In this sample, central sleep apnea was six times more common in patients with a history of bulbar polio, and central sleep apnea was more common during non-REM (NREM) sleep than REM sleep.[10] In Hsu and Staats' sample of 35 postpolio patients, sleep apnea was most notable during REM sleep, which they related to decreased skeletal muscle tone during REM sleep.[39] They found snoring and obesity to be correlated with obstructive sleep apnea. Hypoventilation tended to be associated with diffuse neurologic deficits and scoliosis.

For treatment of sleep-disordered breathing, polio survivors should be referred to sleep specialists who will determine the proper nocturnal oxygen supplementation, if needed. Continuous positive air pressure (CPAP) and bilevel positive airway pressure (BiPAP) are sometimes used to improve oxygen levels. Determining proper settings and the best mask type to use are very important. Treatment of sleep apnea can markedly decrease complaints of fatigue.[3,4]

Excessive nocturnal movement can also cause patients to complain of fatigue. In a sample of polio survivors, "63% of the 676 respondents reported that their muscles did twitch and jump during sleep and 52% said that their sleep was disrupted by twitching."[40] Abnormal movements in sleep include restless leg syndrome, periodic limb movements, and generalized random myoclonus. In a sample of normal elderly individuals (64 years), 34% reported abnormal movement in sleep[41] compared with 63% in a sample of polio survivors (with an average age of 52 years).[42] Van Kralingen et al. surveyed polio survivors ($n = 38$) and control subjects ($n = 74$) for sleep complaints.[38] A total of 25% of the polio survivors complained of abnormal sleep movements compared with 3% of control subjects.

Restless leg syndrome (RLS) has been associated with iron deficiency, specifically measured by ferritin levels. Treatment for this is oral iron supplementation to raise the ferritin level above 50 ng/mL.[43] Medications that can be considered for RLS treatment are dopamine agonists, opiates, and neurontin.[43] Short-acting benzodiazepine may also be used to treat patients with abnormal sleep movements in general.[40]

OSTEOPOROSIS, FALLS, AND FRACTURES

Polio survivors are at increased risk for osteoporosis, falls, and subsequent fractures compared with age-matched peers.[3–5,11,12] Enhancing bone mass and decreasing fall risk have been shown to decrease the risk of osteoporotic fractures.[44]

Osteoporosis is important to screen for because of the increased fracture risk associated with low bone mineral density (BMD).[44,45] In the femoral neck, fracture risk is approximately four times increased for the first standard deviation (SD) below young adult mean values for normal bone density; for the second SD below, it is 10 times increased (and < 2 SD, fracture risk increases exponentially).[46]

Interestingly, in premenopausal women, exercise during adolescence and early adulthood was a better indicator of BMD than recent activity.[45] Because many polio survivors had polio during young adulthood, this might be significant. It may indicate increased risk for low BMD, especially for people who had polio during adolescence and early adulthood.

Geusens et al. found that 15% of their sample of postmenopausal women had osteoporosis.[47] Nineteen percent reported one or more falls during the past year, and 1.8% had a fracture during the past year.[47] The women at highest risk for fracture were those who had both osteoporosis and had a fall within the past year.[47] For polio survivors, there may also be additive factors that contribute to fracture risk. Further studies are needed to examine polio survivors and determine what combination of factors represents their greatest fracture risk.

Kawada et al. found that in severely disabled persons, increased BMD was positively correlated with decreased fracture risk.[48] They also found that use of anticonvulsants was linked with low BMD.[48] The findings from Kawada et al.'s study supports increasing BMD as important to decrease fracture risk.

Because BMD is positively correlated with strength,[44,46,49] muscle strengthening is one of the appropriate interventions for osteoporosis. However, strengthening in polio survivors is not always possible because of paralysis, or it may be contraindicated. Treatment recommendations to improve BMD also include weight-bearing exercises, increased dietary calcium and vitamin D, and medication.[45]

A variety of possible appropriate medications may improve BMD. In a case study of a 57-year-old male polio survivor, alendronate sodium (Fosamax) was shown to significantly improve his BMD scans.[50] After approximately 3 years of use, his repeat scans showed a 7% increase in lumbar BMD and the left femoral neck a 4% increase in BMD.[50] This is statistically significant, and research to develop new and improved medications is ongoing.

Iwamoto et al. studied postmenopausal women ($n = 35$) who were given cyclical etidronate treatment after stopping exercising. They found that this prevented or restored bone loss in the absence of exercise.[51] Because polio survivors may have a limited ability to exercise, this medication may be considered for them as well.

A dangerous combination is falling and osteoporosis. According to the National Center for Injury Prevention and Control, falls rank first as the cause of injury related death for people older than 65 years in the United States.[52] The force generated by a fall from a standing position is two to three times greater than necessary to fracture the hip of an average person older than age 65 years.[53] Osteoporotic fractures are associated with high health costs, marked disability, and increased risk of death.[54–57] One year after hip fracture, 40% of people are not able to walk independently as they did before the fracture.[58]

Silver and Aiello found polio survivors ($n = 233$) at high risk of falls. Sixty-four percent reported falling within the past year, and 35% reported a history of at least one fracture caused by a fall.[11] Comparatively, in community-dwelling elders (age > 65 years), approximately 30% fall each year; of those falls fewer than 1 in 10 results in a fracture.[59] This is a significant difference, especially because the average age of Silver and Aiello's study participants was 58 years.[11]

Decreased single leg stance time, decreased sit-to-stand time, and lower extremity weakness have been associated with falling in community-dwelling elders.[60] Both intrinsic and extrinsic factors contribute to fall risk in polio survivors.[61] Extrinsic factors are primarily home hazards such as a wet floor or a raised doorway threshold.[61] Tripping has been found to be predictive of falling in polio survivors.[11] Lower extremity weakness and increased postural sway on foam (with eyes open) were also correlated with falling in polio survivors.[62] Therefore, interventions to reduce falls in polio survivors should include exercise prescription; gait and balance training; orthotic assessment; and patient education, including home safety.[3,4,5,11,61] Education for safety may include a videotape such as *Safe at Home* that explains some basic home modifications.[63]

Day et al. studied community-dwelling elders and found group exercise to be the best intervention to decrease fall risk.[64] Home hazard management and vision management also decreased fall risk.[64] A study by Robertson et al. found individualized home exercise programs reduced falls in elderly individuals by 35%.[65] It is recommended that several treatment options be addressed to aid in minimizing fall risk.

Fall prevention is a key to minimize fracture risk. But if a person does fall, what decreases fracture risk? As already discussed, increased BMD decreases fracture risk. Recently, there has been a great deal of discussion regarding the possible effectiveness of hip protectors as a measure to decrease fracture rate.

There are two types of hip protectors. One pads the lateral hip area with a soft energy-absorbing material, and the other uses a semirigid material that diverts forces to the surrounding muscles and soft tissue.[66] The soft padded type is the one most commonly in use.

It is estimated that the lifetime risk of hip fracture is approximately 14% in postmenopausal women and about 6% in men. This risk for fracture increases exponentially with increased age.[67] Theoretically, in a fall to the side, padding the lateral hip may reduce fracture risk by helping to dissipate the impact of the fall.[68] In an unprotected fall, the force on the hip is 35% of the body weight.[68] Among nursing home residents, the incidence of falling on the hip is about 290 falls per 1000 person/years, and approximately 24% of these falls lead to hip fractures.[68] Hip protectors have been found to decrease fracture risk in nursing home patients.[66–69] In a nursing home setting, compliance is a staff issue rather than an individual responsibility.[66]

Kannus et al. tested four different hip protectors and recorded different efficacy levels.[70] They concluded that each hip protector device should be individually evaluated and tested in randomized clinical trials to truly assess efficacy.[70] There have been instances of reported fracture in which patients were wearing properly applied hip protectors.[71]

Very little has been done in regard to studying hip protectors in community-based populations. Compliance may be a notable problem. In a study by McAughey, 49 community-dwelling patients with osteoporosis were issued hip protectors.[72] Initially, 59% used the protectors; at the 6-month follow-up, this decreased to only 35% who were at least partially compliant.[72] Reasons for noncompliance with the protectors include discomfort, too much effort, skin irritation, incontinence, too difficult to don and doff, and expenses caused by multiple pairs needed for hygiene.[72,73] Chu et al. evaluated inpatients; 47 patients had hip protectors and 49 control patients did not. Of this test group, 12.8% were compliant and only 21.3% of them wore it most of the time.[74]

Cameron et al. studied community-dwelling elderly women with a history of two falls or one fall requiring hospital treatment in the past year ($n = 69$ intervention/ hip protector and 75 controls).[75] Two adherence nurses were assigned to each intervention patient to personally assist them with compliance strategies. Part of the study design was that the nurses would call and visit more frequently if compliance decreased.[75] The nurses did not call and visit the control subjects with the same regularity. Because this visit regularity was different between the groups, results cannot be attributed to only the hip protector. At completion of the study, the intervention group was less fearful about falling; however, it is unclear what portion is caused by the nursing contact and what is caused by the hip protector use. No determination could be made about decreased fracture risk based on this study. At the 4-month follow-up, compliance was an issue. A total of 9% of subjects dropped out of the study, 8% of the subjects were completely noncomplaint, and the others were in partial compliance.[75] Partial compliance was not clarified.

Compliance with hip protector use is a problem. It may be more of an issue for community-dwelling elders who must be responsible themselves compared with caregivers in nursing home settings. Also, hip fractures are often caused by external rotation force on the neck of the femur, and hip protectors will likely not have an effect on that.[76]

There is no evidence that hip protectors decrease fracture risk in community-dwelling elders, but the theory of their absorbing impact in a lateral fall is reasonable. When taking a fall history, if a patient has a tendency to fall sideways, a hip protector may be a possible option to try to decrease fracture risk. This is an area that warrants further study. In polio survivors, fall pattern is often related to falling forward because of tripping or knee buckling or falling backward because of a loss of balance.[61] Thus, the indication for hip protector use in polio survivors may be limited.

DEPRESSION

Depression is associated with fatigue; therefore, it is an important comorbidity to rule out in polio survivors. Schanke et al. surveyed polio survivors ($n = 276$) with complaints of mild fatigue compared with severe fatigue. They discovered that patients with complaints of severe fatigue were more likely to have psychological comorbidities.[77] (For a more detailed discussion, refer to Chapter 18.)

The Short-Form 36 indicated no significant difference between polio survivors and normative scores for mental health.[59,78] Therefore, although lower scores for physical functioning have been linked to depression,[79] this is not necessarily true of polio survivors.[59,78]

CONCLUSION

For people with a history of polio, aging is more challenging. They have an increased risk for comorbidities. Additionally, significant pathophysiological changes occur in the muscle that impair function.

A comprehensive team approach to treating polio survivors is important. Both intrinsic and extrinsic factors should be addressed to optimize health. Fall prevention is a key issue for this patient population.

References
1. Hubert HB, Bloch DA, Fries JF: Risk Factors for physical disability in an aging cohort: the NHANES I Epidemiologic Followup Study. J Rheumaol 20:480–488, 1993.
2. Klein MG, Whyte J, Keenan MA, et al: Changes in strength over time in polio survivors. Arch Phys Med Rehabil 81:1059–1064, 2000.
3. Silver JK: Post-Polio Syndrome: A Guide for Polio Survivors and Their Families. New Haven, CT, Yale University Press, 2001.
4. Silver JK, Aiello DD: Post-polio syndrome. In Frontera WR, Silver JK (eds): Essentials of Physical Medicine and Rehabilitation. Philadelphia, Hanley & Belfus, 2001, pp 678–686.
5. Silver JK, Aiello DD: What internists need to know about post-polio syndrome. Clevel Clin J Med 69:704–712, 2002.
6. Jones B, Bucholz DW, Ravich WJ, Donner MW: Swallowing dysfunction in the postpolio syndrome: A cinefluorographic study. Am J Roentgenol 158:283–286, 1992.
7. Mahgoub A, Cohen R, Rossoff LJ: Weakness, daytime somnolence, cough, and respiratory distress in a 77-year-old man with a history of childhood polio. Chest 120:659–661, 2001.
8. Bach JR, Alba AS: Pulmonary dysfunction and sleep disordered breathing as post-polio sequelae: Evaluation and management. Orthopedics 14:1329–1337, 1991.
9. Labanowski M, Schmidt-Nowara W, Guilleminault C: Sleep and neuromuscular disease: Frequency of sleep-disordered breathing in a neuromuscular disease clinic population. Neurology 47:1173–1180, 1996.
10. Dean AC, Graham BA, Dalakas M, Sato S: Sleep apnea in patients with post-polio syndrome. Ann Neurol 43:661–664, 1998.
11. Silver JK, Aiello DD: Polio survivors: Falls and subsequent injuries. Am J Phys Med Rehabil 81:567–570, 2002.
12. Silver JK, Aiello DD: Polio survivors: Low bone mineral density in males [unpublished]. 2003.
13. Alba A, Block E, Adler JC, Chikazunga C: Exercise testing as a useful tool in physiatric management of the post-polio survivor. Birth Defects 23:301–313, 1987.
14. Nollet F, Beelen A, Prins MH, et al: Disability and functional assessment in former polio patients with and with-out post-polio syndrome. Arch Phys Med Rehabil 80:136–143, 1999.

15. Halstead LS, Rossi CD: New problems in old polio patients: Result of survey of 539 polio survivors. Orthopedics 8:845–850, 1985.

16. Owen RR, Jones DD: Polio residuals clinic: Conditioning exercise program. Orthopedics 8:882–883, 1985.

17. Agre JC: The role of exercise in the patient with post-polio syndrome. Ann N Y Acad Sci 753:321–334, 1995.

18. Jones DR, Speier J, Canine K, et al: Cardiorespiratory responses to aerobic training by patients with postpoliomyelitis sequelae. JAMA 261:3255–3288, 1989.

19. Agre JC, Rodriguez AA, Sperlina KB: Plasma lipid and lipid concentrations in symptomatic post-polio patients. Arch Phys Med Rehabil 71:393–394, 1990.

20. Thompson LV: Skeletal muscle adaptions with age, inactivity and therapeutic exercise. J Orthop Sports Phys Ther 32:44–57, 2002.

21. Williams GN, Higgins MJ, Lewek MD: Aging skeletal muscle: Physiologic changes and the effects of training. Phys Ther 82:62–68, 2002.

22. Warren GL, Ingalls CP, Lowe DA, Armstrong RB: What mechanism contribute to the strength loss that occurs during and in the recovery from skeletal muscle injury? J Orthop Sports Phys Ther 32:58–64, 2002.

23. Grimby G, Hedberg M, Henning G: Changes in muscle morphology, strength and enzymes in a 4–5 year follow-up of subjects with poliomyelitis sequelae. Scand J Rehabil Med 26:121–130, 1994.

24. Halstead LS: Managing Post-Polio: A Guide to Living Well with Post-Polio Syndrome. Washington, DC, NRH Press, 1998.

25. Nordgren B, Falck B, Stalberg E, et al: Postpolio muscular dysfunction: Relationships between muscle energy metabolism, subjective symptoms, magnetic resonance imaging, electromyography and muscle strength. Muscle Nerve 20:1341–1351, 1997.

26. Gandevia SC, Allen GM, Middleton J: Post-polio syndrome: Assessments, pathophysiology and progression. Disabil Rehabil 22:38–42, 2000.

27. Maselli RA, Wollmann R, Roos R: Function and ultra-structure of the neuromuscular junction in post-polio syndrome. Ann N Y Acad Sci 753:129–137, 1995.

28. Grimby L, Tolback A, Muller U, Larsson L: Fatigue of chronically overused motor units in prior polio patients. Muscle Nerve 19:728–737, 1996.

29. Allen GM, Gandevia SC, Neering IR, et al: Muscle performance, voluntary activation and perceived effort in normal subjects and patients with prior poliomyelitis. Brain 117:661–670, 1994.

30. Dalakas MC: Pathogenetic mechanisms of post-polio syndrome: Morphological, electrophysiological, virological, and immunological correlations. Ann N Y Acad Sci 753:167–185, 1995.

31. Cashman NR, Maselli R, Wollmann RL, et al: Late denervation in patients with antecedent paralytic poliomyelitis. N Engl J Med 317:7–12, 1987.

32. Tam SL, Archibald V, Tyreman N, Gordon T: Effect of Exercise on stability of chronically enlarged motor units. Muscle Nerve 25:359–369, 2002.

33. Dowlaniuk M, Schentag C: Dysphagia in individuals with no history of bulbar polio. Ann NY Acad Sci 753:405–407, 1995.

34. Siegel H, McCutchen C, Dalakas MC, et al: Physiologic events initiating REM sleep in patients with the post-polio syndrome. Neurology 52:516–522, 1999.

35. Chasens ER, Umlauf M, Valappil T, Singh KP: Nocturnal problems in post-polio syndrome: Sleep apnea symptoms and nocturia. Rehabil Nurs 26:66–71, 2001.

36. Attarian H: Sleep and neuromuscular disorders. Sleep Med 1:3–9, 2000.

37. Cosgrove JL, Alexander MA, Kitts EL, et al: Late effects of Poliomyelitis. Arch Phys Med Rehabil 68:4–7, 1987.

38. Van Kralingen KW, Ivanyi B, van Keimpema AR, et al: Sleep complaints in post-polio syndrome. Arch Phys Med Rehabil 77:609–611, 1996.
39. Hsu AA, Staats BA: "Postpolio" sequelae and sleep-related disordered breathing. Mayo Clin Proc 73:216–224, 1998.
40. Bruno RL: Abnormal movements in sleep as a post-polio sequelae. Am J Phys Med Rehabil 77:339–343, 1998.
41. Ancoli-Israel S, Kripke DF, Mason W, Kaplan OJ: Sleep apnea and periodic limb movement in an aging sample. J Gerontol 40:419–425, 1985.
42. Lugaresi E, et al: Good and poor sleepers: An epidemiological survey. In Guilleminault C, Lugaresi E (eds): Sleep/wake Disorders: Natural History, Epidemiology, and Long-Term Evolution. New York, Raven Press, 1983, pp 145–155.
43. Allen RP, Earley CJ: Restless legs syndrome: A review of clinical and pathophysiologic features. J Clin Neurophysiol 18:128–147, 2001.
44. NIH Consensus Development Panel on Osteoporosis: Osteoporosis prevention, diagnosis and therapy. JAMA 285:785–795, 2001.
45. Brecher LS, Pomerantz SC, Snyder BA, et al: Osteoporosis prevention project: A model multidisciplinary educational intervention. J Am Osteopath Assoc 102:327–335, 2002.
46. World Health Organization: [Information pamphlet]. Geneva, WHO, 2000.
47. Geusens P, Autier P, Boonen S, et al: The relationship among history of falls, osteoporosis, and fractures in postmenopausal women. Arch Phys Med Rehabil 83:903–906, 2002.
48. Kawada T: Factors influencing bone fractures in severely disabled persons. Arch J Phys Med Rehabil 81:424–428, 2002.
49. Gazit D, Zilberman Y, Ebner R, Kahn A: Bone loss (osteopenia) in old male mice results from diminished activity and availability of TGF-B. J Cell Biochem 70:478–488, 1998.
50. Silver JK, MacNeil JR, Aiello DD: Effect of Fosamax on bone density in a male polio survivor: A case report [abstract]. Arch Phys Med Rehabil 81:1329, 2001.
51. Iwamoto J, Takeda T, Ichimura S: Beneficial effect of etidronate on bone loss after cessation of exercise in postmenopausal osteoporotic women. Am J Phys Med Rehabil 81:452–457, 2002.
52. Cook As, Baldwin M, Polissar NL, Gruber W: Predicting the probability for falls in community-dwelling older adults. Phys Ther 77:812–819, 1997.
53. Birge SJ: Can falls and hip fracture be prevented in frail older adults? J Am Geriatr Soc 47:1265–1266, 1999.
54. Kannus P, et al: Genetic factors and osteoporotic fractures in elderly people: Prospective 25-year follow-up of a nationwide cohort of elderly Finnish twins. Br Med J 319:1334–1337, 1999.
55. Melton LJ 3d: Hip fractures: A worldwide problem today and tomorrow. Bone 14:51–58, 1993.
56. Cooper C, Atkinson EJ, Jacobsen SJ, et al: Population-based study of survival after osteoporotic fractures. Am J Epidemiol 137:1001–1005, 1993.
57. Kannus P, Parkkari J, Niemi S: Age-adjusted incidence of hip fractures. Lancet 346:50–51, 1995.
58. Ioannidis G, Papaioannou A, Adachi JD: Quality of life impacts osteoporotic fracture outcomes. Biomechanics (June):27–34, 2002.
59. Gillespie LD, Gillespie WJ, Robertson MC, et al: Interventions for preventing falls in elderly people. Cochrane Database Syst Rev (3):CD000340, 2001.
60. MacRae PG, Lacourse M, Moldavon R: Physical performance measures that predict faller status in community-dwelling older adults. JOSPT 16:123–128, 1992.

61. Aiello DD: Polio Survivors: A Comparison of Fallers versus Non-fallers on a Functional Task and a Disability Measure. Ann Arbor, MI, UMI Dissertation Services, Bell & Howell Company, 2001, pp 1–49.

62. Lord SR, Allen GM, Williams P, Gandevia SC: Risk of falling: Predictors based on reduced strength in persons previously affected by polio. Arch Phys Med Rehabil 83: 757–763, 2002.

63. Safe at Home [videotape]. Framingham, MA, IRCP, 2002. Available online at www. bobvila.com or www.polioclinic.org.

64. Day L, Fildes B, Gordon I, et al: Randomised factorial trial of falls prevention among older people living in their own homes. Br Med J 325:1–6, 2002.

65. Robertson MC, Campbell AJ, Gardner MM, Devlin N: Preventing injuries in older people by preventing falls: A meta-analysis of individual-level data. J Am Geriatr Soc 50: 905–911, 2002.

66. Cameron IA: Hip protectors: Prevent fractures but adherence is a problem. Br Med J 324:375–376, 2002.

67. Lauritzen JB: Hip fractures: incidence, risk factors, energy absorption, and prevention. Bone 18(Suppl):65–75, 1996.

68. Lauritzen JB: Hip fractures: Epidemiology, risk factors, falls, energy absorption, hip protectors and prevention. Dan Med Bull 44:155–168, 1997.

69. Srivastava M, Deal C: Osteoporosis in elderly: Prevention and treatment. Clin Geriatr Med 18:529–555, 2002.

70. Kannus P, Parkkari J, Poutala J: Comparison of force attenuation properties of four different hip protectors under simulated falling conditions in the elderly: An in vitro biomechanical study. Bone 25:229–235, 1999.

71. Cameron ID, Kurrle SE, Cumming RG, Quine S: Proximal femoral fracture while wearing correctly applied hip protectors. Age Ageing 29:85–86, 2000.

72. McAughey JM: Acceptability of hip protectors. Br Med J 324:1454, 2002.

73. Van Schoor NM, Deville WL, Bouter LM, et al: Acceptance and compliance with external hip protectors: a systemic review of the literature. Osteoporos Int 13:917–924, 2002.

74. Chu LW: Compliance with hip protectors is a problem for Chinese geriatric patients in Hong Kong. Br Med J 324:7334, 2002.

75. Cameron ID, Stafford B, Cumming RG, et al: Hip protectors improve falls self-efficacy. Age Ageing 29:57–62, 2000.

76. Thakur R: Hip protectors: An orthopedic perspective. Br Med J 324:7335, 2002.

77. Schanke AK, Stanghelle JK, Anderson S, et al: Mild versus severe fatigue in polio survivors: Special characteristics. J Rehabil Med 34:134–140, 2002.

78. Ware JE, Snow KK, Kosinski M, Gandek B: SF-36 Health Survey: Manual and Interpretation Guide. Boston, The Health Institute, 1993.

79. Carson AJ, Ringbauer B, MacKenzie L, et al: Neurological disease, emotional disorder, and disability: They are related: A study of 300 consecutive new referrals to a neurology outpatient department. J Neurol Neurosurg Psychiatry 68:202–206, 2000.

Psychological Well-being of Polio Survivors

Claire Z. Kalpakjian, PhD, Sunny Roller, MA, and
Denise G. Tate, PhD

Before the late 1980s, comparatively little was written on polio's psychological effects. Millions of children and adults had to live with its devastating long-term consequences, yet pedagogic interests lay elsewhere. Literature written before the advent of the polio vaccines recognized the psychological impact of polio and the resilience of polio survivors. However, a brief search of three academically prominent databases (e.g., Web of Science, Medline, Psychinfo) from 1900 to 2002 using key words *psychological* and *psychosocial* reveals a paucity of peer-reviewed publications from the mid-1950s until the early 1980s.

This gap reflects what many polio survivors believe is a lack of interest in their lifelong disability experience after the advent of the Salk vaccine in 1955. As reported by Halstead, with the declaration that polio had been conquered, its survivors began to fade from national awareness in the United States.[1] The belief that polio was a static disease also fueled dismissal of problems by the medical community. Many polio survivors who appeared on their doctors' doorsteps in the early 1980s with reports of new pain, weakness, and unaccustomed fatigue were told their complaints were "all in their heads." Thus, they faced a double burden—not only did their complaints fall on deaf ears, but the loss of often hard-won physical functioning and independence was unexpected and frightening.[2]

Interest in the psychological well-being of polio survivors experiencing later effects of the disease began to reemerge in the late 1980s after many of them coalesced both nationally and internationally to demand recognition. They had initiated a robust sociopolitical movement to address their new, unexpected issues, building local support groups, state-level nonprofit organizations, and an International Polio Network in St. Louis, Missouri.

One important result of polio survivors' collective rally for validation was that key physicians, now known as medical pioneers in the postpolio field, agreed to give a name to this new constellation of symptoms (e.g., pain, weakness, and fatigue). These medical designations have become known as *polio sequelae, the late effects of polio,* or *postpolio syndrome* (PPS). In concert with validation from the medical community, studies on the psychological reactions to postpolio problems began to appear more frequently. Today, these empirical investigations are still relatively few, but their importance to the field of rehabilitation as a theoretical model for adjustment to other chronic illnesses and disability has been widely recognized (Fig. 1).

Well-being refers to optimal psychological functioning and experience.[3] Psychological well-being, in theory, can encompass low levels of emotional distress, high levels of life satisfaction, and the use of effective coping strategies in adapting to change. *Coping* denotes goal-directed behavior in response to a situation that is perceived as threatening, harmful, or challenging. *Emotional distress* (ED) refers to negative affect or mood states, such as depression, dysphoria, and anxiety, or a negative coping response to stress. *Life satisfaction* (LS) refers to the cognitive, subjective assessment of one's life. Disturbance in these areas has the potential to compromise both the psychological and physical health and coping of polio survivors.

This chapter reviews the body of literature related to the psychological well-being of polio survivors, including the original polio experience, psychological characteristics and issues, coping and adaptation strategies, and psychological treatment and interventions. The following is presented with an emphasis on quantitative and qualitative empirical research conducted during the past 20 years. Some early work during the epidemics of the mid-20th century is also referenced to give a contextual framework for current research. Although this chapter focuses on empirical research, commentaries and anecdotal literature are highlighted when they provide critical insight into polio survivors' psychosocial experience.

THE ORIGINAL POLIO EXPERIENCE

Early commentaries written during the polio epidemics of the 1940s and 1950s reflect a deep understanding of the emotional impact of polio on acutely ill patients.[4,5] Anecdotal reports and case histories describe powerful and traumatic early polio experiences of many survivors. For example, 75% of the participants in Wen-

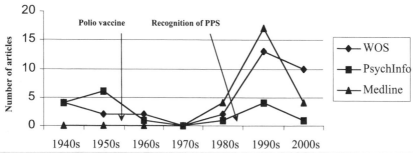

Figure 1. Articles found in databases with focus on psychological aspects of polio. WOS = Web of Science, 1945 to present; PsychoInfo, 1900 to present; Medline, 1966 to present.

nenberg and Ahlstrom's qualitative study said that the sudden separation from their loved ones, illness, and rehabilitation were traumatic.[6] The reemergence of a disease once thought to have been conquered and its potential to trigger early memories of it has been cited as making a substantial contribution to diminished psychological well-being experienced by polio survivors,[2,7–10] yet few empirical studies account for this.[11]

Silver suggests that early repression of anger, self-pity, and grief propelled polio survivors to move forward, but a return of problems later in life can bring these feelings to the surface.[12] The emergence of these early memories has also been described as evoking feelings of despair, guilt, and powerlessness.[13] For example, Kohl[14] observed that polio survivors in her study formed early associations between productivity and love and acceptance. Reducing productivity demanded by changes in physical functioning often elicited feelings of worthlessness, fear of abandonment, and loss of love.[14]

Many polio survivors have reluctantly embraced adapting to new, unexpected health problems after years of stability. Responses to this challenge have ranged from initial expressions of outrage and alarm at having to deal with this often difficult turn of events[15] to the international, sociopolitical postpolio movement and formation of a currently documented 180 polio survivor support groups providing instrumental assistance and emotional encouragement.

PSYCHOLOGICAL CHARACTERISTICS AND ISSUES

Before World War II, psychology's primary missions were curing mental illness, making people's lives more productive, and nurturing talent. But after the war, it concerned itself almost exclusively with pathology and healing.[16] Because of this, not only has the study of well-being been neglected,[3] but so have strength, resilience, and perseverance in managing the challenges imposed by chronic illness and disability. However, there has been a renewed interest in the promotion of well-being and human growth.[3,16]

Polio survivors have much to offer in furthering understanding of the relationship between well-being and disability. They have often been characterized as determined, hard working, and capable of overcoming a multitude of barriers to achieve both personal and professional success.[6,12,17,18] Scheer and Luborsky note that polio survivors learned determination, consistency, and problem solving early in adapting to disability. They suggest that "polio traditions" characterized by the expectation that polio survivors would return to the mainstream of American life facilitated this determination and drive.[18] Silver comments that Franklin Delano Roosevelt's success as a polio survivor exerted enormous pressure on other survivors to become successful, despite his taking great pains to hide his disability.[12] Wennenberg and Ahlstrom found that their sample had overwhelmingly believed that they had accomplished their ambitions in work and family life, showing "enormous determination" to overcome barriers.[6]

In discussing psychological well-being among polio survivors, two important domains should be highlighted: ED and LS.

CONCEPTUALIZATION OF EMOTIONAL DISTRESS

Emotional distress refers to negative mood states, such as depression and anxiety, that can accompany the onset or exacerbation of a chronic illness or disability. This relationship is bidirectional in that ED also can amplify the effects of medical illness.[19] In the context of chronic illness and disability, ED is typically characterized by a negative orientation toward loss that pervades the literature and clinical approaches.[20,21] As a result, few studies come from a positive perspective; although strength and resilience are acknowledged in studies of polio survivors, they seem more an afterthought in the interpretation of findings.

Negative expectations also can have a bearing on approaches to care,[22] such as health care providers expecting or even encouraging ED.[23,24] One example of this negative orientation is Kuehn and Winter's suggestion that low rates of ED in their sample might be attributed to denial, with no attempt to give a positive interpretation.[25] Acknowledging this negative perspective, Liechty calls for learning more about polio survivors' strengths, adaptive coping, and effective lifestyle modifications.[26]

METHODOLOGIC CONSIDERATIONS

The definition or operationalization of ED in studies of polio survivors has been inconsistent and in some cases is even absent.[26] The importance of a clear definition and criteria for "caseness" (i.e., identifying those who meet criteria for mood disorder) cannot be overstated when attempting to establish prevalence rates. In fact, overestimations or underestimations of depression or anxiety (or both), coupled with a negative bias, have the potential to substantially impact the recognition and treatment of ED in polio survivors.

The diversification among the types of measures of mood states used also complicates the assessment of ED. Many mood measures are developed on nondisabled samples and include somatic symptoms such as poor appetite, weight loss or gain, or sleep disturbance. However, many of these somatic complaints can also be directly related to the disabling condition or the disease itself and not to mood states,[27,28] and scores on measures that contain such items can be misleading when assessing ED among polio survivors.[26] Supporting this contention, Frank and colleagues found that the core element of depression among a sample of individuals with chronic illness and disability and a nondisabled control group was negative self-evaluation, depressed affect, and suicidal ideation—not somatic complaints.[27]

Representativeness of samples is another important consideration in interpretation of findings. Many samples are drawn from postpolio clinics and may not be representative of the broader spectrum of polio survivors, particularly those who are not experiencing problems.[26] Similarly, the use of nondisabled comparison groups is a useful way of understanding the unique contribution of PPS to ED. For example, Kemp et al. found no difference between polio survivors and age-matched, nondisabled control subjects on a depression questionnaire.[28]

Early studies of psychological reactions of polio survivors to PPS symptoms were conducted at a time when PPS was new and poorly understood, which by itself could influence psychological reactions.[8,29] As such, the timing of a study has been cited as an important consideration in the assessment of the emotional response to PPS.[26,29] Timing is particularly problematic in cross-sectional studies because individuals may experience less distress over time as they gradually adapt to new limitations.[30] Longitudinal studies provide a more comprehensive assessment of ED in polio survivors given the dynamic nature of PPS.[6]

A few studies have used a longitudinal design to assess ED in polio survivors across time. Schanke followed individuals who had initially been inpatients in a postpolio program and who were now living in the community.[29] At 3–5-year follow-up, they had lower levels of overall ED, a majority had an improved attitude toward their situation, and approximately 50% thought that their psychological well-being had improved. Those reporting improved psychological well-being were significantly younger, reported more invisible disability, and had experienced greater distress 5 years earlier. Westbrook and McIlwain similarly found lower levels of anxiety, uncertainty, depression, and helplessness at a 5-year follow-up.[31]

PREVALENCE AND CORRELATES OF EMOTIONAL DISTRESS

Despite the fact that ED has received the most attention in the psychosocial polio literature,[26] prevalence estimates of ED have varied substantially. For example, Clark and colleagues[10] did not find abnormal psychological symptoms or personality characteristics in their sample, nor did Schanke.[29] However, Mullins and colleagues found that more than 50% of their sample evidenced clinically significant levels of ED.[32] Others have found rates of 11% possible depression and 24% anxiety,[33] 15% significant depressive symptoms,[34,35] and 23% mild to moderate depressive symptoms.[36] In studies using self-report data (e.g., "Do you feel you are depressed?") versus a standardized instrument, rates of 49%[37] and 50%[8] for depression and 44%[37] and 46%[8] for anxiety have been reported.

Findings on the relationship between PPS symptoms and ED have been mixed. Some studies have found no association between PPS symptoms and ED.[8,10,28] In others, symptoms such as fatigue,[33] pain,[35,38,39] low energy,[36] poor health rating,[35] more somatic complaints,[39] and diminished physical mobility[38] were associated with elevated levels of ED. Hazendonk and Crowe compared control subjects with polio survivors with and without PPS and found that survivors with PPS had significantly higher levels of ED than did control subjects and survivors without PPS.[40] Polio survivors with and without PPS also reported significantly more feelings of anger and interpersonal conflict than controls.[40] In Westbrook and McIlwain's study, those who focused on their symptoms had more prominent feelings of helplessness, depression, and anger.[31] Polio survivors who had less initial visible disability were the most distressed with the onset of new problems.[29,41]

It is important to note that ED and PPS symptoms can have a bidirectional relationship; higher levels of ED can influence symptom reporting[10] and amplify symptoms.[19] For example, Bruno and Frick found that emotional stress was the second most frequently reported cause of fatigue and the third most frequently reported cause of muscle pain.[17] Some evidence suggests that female polio survivors may have more somatic complaints than male polio survivors,[6,10] suggesting that gender also may indirectly influence ED in polio survivors.

Schanke and colleagues found that 27% of their sample reported having been psychologically harmed by the treatment they received during acute illness.[11] They were significantly younger at polio onset, had been hospitalized longer, and had fewer parental visits and less support. Many years later, they reported significantly more pain; took more analgesics and sedatives; and had more fatigue, sleep disturbance, and nightmares. They also reported significantly higher ED, lower LS, and had less social support from their spouse or children. They also reported less efficacy in coping with PPS symptoms, were more likely to have had psychological counseling in the past, and more likely to think they would need it in the future.[11]

These mixed findings suggest that more than physical status has influence over emotional states. In fact, individual perception, attribution, and meaning have been found to be more powerful predictors of ED than objective findings in the context of illness and disability.[8,42] The unpredictability of problems associated with polio can also have an important impact on emotional adaptation.[32] For example, Tate et al. found that self-perceived lack of control over health was significantly associated with depression.[39]

Coping resources have also been associated with ED in polio survivors. Kuehn and Winters found that those who had greater coping resources evidenced lower ED.[25] Tate and colleagues similarly found that lower coping scores were associated with higher ED.[35] Other psychosocial factors such as lower satisfaction with social relationships,[29] living alone,[35] an increased number of life stressors,[29] and seeking professional[35] help also have been associated with ED. Distrust of medical personnel during acute illness[13] and a lack of understanding and support from medical personnel[8] have been associated with elevated ED.

In a recent study on the effects of a comprehensive treatment program for polio survivors, Strumse et al. found that, after completing a similar treatment program, participants in a warmer climate reported significantly less ED than those in a colder climate (both groups had significantly improved).[43] The authors suggest that a warmer climate may facilitate socialization, thereby increasing psychological well-being. Because of the mixed findings of these studies, it is difficult to reach a definitive conclusion about the relationship of ED to PPS symptoms and loss of physical functioning. However, the body of literature suggests that physical, psychological, and social or environmental factors impact ED in polio survivors; these are summarized in Table 1.

CONCEPTUALIZING LIFE SATISFACTION

More recently, psychologists adopting a positive view of health and wellness after disability have been particularly interested in studying the concept of LS of polio survivors. Diener and colleagues argue that peoples' evaluation of their lives is an indispensable aspect of positive mental health.[44] Life satisfaction's fundamental premise is that, in order to understand the well-being of an individual, it is important to directly

	Table 1. CORRELATES OF EMOTIONAL DISTRESS IN POLIO SURVIVORS	
PHYSICAL	**PSYCHOLOGICAL**	**SOCIAL OR ENVIRONMENTAL**
Fatigue[33,36]	Attributional style[66]	Living alone[35]
Pain[33,35,38,39]	Lack of perceived control	Warmer climate[43]
Poor health rating[35]	over health[35]	Lack of understanding by
Reduced physical	Low satisfaction with	medical personnel[8,13]
mobility[38]	social relationships[29]	Seeking professional help[35]
History of "hidden"	Increased number of life	
disability[11,54]	stressors[29]	
Somatic complaints[35]	Traumatic early polio	
Focus on PPS	experience[11,12]	
symptoms[31]	Coping resources[25,35]	

measure cognitive and affective reactions to his or her life.[45] In other words, LS is primarily concerned with an internal judgment of well-being, rather than objective factors. Nonetheless, early efforts to define LS in relation to disability and rehabilitation typically involved health status. These objective indicators have included impairment, disability, societal participation, independent living, and employment.[46] Research has shown, however, that objective factors alone do not account for LS among those with chronic illness or disability and, specifically, those who had polio.[22] Life satisfaction has also been shown to be influenced by personality factors such as temperament, extroversion or introversion, and optimism, as well as personality and environmental interactions.[47]

METHODOLOGIC CONSIDERATIONS

Unlike the well-established, standardized instruments typically (though not exclusively) used to measure mood states, LS instruments are highly variable in standardization. These measures vary in the combination of subjective and objective factors; length (ranging from a single item to a lengthy questionnaire); and the use of either a single global rating, individual domain ratings (e.g., financial, health, relationship), or a composite of domains. Debates exist concerning whether LS instruments capture the domains deemed important to the particular individual or whether relevant domains have been omitted. Not surprisingly, given this variability, of the eight studies on LS in polio survivors reviewed for this chapter, no two used the same instrument. Also, the quality of instrumentation ranged from being well established and standardized to not even being specified.

Comparison groups can provide a useful yardstick against which the unique impact of PPS on LS is measured, although these findings have also been mixed. For example, compared with polio survivors, control subjects had reported higher overall health and economic satisfaction.[28] Polio survivors have also reported a significantly lower LS than their nondisabled, same-gender siblings.[48] On the contrary, LS was similar between ventilator-assisted polio survivors and a control group of health care personnel and control subjects significantly underestimated survivors' LS and overestimated the burden the survivors experienced.[22]

CORRELATES OF LIFE SATISFACTION AMONG POLIO SURVIVORS

One of the first empirical studies of the psychosocial effects of polio was conducted in 1947 by Lowman and Seidenfeld.[49] They interviewed 537 individuals who had had polio as children and were currently receiving follow-up care. The majority of them were satisfied with their social lives, and those who were employed enjoyed better social adjustment in general. A minority of participants believed that their physical disability had unfavorably altered their marital plans, but the vast majority of the sample was married and engaged in productive activity.[49]

Some studies have found no relationship between lower overall LS and PPS or the level of disability caused by polio.[34] Others have found factors such as muscle and joint pain[50] and number of new health problems[51] associated with lower LS. Psychosocial factors such as social support and acceptance of disability have also been associated with LS.[29,34] Within specific domains, lower satisfaction with health,[34] physical functioning,[52] and financial situation[51] have been reported.

Although compared with control subjects, polio survivors may report lower levels of LS,[28,52] these levels themselves are not necessarily low. For example, high levels of satisfaction in domains of family life[34,52] and sexual functioning[52] have been found, and a number of studies have found generally high levels of LS and happiness among polio survivors.[21,22,49,53] The variability and relatively low number of empirical studies of LS among polio survivors make it difficult to reach definitive conclusions about factors that diminish or enhance LS, other than to say that a multiplicity of factors influences LS and more research is needed to better understand them.

COPING STRATEGIES AND ADAPTATION

Coping with polio has become a two-part process for survivors: dealing with the acute phase of polio and then, years later, dealing with the postpolio phase, which often involves a different repertoire of coping strategies than those used during the acute phase of illness.[53] This adaptation process often requires returning to rehabilitation after 20–40 years of physical stability and is sometimes referred to as postpolio "re-rehabilitation."[54]

The variability of coping styles used by polio survivors was recognized in the early polio literature. For example, in 1961, Vitsotsky and colleagues observed the coping behavior of 81 polio survivors during the acute illness through rehabilitation and follow-up.[55] Among the various strategies commonly used during these periods were tapping emotional support from friends and family, finding hope, and building relationships with other polio patients.[55]

Coping strategies reflected in both the empirical and consumer literature can generally be organized into two primary categories: problem focused and emotion focused. In addition, polio survivors have used other strategies, such as social support and spirituality-focused coping. Models of adaptation have been proposed to understand adaptation of polio survivors to PPS.[2,56] Adaptation to change also can be hampered by belief systems and ideologies formed during the early polio experience. Although more research is warranted, empirical studies, both qualitative and quantitative, suggest that polio survivors can successfully use various coping strategies to maintain and improve their health and psychological well-being.[29,53] The following sections summarize findings related to specific coping strategies reported in the literature.

PROBLEM-FOCUSED COPING

Problem-focused coping is characterized by the use of strategies to solve problems. These strategies are typically aimed at defining a problem; generating alternative solutions; weighing the costs and benefits of alternatives; choosing among them; and, finally, acting on them.[57] It differs from emotion-focused coping in that its efforts are aimed toward changing the situation rather than the perception of the situation. In general, polio survivors have been shown to use a high level of problem-focused coping.[29,58] For example, reading about PPS, subscribing to a polio survivor newsletter, and making lifestyle changes, such as home modifications, are effective coping strategies that have been used.[31]

One commonly recommended problem-focused strategy is *selection,* or restricting activity because of lost capacity. In fact, this is perhaps the most widely prescribed way of managing PPS symptoms. For example, pacing, reducing physical activity, resting,[31] and restricting leisure activities[59] have been used as effective ways of coping with new limitations. *Compensation* is meeting goals in a new way, such as by changing behaviors or using assistive devices.[60] Natterland and Ahlstrom found that, in order to successfully adapt to new limitations, a majority of their participants used new devices and "tricks" for personal care routines, mobility, and transportation needs.[61] Strategies included performing activities in a new way such as using different muscles for the same activity, using technical aids such as adapted driving controls or other assistive devices, and accepting new help from others in home management tasks.[61] Using household help and buying special furniture or equipment were very helpful.[31] Planning ahead and using new aids such as walkers and orthoses are other examples of coping strategies for polio survivors with PPS.[53]

Optimization refers to active efforts, such as exercising, to enrich one's physical reserves in order to continue functioning.[62] Comprehensive and integrated wellness programs have been suggested as a viable intervention for polio survivors to optimize their health.[63] In Strumse et al.'s dual-site study in Norway and the Canary Islands, a positive effect of a 4-week wellness program on polio survivor's emotional and physical health was found.[43] This program involved one to two sessions per week in which participants took part in adapted swimming, gymnastics, and relaxation techniques.[43]

Despite the efficacy of treatment programs for improving physical functioning, some polio survivors have been unwilling to make lifestyle changes to accommodate new limitations, which is one of the most common reasons for treatment failure.[64] Some have suggested that coping behavior adopted early in the polio experience that had bolstered determination may now prove maladaptive when there is a need to slow down and make lifestyle changes to accommodate changing capabilities.[29]

EMOTION-FOCUSED COPING

Emotion-focused coping is characterized by cognitive strategies directed at reducing ED by changing perception rather than the situation itself.[62] *Avoidance, denial,* and *distancing* have been cited as being beneficial early in coping with polio to avoid being overwhelmed, but they are less useful in later life.[55] Ahlstrom and Wennenberg found that polio survivors used distancing significantly more than a nondisabled control group,[58] but Schanke found that avoidance was one of the least used coping strategies in her sample of polio survivors.[29] Although beneficial in early adaptation, avoidance and denial can become maladaptive when polio survivors resist making lifestyle changes to accommodate their new limitations.[65]

One of the most widely used strategies of emotion-focused coping is *reappraisal.* Making positive interpretations of negative events can be an effective buffer against ED for polio survivors.[66] Those in Hansson and Ahlstrom's study coped by making great efforts to make the best out of everyday life situations.[53] Schanke found frequent use of positive reappraisal as a means of coping.[29] Tate and colleagues found that those with low ED tended to endorse positive self-acceptance and an optimistic outlook on their lives.[35]

Response shift posits that when individuals undergo changes in their health status, they may change their internal standards, values, or conceptualizations of quality of life in order to successfully manage a new disability.[67] In Westbrook and McIlwain's study, appreciation of new values and expanding life philosophies were used as a way of coping with postpolio problems.[31] Kuehn and Winters similarly found that polio survivors evidenced higher levels of philosophical coping than a nondisabled, normative sample.[25]

The influence of belief systems, often formed early in life, has the potential to hamper polio survivors' coping with lifestyle changes to accommodate functional losses. Locker and colleagues suggest that "ideologies" about disability and coping strategies established early will impact later use of technology.[68] For example, the use of crutches and braces can have significant symbolic meaning[14]; as a result, there can often be great resistance to using adaptive devices despite their beneficial impact.[64]

ADDITIONAL COPING STRATEGIES USED BY POLIO SURVIVORS

Maynard and Roller identified three coping styles polio survivors developed during acute illness, based on clinical observation and attitude surveys.[54] Although these coping styles have yet to be empirically tested and are subject to overgeneralization, anecdotal reports suggest that these descriptions resonate with many polio survivors and are worthy of further investigation. Their model describes polio survivors as *passers, minimizers,* and *identifiers,* labels that characterize typical attitudes and behaviors adopted in order to cope with mild, moderate, or severe disability. Polio survivors with a mild disability could "pass" for normal and became invested in doing so. Individuals with a more obvious disability adapted by downplaying or "minimizing" the apparent effects of the disease, such as using braces or crutches. Those who used wheelchairs or ventilators were forced to fully "identify" with their disability in order to face attitudinal and architectural barriers.

Tate and colleagues found three coping factors reflected in the strategies used by their sample of polio survivors: positive self-acceptance, information exchange, and social activism.[35] Positive self-acceptance was characterized by self-esteem, optimism, and adjustment. Information exchange reflected seeking and providing information about disability and being aware of personal needs. Social activism was characterized by participating in social activities and self-advocacy.[35]

Spiritually focused coping has received comparatively less attention in the rehabilitation literature, but interest in its salutatory effects on well-being are growing. This form of coping involves trusting and having a harmonious relationship with a transcendent dimension or "Ultimate Other" and can be nurtured by or be independent of religion.[69] In this framework, when individuals reconcile a new disability and discover their own inner resources and strengths, they realize their own inherent sense of wholeness and unity and experience a deeper meaning, sense of self, and spirituality within their lives.[70]

Although not extensively studied, some evidence suggests that polio survivors may uses spiritually focused coping. For example, Woods-Smith found that polio survivors reported a significantly greater level of spirituality than a nondisabled comparison group. Additionally, there was a significant relationship between their level of spirituality and belief in their capacity to change.[71] Sixty-two percent of Westbrook and McIlwain's sample reported that, in order to cope, they had become more spiritual people.[31]

Problems in social life have been associated with more distress in pain, physical mobility, energy, emotional reaction, and social isolation.[14,38] Kohl suggests that support systems have played an important role in adapting to polio.[14] Participants in Hansson and Ahlstrom's study noted the importance of seeking social support in coping with PPS.[53] Gender differences in social support have also been found. For example, male polio survivors have reported significantly greater social isolation than women.[10] Family members also can serve as an especially important source of both instrumental and emotional support.[53]

However, not all polio survivors are willing or able to seek emotional support from those around them. For example, many in the Westbrook and McIlwain study were reluctant to talk about postpolio issues with other people.[31] In Ahlstrom and Wennenberg's study, they were significantly less likely to seek social support compared to nondisabled control subjects.[6] Schanke and colleagues found that individuals who reported being psychologically harmed by their early polio experiences were significantly less likely to talk about polio with family and felt less supported by their spouses or children.[11]

Unfortunately, many polio survivors may not view the medical community as a useful source of social support.[7,32] Often, medical professionals are seen as lacking knowledge about the late effects of polio and experience needed to provide effective care and support. Attitudes toward the medical community as a barrier to improved health are not typically taken into account in the empirical literature, but the topic is widely discussed in the anecdotal and consumer literature and is worthy of empirical investigation. As with psychological characteristics, polio survivors display a significant variety of coping strategies, many of which contribute to their perception of well-being and positive LS. Examples of these strategies are given in Table 2.

MODELS OF ADAPTATION FOR POLIO SURVIVORS

Adjustment models are commonly used to describe the process of adaptation to chronic illness and disability. Many of these models are based on the bereavement literature, which postulates that in response to a loss, individuals pass through a linear progression of stages to a final stage of adjustment. Failure to proceed through these stages signals denial, and lock-step progression signals successful adjustment.[24]

Hollingsworth and colleagues[2] and Frick[56] describe stage models of psychological adjustment to PPS, based largely on other models of adaptation and disability. Initial shock and denial followed by a period of devaluation and sadness characterize these models. Eventually, values are reassessed and a new self-concept is shaped, culminating in a final stage of reintegration and adaptation.

Although these stage models proposed by Hollingsworth et al. and Frick may provide some guidance in understanding adjustment to PPS, similar to other stage models, they suffer from a lack of empirical validation.[20,23,29] Additionally, models based on the bereavement literature are problematic in the direct application to disability because losses associated with death are not necessarily the same as those associated with disability.[72] Similarly, Westbrook and McIlwain argue that because of the progressive and dynamic nature of PPS, "reaching acceptance of disability" or having "adjusted" postulated as an endpoint of adjustment models should be revised because adjustment is an ongoing process.[31]

Table 2. EXAMPLES OF COPING STRATEGIES USED BY POLIO SURVIVORS

PROBLEM-FOCUSED STRATEGIES	EMOTION-FOCUSED AND OTHER STRATEGIES
Reading about PPS[31]	Avoidance or denial[29,58]
Subscribing to a PPS newsletter[31]	Distancing[58,65]
Home modifications[31]	Positive reappraisal[29,35,53,66]
Lifestyle changes	Adopting or reevaluating values[25,31]
Restricting activity[31,61]	Spirituality[31,71]
Using assistive devices[61]	Expanding life philosophy[31]
Employing household help[31]	Information exchange[12,14]
Planning ahead[53]	Social activism[35]
Exercise[43]	Relationships with others; social support[14,53]
Joining a support group[31]	Relaxation and imagery[75]
Accepting help from others[61]	

Three empirical studies describe models of adaptation based on polio survivors' direct experience and not on traditional stage models. Using a qualitative method, Thoren-Jonsson describes a model characterized by a *gradual realization* of a change in abilities.[65] Initially, inattentiveness to physical changes in the body leads to *overloading* signaled by fatigue, muscle and joint pain, and anxiety. A *vicious circle* could then ensue because of continued overloading or if other ways of carrying out daily responsibilities cannot be identified. Some individuals *withdraw* when they are no longer able to maintain their usual social and occupational roles. Gradually, individuals begin to make alterations in the way they perform, facilitating flexibility and culminating in *insight* and *reorganization* of self-concepts. Thoren-Jonsson cautions that a myriad of factors influence adjustment in each individual, and as such, not every polio survivor experiences all of these phases of adjustment.[65]

Scheer and Luborsky describe a "polio trajectory" based on ethnographic research with polio survivors.[18] This trajectory refers to the natural history of polio: (1) acute infection, (2) recovery or rehabilitation, (3) functional stability, and (4) onset of secondary disability. The "polio biography" reflects a view of the individual within the context of his or her own lifetime experience and polio traditions. In this model, functional loss is not an isolated event; rather, it rests within the context of the individual's experience and is infused with meaning that is unique to that person.

In contrast to stage models, this polio trajectory is characterized by individual experience within the larger context of culture and polio traditions. Early polio traditions are characterized by viewing disability as primarily a medical problem. Polio survivors were expected to get on with their lives and return to mainstream American life. Late polio traditions are characterized by a broader understanding of the social and psychological demands of aging with polio. For many polio survivors, transition across these traditions requires examination of belief systems and expectations.[18]

Wennenberg and Ahlstrom[6] found support for Scheer and Luborsky's[18] polio trajectory in their qualitative study of 15 polio survivors and their lifetime illness experience. The polio trajectory is reflected in the temporal sequence of the illness experience described by their sample: (1) acute illness, (2) rehabilitation and restoration, (3) stability, (4) transition and functional loss, (5) living with PPS today, and (6) apprehension about the future and memories of the past. They acknowledge that although these phases represent more of the physical dimension of polio, function and psychosocial and cultural dimensions also exert their influence over them.[6]

Models arising directly out of polio survivors' experience, such as those of Thoren-Jonsson,[65] Scheer and Luborsky,[18] and Wennenberg and Ahlstrom,[6] provide an important foundation for further development of adjustment to PPS models. They are superior to stage models because of their inclusion of early polio experience and belief systems at both the individual and cultural levels. In addition, they are fluid in their application and do not require individuals to progress or lock-step through the phases. Instead, they emphasize individual experience and recognize the influence of a myriad of physical, psychological, social, and cultural factors.

Despite advancements over the more widely used stage models, these models also require further empirical validation before they can confidently be used to understand

and describe the adaptation of polio survivors. It is also important to note that mis-application of any adjustment model can hamper efforts to facilitate effective coping and reduce ED by drawing attention away from individual experience.

PSYCHOSOCIAL INTERVENTIONS AND IMPLICATIONS FOR CLINICAL PRACTICE

Early commentaries reflect an understanding that individuals with polio required not only treatment of the disease but also a holistic approach to care.[4,5,73] In 1948, Cohen asserted that the care of the whole patient, not just the disease itself, was the primary aim of the treatment team, noting a lack of attention by an overwhelmed hospital staff to the emotional needs of young polio patients.[5] In 1953, Ignatus, a self-described "ordinary priest," suggested that a rigid hierarchy, with physicians at the top and patients at the bottom, and an "exaggerated" fear that any accommodation would "spoil" polio patients only amplified their sense of helplessness.[73] He asserted that the hospital chaplain was an integral part of the treatment team helping to ensure that all efforts were directed at maximum recovery.[73] In 1955, Wendland described a psychotherapeutic group for spouses of polio patients whose own adjustment needs were being neglected.[74]

Despite this early recognition of polio's impact on psychosocial well-being, nearly 60 years later, few empirical studies have addressed psychological or psychosocial interventions to help reduce ED, improve LS, and enhance the coping skills of polio survivors.[26] Agre and colleagues suggest that psychological assessment and intervention are important for polio survivors who have difficulty making the lifestyle changes necessary for their health and well-being,[37] but Kemp et al.[28] and Kemp and Krause[34] note an "appalling" lack of treatment for polio survivors with probable depressive disorders. For example, efficacy of antidepressant medication has not been studied, nor has the effectiveness of psychotherapy. Westbrook and McIlwain found that only 8% of their sample had used counseling as a means of coping, and the majority of those found it only of "some help."[31]

Some evidence suggests that certain techniques help to reduce ED in polio survivors. For example, Tate and colleagues[75] developed a wellness program for postmenopausal polio survivors that focused on stress management techniques. Teaching relaxation and positive imagery was found to have an impact on participants' perceived sense of well-being as these skills were incorporated into their repertoire of newly acquired health behaviors.[75]

Strategies for improving psychological well-being among polio survivors, such as participation in support groups and informational networks, are frequently discussed as valuable resources in commentaries and consumer literature.[12,76] Westbrook and McIlwain found that a majority of their sample had joined a support group and found this of some help or very helpful in coping with PPS.[31] Although the efficacy of support groups in facilitating coping and reducing ED has not received much empirical investigation in the polio literature,[31] Natterlund and Ahlstrom found that individuals with muscular dystrophy experiencing progressive muscle weakness benefited from the social support of a treatment program by meeting others with the same condition and gaining a better understanding of their condition.[77] However, Kohl[14] cautions that referrals to support groups should coincide with an individual's capacity and readiness for learning.

The dearth of empirical studies on psychosocial interventions may be attributed to various factors. It may simply be the relative infancy of this line of research resumed in the late 1980s. It may be influenced by the predominant use of a medical model in PPS management, with the expectation that amelioration of physical symptoms will necessarily improve psychological well-being. Many survivors may also be resistant to change and, thus, less likely to seek help, perhaps compounded by the lack of support given to polio survivors by the medical community. This scarcity of intervention studies may also reflect Halstead's contention that polio survivors have faded from national consciousness.[1]

Sensitivity to the complex dynamics of many factors that can influence polio survivors' psychological well-being is perhaps the most important message gleaned from this body of literature. Understanding both the larger social and historical context of polio and individual experiences are critical considerations for clinicians. Scheer and Luborsky suggest that clinicians be aware of the individual's "polio biography" and the meaning he or she assigns to new functional losses.[18] Awareness of the vulnerability to the resurgence of early and potentially traumatic memories is equally critical for clinicians.[6] For example, a therapist recommending an assistive device who may not recognize the symbolic meaning of a crutch or brace can misinterpret resistance to reflect a lack of motivation or denial. A physician discussing treatment options may be suddenly faced with a patient's emotional reaction that appears to be out of proportion to the information presented.

Similarly, clinicians should also view new functional losses in the context of developmental tasks.[18] For example, a decline in energy will have different implications for someone with numerous family and work obligations than for someone who is retired with few family responsibilities. Superimposed on this developmental path is the impact of functional loss on social roles and the pursuit of present and future goals.[18] Kohl also cautions clinicians to pay close attention to the language used by the individual in describing both their experiences and themselves; by using the same kind of language, clinicians can facilitate communication without unnecessarily increasing ED.[14] Failure to recognize the influence of early polio experiences and related belief systems in situations such as these can attenuate clinicians' effectiveness.

Because of the impact of PPS symptoms on many areas of life, a comprehensive, holistic, and multidisciplinary approach to treatment is typically recommended.[2,37,52,65] Comprehensive treatment programs should also include a strong psychological component[37] because the empirical literature demonstrates that more than physical functioning and health status influence psychological well-being. Unfortunately, empirical studies suggest that few polio survivors avail themselves of psychological counseling,[31] although the reasons for this are not entirely clear. Peach and Olejnik note that polio survivors who are resistant to change may also resist psychological support to help them make beneficial changes in lifestyle.[64] That polio survivors do not use make use of psychological services in greater numbers may be related, in part, to feelings of distrust of those connected with the medical community. It may also be a matter of availability of psychologists with expertise in addressing their unique concerns.

Coping strategies used by polio survivors have been remarkably flexible; appreciating this range of strategies is important for clinicians in encouraging their use.[53,54] Scheer and Luborsky suggest that the same determination, steadfastness, consistency, and problem solving learned early by many polio survivors can be used to help them adapt to new polio-related problems.[18] Kohl offers some techniques for making lifestyle changes culled from participants, their families, and staff members.[14] They include acknowledging that a decrease in activity is a testament to self-care, rather than failure, documenting accomplishments to increase awareness of energy expenditure, and increasing direct communication with others.[14] Silver suggests that expecting to experience a range of emotions, accepting less than perfection, and taking back control are useful coping strategies.[12]

Studies of other progressive and disabling conditions have shown that having information before a change in health status, such as in progressive disease, facilitates adjustment to that change,[30] which has particular importance for polio survivors at risk for developing PPS. For example, Thoren-Jonsson[65] and Silver[12] emphasize the importance of providing postpolio information in facilitating polio survivors' adaptation to a change in physical functioning associated with late problems. Postpolio networks and support groups can also be one of the most effective avenues for information transfer and instrumental support.

The clinical implications discussed here highlight avenues for future research. From a historical perspective, theoretical models of psychological adaptation to polio can serve as a guide to other chronic conditions and diseases requiring major adaptation to stressful life events. Significant information about positive and maladaptive coping strategies and psychological well-being can be derived from clinical observations and treatment provided to those aging with polio. Research focusing on successful models for coping and outcomes such as quality of life and well-being should be encouraged, particularly because these investigations can provide a longitudinal perspective of factors influencing such outcomes. Similarly, research studying the effect of psychological and social interventions can be very valuable. Such models of treatment can offer innovative perspectives in addressing the needs of those with newly acquired physical limitations such as mobility restrictions and impairments that are caused by aging.

SUMMARY AND CONCLUSION

This chapter has reviewed the available empirical literature on the polio experience, psychological characteristics and issues, coping and adaptation strategies, psychosocial interventions, and clinical implications of the research. This body of literature reflects an intricate dynamic of early polio experience, lifelong behavioral patterns influenced by this early experience and cultural expectations, the complex interaction of physical and psychological factors impacting ED and LS, and a varied repertoire of coping strategies. The findings reviewed here echo Scheer and Luborsky's contention that an individual's response to new losses cannot be understood outside the larger context of the polio experience and cultural influences.[18]

Many polio survivors have requested and required both medical and psychosocial rehabilitation to assist them in maintaining active and productive lives as they grow older with a chronic yet changing disability. As they look to medical professionals for help, several areas of empirical research must continue to expand clinical understanding of the complex and dynamic processes that impact their psychological well-being. The influence of early polio experience is still lacking empirical examination despite its potential to substantially influence later psychological well-being. Proposed models of adaptation to PPS require more scientific testing and validation given their power to influence treatment and conceptualization of the adaptation process. Psychosocial interventions, some of which have been successfully used by many polio survivors and some that have yet to be explored, also warrant empirical study.

Finally, the principles of positive psychology have much to offer in guiding future research on polio survivors' strength, resilience, and perseverance in facing new functional losses. By moving away from negative biases and using a more balanced approach, greater understanding and appreciation of not only the struggle polio survivors face, but also of their adaptive strengths and resilience, can be achieved.

References

1. Halstead L: The lessons and legacies of polio. In Halstead L, Grimby G (eds): Post-Polio Syndrome. Philadelphia, Hanley & Belfus, 1995, pp 199–214.
2. Hollingsworth L, Didelot M, Levington C: Post-polio syndrome: Psychological adjustment to disability. Iss Ment Health Nurs 23:135–156, 2002.
3. Ryan RM, Deci EL: On happiness and human potentials: A review of research on hedonic and eudaimonic well-being. Annu Rev Psychol 52:141–166, 2001.
4. Garber M: Some emotional aspects of poliomyelitis. Public Health Nurs 44:340–344, 363, 1952.
5. Cohen E: A medical-social workers approach to the problem of poliomyelitis. Am J Public Health 38:1092–1096, 1948.
6. Wennenberg S, Ahlstrom G: Illness narratives of persons with post-polio syndrome. J Adv Nurs 31:354–361, 2000.
7. Bruno RL, Frick NM: The psychology of polio as prelude to postpolio sequelae: Behavior-modification and psychotherapy. Orthopedics 14:1185–1193, 1991.
8. Conrady LJ, Wish JR, Agre JC, et al: Psychologic characteristics of polio survivors: A preliminary report. Arch Phys Med Rehabil 70:458–463, 1989.
9. Wenneberg S, Ahlstrom G: Illness narratives of persons with post-polio syndrome. J Adv Nurs 31:354–361, 2000.
10. Clark K, Dinsmore S, Grafman J, Dalakas MC: A personality profile of patients diagnosed with postpolio syndrome. Neurology 44:1809–1811, 1994.
11. Schanke AK, Lobben B, Oyhaugen S: The Norwegian Polio Study 1994 part II: Early experiences of polio and later psychosocial well-being. Spinal Cord 37:515–521, 1999.
12. Silver J: Post-Polio Syndrome: A Guide for Polio Survivors and their Families. New Haven, CT, Yale University Press, 2001.
13. Backman M: The post-polio patient: psychological issues. J Rehabil 53:23–26, 1987.

14. Kohl S: Emotional response to the late effects of poliomyelitis. In Halstead L, Wiechers D (eds): Research and Clinical Aspects of the Late Effects of Poliomyelitis. White Plains, NY, March of Dimes Birth Defects Foundation, 1986, pp 135–143.

15. Roller A: Post-polio. Accent Liv 35:72, 1990.

16. Seligman MEP, Csikszentmihalyi M: Positive psychology: An introduction. Am Psychol 55:5–14, 2000.

17. Bruno R, Frick N: Stress and "type A" behavior as precipitants of post-polio sequelae: The Felician/Columbia Survey. In Halstead L, Wiechers D (eds): Research and Clinical Aspects of the Late Effects of Poliomyelitis. White Plains, NY, March of Dimes Birth Defects Foundation, 1986, pp 145–155.

18. Scheer J, Luborsky MR: The cultural context of polio biographies. Orthopedics 14: 1173–1181, 1991.

19. Gaynes BN, Burns BJ, Tweed DL, Erickson P: Depression and health-related quality of life. J Nerv Ment Dis 190:799–806, 2002.

20. Elliott TR, Kurylo M, Rivera P: Positive growth following acquired physical disability. In Snyder CR, Lopez S (eds): Handbook of Positive Psychology. New York, Oxford University Press, 2002.

21. Ahlstrom G, Karlsson U: Disability and quality of life in individuals with postpolio syndrome. Disabil Rehabil 22:416–422, 2000.

22. Bach JR, Campagnolo DI: Psychosocial adjustment of postpoliomyelitis ventilator assisted individuals. Arch Phys Med Rehabil 73:934–939, 1992.

23. Wortman CB, Silver RC: The myths of coping with loss. J Consult Clin Psychol 57: 349–357, 1989.

24. Kendall E, Buys N: An integrated model of psychosocial adjustment following acquired disability. J Rehabil 64:16–20, 1998.

25. Kuehn A, Winters R: A study of symptom distress, health locus of control and coping resources of aging post-polio survivors. IMAGE. J Nurs Scholarship 26:325–331, 1994.

26. Liechty J: Psychosocial issues and post-polio: A literature review of the past thirteen years. In Halstead L, Grimby G (eds): Post-Polio Syndrome. Philadelphia, Hanley & Belfus, 1995, pp 199–214.

27. Frank RG, Chaney JM, Clay DL, et al: Dysphoria: A major symptom factor in persons with disability or chronic illness. Psychiatry Res 43:231–241, 1992.

28. Kemp BJ, Adams BM, Campbell ML: Depression and life satisfaction in aging polio survivors versus age-matched controls: Relation to postpolio syndrome, family functioning, and attitude toward disability. Arch Phys Med Rehabil 78:187–192, 1997.

29. Schanke HK: Psychological distress, social support and coping behaviour among polio survivors: A 5-year perspective on 63 polio patients. Disabil Rehabil 19:108–116, 1997.

30. Erdal KJ, Zautra AJ: Psychological impact of illness downturns: A comparison of new and chronic conditions. Psychol Aging 10:570–577, 1995.

31. Westbrook MT, McIlwain D: Living with the late effects of disability: A five-year follow-up survey of coping among post-polio survivors. Aust Occup Ther J 43:60–71, 1996.

32. Mullins LL, Chaney JM, Hartman V, et al: Cognitive and affective features of postpolio syndrome: Illness uncertainty, attributional style and adaptation. Int J Rehabil Health 1:211–222, 1995.

33. Schanke A, Stangelle J: Fatigue in polio survivors. Spinal Cord 39:243–251, 2001.

34. Kemp BJ, Krause JS: Depression and life satisfaction among people ageing with postpolio and spinal cord injury. Disabil Rehabil 21:241–249, 1999.

35. Tate D, Kirsch N, Maynard F, et al: Coping with the late effects: Differences between depressed and nondepressed polio survivors. Am J Phys Med Rehabil 73:27–35, 1994.

36. Berlly MH, Strauser WW, Hall KM: Fatigue in postpolio syndrome. Arch Phys Med Rehabil 72:115–118, 1991.
37. Agre J, Rodriquez AA, Sperling KB: Symptoms and clinical impressions of patients seen in a postpolio clinic. Arch Phys Med Rehabil 70:367–370, 1989.
38. Thoren-Jonsson AL, Hedberg M, Grimby G: Distress in everyday life in people with poliomyelitis sequelae. J Rehabil Med 33:119–127, 2001.
39. Tate DG, Forchheimer M, Kirsch N, et al: Prevalence and associated features of depression and psychological distress in polio survivors. Arch Phys Med Rehabil 74:1056–1060, 1993.
40. Hazendonk KM, Crowe SF: A neuropsychological study of the postpolio syndrome: Support for depression without neuropsychological impairment. Neuropsychiatry Neuropsychol Behav Neurol 13:112–118, 2000.
41. Maynard F, Julius M, Kirsch N, et al: The late effects of polio: A model for identification and assessment of preventable secondary conditions. Ann Arbor, MI, Department of Physical Medicine and Rehabilitation, University of Michigan, 1991.
41. Cooper AF: Whose illness is it anyway? Why patient perceptions matter. Int J Clin Pract 52:551–556, 1998.
43. Strumse Y, Stanghelle JK, Utne L, et al: Treatment of patients with postpolio syndrome in a warm climate. Disabil Rehabil 25:77–84, 2003.
44. Diener E, Sapyta J, Suh E: Subjective well-being is essential to well-being. Psychol Inq 9:33–37, 1998.
45. Diener E, Suh E: Measuring quality of life: Economic, social and subjective indicators. Soc Indicators Res 40:189–216, 1997.
46. Tate D, Kalpakjian C, Forchheimer M: Quality of life issues in individuals with spinal cord injury. Arch Phys Med Rehabil 83(suppl 2):1–8, 2002.
47. Diener E, Suh E, Lucas R, Smith H: Subjective well-being: Three decades of progress. Psychol Bull 125:276–302, 1999.
48. Farbu E, Gilhus N: Former poliomyelitis as a health and socioeconomic factor: A paired sibling study. J Neurol 249:404–409, 2002.
49. Lowman CL, Seidenfeld MA: A preliminary report of the psychosocial effects of poliomyelitis. J Consult Psychol 11:30–37, 1947.
50. Vasiliadis H, Collet J, Shapiro S, et al: Predictive factors and correlates for pain in postpoliomyelitis syndrome patients. Arch Phys Med Rehabil 83:1109–1115, 2002.
51. Burger H, Marincek C: The influence of post-polio syndrome on independence and life satisfaction. Disabil Rehabil 22:318–322, 2000.
52. Kling C, Persson A, Gardulf A: The health-related quality of life of patients suffering from the late effects of polio (post-polio). J Adv Nurs 32:164–173, 2000.
53. Hansson B, Ahlstrom G: Coping with chronic illness: A qualitative study of coping with postpolio syndrome. Int J Nurs Stud 36:255–262, 1999.
54. Maynard F, Roller A: Recognizing typical coping styles of polio survivors can improve rehabilitation: A commentary. Am J Phys Med Rehabil 70:70–72, 1991.
55. Visotsky HM, Goss ME, Lebovits BZ, Hamburg DA: Coping behavior under extreme stress: Observations of patients with severe poliomyelitis. Arch Gen Psychiatry 5:423–448, 1961.
56. Frick N: Post-polio sequelae and the psychology of second disability. Orthopedics 8:851–853, 1991.
57. Lazarus R, Folkman S: Stress, Appraisal and Coping. New York, Springer Publishing, 1984.
58. Ahlstrom G, Wenneberg S: Coping will illness-related problems in persons with progressive muscular diseases: The Swedish version of the Ways of Coping Questionnaire. Scand J Caring Sci 16:368–375, 2002.

59. Natterlund B, Gunnarsson LG, Ahlstrom G: Disability, coping and quality of life in individuals with muscular dystrophy: A prospective study over five years. Disabil Rehabil 22:776–785, 2000.

60. Gignac MAM, Cott C, Badley EM: Adaptation to disability: Applying selective optimization with compensation to the behaviors of older adults with osteoarthritis. Psychol Aging 17:520–524, 2002.

61. Natterlund B, Ahlstrom G: Problem-focused coping and satisfaction with activities of daily living in individuals with muscular dystrophy and postpolio syndrome. Scand J Caring Sci 13:26–32, 1999.

62. Folkman S, Moskowitz T: Positive affect and the other side of coping. Am Psychol 55: 647–654, 2000.

63. Roller A: Health promotion for people with chronic neuromuscular disabilities. In Krotoski D, Nosek M, Turk M (eds): Women with Physical Disabilities: Achieving and Maintaining Health and Well-being. Baltimore, Paul H. Brookes Publishing, 1996, pp 431–439.

64. Peach P, Olejnik S: Effect of treatment and noncompliance on post-polio sequelae. Orthopedics 14:1199–1203, 1991.

65. Thoren-Jonsson AL: Coming to terms with the shift in one's capabilities: A study of the adaptive process in persons with poliomyelitis sequelae. Disabil Rehabil 23:341–351, 2001.

66. Peterson C, Kirsch N, Tate D: Coping with post-polio III: Optimism and cognitive style. Arch Phys Med Rehabil 70(Suppl A):25, 1989.

67. Schwartz C, Sprangers M: Adaptation to Changing Health: Response Shift in Quality-of-Life Research. Washington, DC, American Psychological Association, 2000.

68. Locker D, Kaufert P, Kirk B: The impact of life support technology upon psychosocial adaptation to the late effects of poliomyelitis. In Halstead L, Wiechers D (eds): Research and Clincal Aspects of the Late Effects of Poliomyelitis. White Plains, NY, March of Dimes Birth Defects Foundation, 1986, pp 157–171.

69. Smith DW: Power and spirituality in polio survivors: A study based on Rogers science. Nurs Sci Q 8:133–139, 1995.

70. DoRozario L: Spirituality in the lives of people with disability and chronic illness: A creative paradigm of wholeness and reconstitution. Disabil Rehabil 19:427–434, 1997.

71. Woods-Smith DW: Power and spirituality in polio survivors: A study based on Rogers science. Nurs Sci Q 8:133–139, 1995.

72. Niemeier JP, Burnett DM: No such thing as "uncomplicated bereavement" for patients in rehabilitation. Disabil Rehabil 23:645–653, 2001.

73. Ignotus P: Some psychological and spiritual aspects of acute anterior poliomyelitis. Ment Health 7:95–98, 1953.

74. Wendland L: A therapeutic group with husbands and wives of poliomyelitic patients. Group Psychother 8:25–32, 1955.

75. Tate D, Forchheimer M, Roller A: A wellness and health promotion program for women with polio [unpublished report]. Ann Arbor, MI, Department of Physical Medicine and Rehabilitation, University of Michigan, 1998.

76. Hoffman C, Maynard F: A pilot program of nutrition and exercise for polio survivors: A community-based model for secondary disability prevention. Top Clin Nutr 7:69–80, 1992.

77. Natterlund B, Ahlstrom G: Experience of social support in rehabilitation: A phenomenological study. J Adv Nurs 30:1332–1340, 1999.

INDEX

Page numbers in **boldface type** indicate complete chapters.